The Politics of Breastfeeding

to my family

Gabrielle Palmer is a nutritionist and a campaigner. She was a breastfeeding counsellor in the 1970s and helped establish the UK pressure group Baby Milk Action. In the early 1980s she worked as a volunteer in Mozambique. She has written, taught and campaigned on infant feeding issues, particularly the unethical marketing of baby foods. In the 1990s she co-directed the International Breastfeeding: Practice and Policy Course at The Institute of Child Health in London until she went to live in China for two years.

She has worked independently for various health and development agencies, including serving as HIV and Infant Feeding Officer for UNICEF New York. She recently worked at The London School of Hygiene and Tropical Medicine where she had originally studied nutrition.

She is a mother and a grandmother.

The Politics of Breastfeeding

WHEN BREASTS ARE BAD FOR BUSINESS

GABRIELLE PALMER

pinter
&
martin

PINTER & MARTIN
The Politics of Breastfeeding
When breasts are bad for business

First published by Pandora Press 1988
This third updated and revised edition
first published by Pinter & Martin Ltd 2009, reprinted 2009, 2011

ISBN 978-1-905177-16-5 (paperback)

British Library Cataloguing-in-Publication Data
A catalogue record for this book is available from the British Library.

Set in Garamond

This book has been printed on paper that is sourced and
harvested from sustainable forests and is FSC accredited.

Printed in the UK by TJ International Ltd, Padstow, Cornwall

Pinter & Martin Ltd
6 Effra Parade
London SW2 1PS

www.pinterandmartin.com

contents

illustrations

preface to the third edition

I wish I were not writing this preface. There should be no need for this book. In a world beset by overwhelming problems, here is a resolvable issue. Twenty years ago when I was writing the first edition, more than three thousand babies were dying every day from infections triggered by lack of breastfeeding and by the use of bottles, artificial milks and other risky products. This is still happening.

In the first and second editions I described the pressures on women, on health workers and on governments. I wrote about the culture of artificial feeding and the collusion between the baby food companies and the medical, nutritional and healthcare establishments. They have all promoted products and practices which have contributed to the suffering, illness and death of millions of babies and often their mothers too. This is still happening.

This third edition is necessary because some things have changed. Scientific research has revealed more amazing facts about breastfeeding. It is now known that even in a rich country, a millionaire's baby who is artificially fed is less healthy than the exclusively breastfed baby of the most disadvantaged mother. Long term health problems such as high blood pressure and diabetes are influenced by how babies are fed, and breastfeeding women reduce their own risk of breast cancer. Better understanding of women's bodies shows how adaptable they are and what a resilient process breastfeeding is when it is not sabotaged from the start.

Knowledge serves no purpose if it is not spread around. As the poor get poorer and the rich get richer, an entrenched ignorance is kept in place through a culture created and maintained by commercial interests. This new edition shows how the baby food and bottle companies use ever more aggressive promotion. Challenged by the new evidence, they work harder and pour more resources into more sophisticated marketing strategies; they manipulate the media, influence governments' policies and infiltrate the very agencies that are supposed to protect health.

Those who work to combat these influences have become more skilled, but progress is undermined by widespread misinformation and lack of awareness. I am so impressed by the talents of groups who struggle for human welfare: the women who support each other, the campaigners and those health workers who strive to cure their colleagues of the nonsense they learn from outdated training and text books and misleading promotional information. This book is not written for mothers, but for everyone; man or woman, parent or childless, old or young, because this issue concerns us all. I have added some facts and updated others, but the main theme remains unchanged. I hope that this will be my last preface and that this book will become merely the record of a tragically foolish phase in human history.

1 why breastfeeding is political

"From politics it was an easy step to silence."
Jane Austen, Northanger Abbey, 1818

If a multinational company developed a product that was a nutritionally balanced and delicious food, a wonder drug that both prevented and treated disease, cost almost nothing to produce and could be delivered in quantities controlled by consumers' needs, the announcement of this find would send its shares rocketing to the top of the stock market. The scientists who developed the product would win prizes and the wealth and influence of everyone involved would increase dramatically. Women have been producing such a miraculous substance, breastmilk, since the beginning of human existence, yet they form the least wealthy and the least powerful half of humanity.

As subjects of research, breastfeeding and breastmilk have attracted much attention during recent decades, yet as academic careers thrive on discoveries[1] of how breastfeeding works and what breastmilk contains, women and their babies are still prevented from fulfilling this unique relationship. As knowledge about breastfeeding increases, so do global sales of artificial milks and feeding bottles. This may surprise those who live where breastfeeding is still part of the culture or where well-educated women have access to support, information and their babies. There are policy documents, promotional initiatives and media attention in many countries. However, all over the world women are impeded from protecting their own and their babies' health, and often survival, because of factors beyond their control.

Why, after about a million years of survival, has one of the principal evolutionary characteristics by which we identify ourselves as mammals become so damaged? Have women been freed from a time-wasting biological tyranny to lead nobler, more fulfilling and more equal lives? In this book I examine the political reasons for a situation which has a profound effect on the whole world from the major economic effects of squandering a natural resource to the individual misery of a sick child or an unhappy woman.

Why is it that whether we were breastfed ourselves, or breastfeed our own children, depends on our social and economic position? How is it that in many societies, 100% of poor, undernourished women all breastfeed easily, while in others, groups of privileged, well-nourished women believe they cannot? Why is the right to breastfeed fought for so vehemently by some women and rejected so forcefully by others, often according to their class, education or society? And why, if women participate in the modern economic structures which are claimed to be for the benefit of us all, must the breastfeeding relationship be curtailed and restricted? For many women, what could be a simple compromise becomes an agonising decision.

power and sex

'Politics' does not only refer to economic and territorial power structures, it also means sexual politics. The fact of women's separate biological capacities has been used as a pretext for excluding women from the centres of power. But even as women's reproductive functions come to be controlled, both by themselves and others, in general there is little change in predominant male control. At the family level men still have a strong influence over women's decisions about their bodies. Despite some real progress and several notable exceptions, most major organisations, whether governments, big business or international bodies of experts, are dominated by men.* Sometimes, the very men who have discovered the excellence of breastfeeding and recommend it wholeheartedly, will object if employees bring their babies to work. They do little to establish facilities in the workplace or advocate the financial benefits and flexible schedules needed for women who must, or choose to, participate in the wage-earning world.

In most of the industrialised world, and increasingly in the so-called 'developing' world, a woman working in a paid job must not flaunt any signs of lactation. If her breasts are functioning she must discreetly withdraw to feed her baby or express her milk. Is this because to suckle a baby in daily public life is too disturbing a sight for some colleagues? Do both men and women feel shocked, disapproving or even disgusted? Away from the workplace these same workers might pay to watch a woman expose her breasts for the sexual stimulation of strangers. They might pay more for food served by bare-breasted women. Though any part of a woman's body can be a focus of eroticism, our era is the first in recorded history where the breast has become a public fetish for male sexual stimulation, while its

* Even in the supposedly equal society of Sweden only 26.9% of women are company directors on boards. In the USA, it is just 14.8%, the UK 11.5%, France 7.6% and Portugal 0.8%. Source: The Guardian, 17.11.08.

When children's author and illustrator Jan Pienkowski brought out the large format version of The Fairy Tales in 2005, the US publishers wanted the nipples removed from Sleeping Beauty's breasts, even though in the illustration she had just given birth to her baby. "I averted my gaze while that was done," said Pienkowski.
Joanna Carey, Shapes from the Forest, The Guardian, 4.3.2006; also Midweek, BBC Radio 4, 19.11.2008

primary function has diminished on a vast scale. Perhaps the only parallel is the phenomenon of foot-binding in China, when the primary use of a part of the body was sacrificed to serve the cult of a sexual fetishism which celebrated female helplessness.

In the 20th century, women were presented with an illusion of liberation through the artificial feeding of babies, only to find their breasts appropriated by men and popular culture. This continues in the 21st century. This has been expressed both privately, when men pressure their sexual partners not to breastfeed, and publicly through pornography and the mass marketing of products and information. Certainly in the dominant culture of the USA, regarding breasts as an ordinary part of the human body seems impossible. When entertainer Janet Jackson's breast popped out at the televised Super Bowl game in Los Angeles, USA, in 2004, it was as though her breast had a life separate from the rest of her. "That was the most disgusting thing I have ever seen at a sports spectacle," said a baseball coach.[2] Viewers could applaud her sexualised dancing, hip movements and song lyrics about passion and desire, all commonplace themes in popular entertainment, but a breast really freaked them out. Why? Viewers, who watch TV series and films with violence and killing essential to their storylines, could not cope with the sight of a breast. Just a few hundred years ago, most human societies found breast exposure in everyday life unremarkable. What has happened to us?

There is still a fundamental racism in attitudes to public breastfeeding. Intrusive cameras turn the lens on hungry women who, during disasters, keep their babies alive with this precious fluid and closeness. As long as the woman is black and devastated, programme makers include the scene, but if a well-dressed, white woman breastfeeds her baby, the camera shot is often edited out.

* * *

market forces

It is not a coincidence that the decline of breastfeeding accelerated as the predominantly male medical profession took over the management of childbirth and infant feeding. Nor was it chance that led to the expansion of the baby milk industry during the late 19th and early 20th centuries when improved techniques and mechanisation of milk-processing led to cows' milk surpluses. When a manufacturer has an excess product his business instinct is to find a way to market it. The development of artificial baby milk has been a marketing success story, not least in the skill with which the competing product has been destroyed. Women are not paid for producing or delivering breastmilk, nor for caring for young humans in this special way. Those who market artificial baby milk, bottles, teats and the essential cleaning materials benefit financially from keeping breastfeeding in check. There is no equivalent vested interest group to protect breastfeeding and it is destroyed for the same reason that forests are destroyed – for immediate profit.

In our modern world, status and often self-esteem come from a person's role in the structures of wealth creation. If a woman joins the modern industrialised economy she must be seen to be like a man and it is taken for granted that she must adapt to this norm, not that social and economic organisation must adapt to all human beings. Women have had to prove (as it happens very successfully) that they are 'as good as' men, but men do not yet have to show that they are as good as women. To gain recognition, striving women must be as tough and competitive as men. New management theories extol women's special skills, but merely for their usefulness in making business more profitable, not because they are good in their own right.

who is left holding the baby?

Women, whatever their nationality or class, still take major responsibility for the care of babies and children. Even in Scandinavia, where legislation and tax-incentives encourage fathers to do more, for the most part mothers remain the principal carers. In most of the world women who have children and who work in the wage economy are expected to delegate and organise the care of their babies, so they can function in a world designed by and for men. In most cases another woman takes on the task and is often underpaid and separated from her own children, or, in the case of relatives, is unpaid. The few men who care for their own or others' children are a minority, perhaps because of the low pay and status. In this struggle for economic and sexual justice a baby's needs are often neglected and, during this crucial phase of physical and emotional development, many are damaged for ever.

who profits?

The global value of baby food sales is projected to reach US$20.2 billion annually of which around two thirds will come from infant formula sales. In 2007 the US infant formula market was estimated at US$3.9 billion. Europe is currently the leading market and sales may reach US$2.1 billion by 2010.[3] Just one British bottle and teat company which exports all over the world had a £90 million annual turnover.[4] Doctors, scientists and nutritionists may be investors and beneficiaries of the industry. A doctor who invents a new artificial milk may get a royalty on each batch sold. Those who support breastfeeding and see a conflict of interest in industry links will rarely get as rich as those who have close ties with a powerful company. Our current economic structure does not encourage the promotion of products or systems which provide long-term benefit and do not make rapid financial profits. As with so many of the biological solutions to the ecological devastation of the planet, the money makers would not benefit immediately if we adopted them, though in the long term the world and all society would be wealthier.

Modern medicine is a wonderful thing and has made life more comfortable and longer for many. Who would want to be without vaccines, modern surgery and anaesthesia? Doctors and manufacturers are not, and mostly have not been, evil individuals consciously planning to appropriate the power of women, though their cultural attitudes to women may have distorted their judgment. Many doctors have been faced with problems of failing lactation or with women not wanting to breastfeed their babies. Because of their own ignorance and misunderstanding they believed artificial feeding to be the answer.

One sad fact of the 20th century was that the more contact mothers had with health workers, the less they breastfed.[5] Industrial society is founded on technological solutions and indifference to the costs of primary extraction; it is often easier, and more lucrative, to work out a stopgap way of alleviating a problem than to discover why it occurred in the first place. Now that researchers have revealed the risks of not breastfeeding, there is no excuse for the medical and commercial promoters of substitute milks to continue their practices, but many are so caught up in the whirlwind of career progress and profit-seeking that they seem unable to stop to review the damage they do.

There has been a curious doublethink among those scientists and manufacturers whose interests lie in the production of breastmilk substitutes. On the one hand there is eagerness to claim that artificially fed babies are just as healthy as breastfed ones and that the choice of feeding method is an equal one; on the other there is the claim to imitate human milk, and to use it as the gold standard to sell the commercial product.

There is still much to find out about breastmilk and breastfeeding and the more research is done the more fascinating and miraculous the process seems. Much research is financed by the baby food industry. There is probably no other manufacturing industry which gains so much free access to the rival product. Drug companies are obsessive about patenting, but all over the world women have unwittingly given away their unique nutrient and medical product to the very people who want to replace it. If society were organised so that the true baby milk manufacturers, women, earned the rewards they deserve for their production, the baby food industry would dwindle and much of the poverty that causes infant disease and death would disappear. Helping and supporting women to breastfeed would save more children's lives than any other public health preventive intervention, more even than immunisation, or improved water and sanitation.[6]

product makers or philanthropists?

Much as they urge us to think otherwise, the infant feeding product companies are not philanthropic organisations, but competitive commercial enterprises. It is in their interests that women find it difficult to breastfeed. Classical economic theory tells us that the invisible hand of the market leads only to the manufacture of products that people need. If this is so, then why do these companies invest millions in promotion to persuade us to use more of their products? These methods are necessary because to sell substantial quantities they must impede the production of the rival product. People may notice the blatant shout of public advertising, but they may be unaware of more subtle tactics. For example, in the 20th century, US-based company Abbott-Ross provided free design-planning for hospitals:

> "The purpose here is to impose a design that literally builds bottle-feeding into the facility by physically separating mother and infant to make bottle-feeding more convenient than breastfeeding for the hospital staff. . . . A single investment in such architectural services can create new sales opportunities for the entire life span of the building."[7]

A company could gain both prestige as a benefactor and create customers, all through a single strategy.

These marketing activities are excellent investments because all parents have one thing in common: whether poor or rich they want their children to live and to be healthy. If a woman's breastfeeding has been sabotaged and she sees artificial milk as the means of her child's survival, she will sacrifice everything to buy it. In most of the world this purchase costs more than half the household income and will impoverish the rest of the family. The more that feeding bottles and artificial milk become acceptable and 'normal' in any society, the more stable are the manufacturers' incomes. Breastmilk substitutes can be useful, life-saving products, just as artificial insulin can save the lives of diabetics, but no honest doctor could advocate the use of insulin unless it were strictly necessary. If a breastmilk substitute is needed, allowing commercial pressure to influence the choice of product is a betrayal of good medical practice, demeaning to the practitioner and a risk to the baby.

the right to choice

The infant feeding issue is often represented as one of individual choice between two parallel methods, 'the breast or the bottle'. Neither the products nor the method are equal and the true cost to society and the individual is seldom mentioned or measured. Women have the right to choose how they use their bodies and they cannot (and should not) be forced to breastfeed, but that does not mean that evidence about the risks of not breastfeeding should be censored. The skilfully managed promotion and public relations of the baby food industry blur and distort the facts, for health workers as much as parents. Informed choice is the mantra of western society and is seen

> *"More than one billion people in the world live on less than one dollar a day. Another 2.7 billion struggle to survive on less than two dollars per day. Poverty in the developing world, however, goes far beyond income poverty. It means having to walk more than one mile every day simply to collect water and firewood; it means suffering diseases that were eradicated from rich countries decades ago. Every year 11 million children die, most of them under the age of five; more than six million of these die from completely preventable causes like malaria, diarrhoea and pneumonia.*
>
> *In some deeply impoverished nations less than half of the children are in primary school and under 20% go to secondary school. Around the world, a total of 114 million children do not get even a basic education and 584 million women are illiterate."*
> Human Development Report 'Fast Facts: The Faces of Poverty',
> United Nations Millennium Development Project, 2005

as a right, but few parents are fully informed. In much of the world the choice between breastfeeding and artificial milk is a choice between infant health and sickness, and too often between life and death.

Much of the medical profession strives to be neutral and to ignore the integration of commercial interests with medical issues. The infant feeding industry provides products, research grants, health information, gifts and sponsorship for conferences: all the activities believed to be essential for progress. When a company donates expensive medical equipment or funds research, the recipients become beholden. That is why the donors invest in these activities. In 1981 the International Code of Marketing of Breastmilk Substitutes was adopted at the World Health Assembly (WHA*) in Geneva. Yet every manufacturer of infant feeding products flouts its provisions, including promoting these products in regions where artificial feeding means playing Russian roulette with a baby's life.

Until the 1990s, even health workers dismissive of breastfeeding in rich societies acknowledged that it was essential in conditions of poverty. But then the Human Immunodeficiency Virus (HIV) became established and there was evidence that breastfeeding could transmit the virus in some cases. Breastfeeding advocates were horrified and there was panic, denial and confusion. At the time there were no drugs to treat HIV infection and it was impossible to predict which

---

* For abbreviations and frequently used terms see page 365.

babies were most at risk. International health organisations struggled to work out policies to protect women and babies and instead created a muddle, mainly because the widening differences between rich and poor in the world led to contradictory messages. Even as compelling evidence emerged showing that breastfeeding was important for rich babies too, the idea was mooted that poor women could 'choose' to feed their babies artificially. The results were tragic as I will explain in Chapter 8.

the widening gap between rich and poor

By the start of this century, in many countries emerging primary healthcare systems had been nipped in the bud by the pincers of 'structural adjustment'.[8] This was the recipe for progress which the international finance bodies, such as the International Monetary Fund (IMF), imposed on poor countries during the 1980s. The message to government leaders was: 'make your people pay for their health and education out of their own pockets and your country will become prosperous; ignore our advice at your peril because we hold the financial reins.' The poor countries were pressured to reform their economies according to a policy which came to be called the 'Washington Consensus'. They had to restrict public spending on public health and education and to open their markets. Ironically, most rich nations had originally invested public spending in health and education as the bedrock for their long-term development. Those same financial institutions did not pressure poor governments to restrict the promotion of products (often imported with scarce foreign currency) which undermined health and drained their economies. Whose interests were they serving? There is now a growing distortion of world food availability and distribution, in part due to these policies. The fact that the powerful men in Washington never counted the most valuable food of all as of economic importance has contributed to the hunger and health crises that many humans are enduring today.

Women have a unique power through breastfeeding to maintain health, life and finite resources. Many might resist this suggestion because it is associated with the oppression of women by limiting them to supposedly traditional roles. When the powerful deny the practice and influence of this activity, and women who do it are kept apart, it is no wonder that confusion reigns. In a shrinking world where the consumption of finite resources and environmental degradation are reaching a breaking point, here is an unacknowledged resource. Until power structures change so that women are recognised and rewarded, gain full access to the means of economic independence and take a real part in decision-making, another natural product remains undervalued and discarded. Just as people have come to realise that forests are not simply a source of firewood or obstacles to the development of land, so economic planners need to learn that human beings are part of the ecosystem and that something as unnoticed as breastfeeding contributes to a saner management of the earth's resources.[9]

> *"Breastfeeding is an unequalled way of providing ideal food for the healthy growth and development of infants; it is also an integral part of the reproductive process with important implications for the health of mothers. As a global public health recommendation, infants should be exclusively breastfed for the first six months of life to achieve optimal growth, development and health. Thereafter to meet their evolving nutritional requirements, infants should receive nutritionally adequate and safe complementary foods while breastfeeding continues for up to two years of age and beyond. Exclusive breastfeeding from birth is possible except for a few medical conditions, and unrestriced exclusive breastfeeding results in ample milk production."*
> WHO/UNICEF The Global Stategy for Infant and Young Child Feeding 2003

2 the right to call ourselves mammals: the importance of biology

"Our class owes its uniqueness to mothering and lactation; indeed that is why it is called 'mammalia', after the mammary glands."
Irene Elia, The Female Animal, Oxford University Press, 1985

I have to start with biology. For a long time I resisted this because I believed that biologists were saying that political ideas could never change our biological destiny; that the forces of natural selection, of competition and of the primal drives for survival made any attempt at the reorganisation of society a meaningless exercise. I now believe that the understanding of nature, of both the planet and our human nature and the links between the two, is vital if we are to have any hope of resolving the problems of people. Just as architects have to understand the qualities of their materials if they are to construct a sound and safe building, nature cannot be disregarded if a system of survival, justice and dignity is to be established.

The biologist Charles Darwin (1809–1882) is famous for his theory of evolution. He observed that animals (including of course humans) survive and reproduce more successfully when they develop characteristics which are suited to their environments. Those who cannot adapt to changing conditions die out. Darwin observed that the better adapted animals are to their surrounding conditions, the greater their chances of survival.

Darwin's theories were misused by 'Social Darwinists' to defend discrimination, and even genocide. For example, sterilisation of the 'feeble minded' was common in the USA and Europe throughout much of the 20th century. This practice was justified by distorted ideas about hereditary traits. Similarly, biological theories are still misused to justify the exploitation of some groups by others. The oppression and exploitation of females is a fact of human society, yet it is not usual in other animal groups. Many women are suspicious of any arguments which glorify motherhood, because they have frequently been used to restrict women and exclude them from positions of power. However, it is those very mothering qualities which have led to highly valued traits such as intelligence, verbal and tactile communication, dexterity, endurance and love, and they are traits of men as well as of women.

In the struggle for power, or simply economic survival in the modern world, many women who have children find that they must curtail mothering, and restricting lactation is part of this. Yet lactation, a process which evolved before gestation, is the very core of our identity. Over the millennia each mammal's milk has become uniquely adapted to its physiological needs, its behaviour and its environment. It is such a spectacular biological strategy that we humans (along with other similar animals) name ourselves after the mammary gland, 'mammals' meaning animals that suckle their young.

Mammals reproduce by what biologists call the 'K-strategy', as opposed to the 'r-strategy'. An example of an r-strategist is the oyster which produces millions of eggs to be fertilised in the sea and does no parenting; K-strategists produce far fewer offspring, but nurture them. If an r-strategist parent dies, the species still survives; indeed some mothers, such as mayflies, die as soon as they have laid their eggs. Humans are of course K-strategists and their young are the most vulnerable and slowest-growing of all mammals. The human baby, supposedly because of its large brain, is considered by some to be born 'prematurely', and therefore called 'the exterogestate foetus'.[1] Breastfeeding provides an intermediate environment of nurturing and security which makes the transference from a mother's womb to the outside world safer and less harsh; a mother's breast gives warmth, food, protection against disease and a learning exercise in interactions.

the physiology of gender relations

Before explaining how lactation works I want to explore the biological explanation of human gender relations. When some people say 'it's natural' for males to dominate females they ignore the behaviour of the majority of species (which are not mammals) where there are as many 'un-motherly' females as there are 'motherly' males. Amongst mammals, most, but by no means all, females do the bulk of the mothering; however, this does not make them vulnerable or oppressed, and in fact many females are stronger than males. Until recently the observers with the status to spread their ideas were usually men and, however intelligent, they could not help but be biased. The Greek philosopher Aristotle (384–322 BCE) assumed the queen bee was male because she was 'king' of the hive. Modern male observers of social animals have described harems as groups of females 'owned' or dominated by one male, but in fact they can also be described as females who form a band to protect those who are pregnant and lactating and who choose to allow one or two males near the band. There are many examples of non-human primates (monkeys and apes) where the female is in charge (such as the siamangs of Asia) or where the sexes are equal and share childcare.

Whenever this subject is discussed someone will say that nevertheless in most human societies males do dominate the females. Even when women do all the work or are extremely strong, men usually have the ultimate political or religious authority and power. Why? One possible explanation is as follows. One survival strategy of human evolution is that humans carry more fat stores in proportion to their body size than any other land mammal, even the pig, and females store more fat than males. Of course an army of researchers look for ways to combat this characteristic, but fat storage is one reason why humans have been so successful in evolutionary terms; they store nourishment in the form of body fat when food is plentiful and draw on those reserves for survival when food is scarce. This is especially useful for females who can support a growing foetus and, after the birth, produce milk to feed it without the need for a dramatic increase in food intake.[2]

If you have a big skeleton, you need more muscle to carry it around and more food to maintain that big body. Girls reach puberty, which accompanies the final phase of skeletal growth, earlier than boys, so that any surplus food eaten towards the end of this phase gets laid down as body fat. Fat does not mean obesity; even slim women have proportionally more body fat than men. The fine tuning of natural selection has resulted in a compromise in women's size. To have a bigger build may mean easier childbirth, but to be too big means that a seasonal food shortage (which was normal for many of our ancestors and still is for subsistence farming families in poor countries) may carry more risk of death than if you are smaller.[3] A smaller body needs less food for basic maintenance, so it can store extra food energy as body fat and these reserves support reproduction and lactation. Adolescent males eating the same amount as adolescent females can just get taller.*

So, human males might have grown bigger because they did not evolve the strategy of fat storage to as great an extent as females, because it made no difference to reproductive capacity. On the principle of power corrupts and absolute power corrupts absolutely the larger males only had to hit out to find that the recipient of the

---

* Modern women in rich societies can be big because they live in a food-abundant environment and being adapted to seasonal hunger has no advantage.

blow fell to the ground. The larger male may have learned the effectiveness of physical violence for dominance which led to its further use. Endocrinologists point to the link between the male hormone testosterone and aggression, and this certainly exists, but not all males are aggressive and some females can be. Observation of primates reveals groups with male dominance are those with the greatest difference of size between the sexes. When the sexes are close in size, as with siamangs and lemurs, there is equality or female dominance.[4]

Extrapolating from 'natural' animal behaviour to human society can be misleading, but I believe there are some links. It is interesting that in Hawaii, where there is a record of extremely tall women, there has been an unusual degree of sexual and political parity with men. It is physical violence or the threat of it which still brings dominance in the modern world. Language reflects the link between size and control, as in the 'superpowers', 'Mr Big' and 'a weighty matter'. People, especially men, buy big cars more for status than convenience. Research shows that taller people are more likely to be successful and in dominant positions. Political strength may now be expressed through sophisticated weapon systems rather than by being tall and muscular, but it is still the fear of being crushed and destroyed that allows certain individuals and groups to be dominated by others. Once dominance is achieved it is hard to take it away. The big male gorilla may let the small female eat bananas if he has a good supply, but if he has taken them all and she tries to snatch one away, woe betide her. The smaller animal soon has to learn other strategies of survival, which may require greater intelligence. In short, I suspect that human males are still in charge because they have been able to use physical coercion, or its implicit threat, both privately and publicly, and this has developed socially into a range of psychological, cultural and economic methods of control.[5] Because of this dominance, most human societies end up being organised by and for men and many particularly female abilities do not earn prestige and rewards. The fact that a woman in power must hide female qualities like lactation, is a measure of continuing male dominance. It is hard to imagine a woman politician with a baby at her breast while making a political speech, yet it would be quite possible. This concept is often met with ridicule, yet I remember an economist and former freedom fighter in Mozambique bringing her new baby with her when she was a speaker at a meeting. She gave a powerful speech and answered questions while breastfeeding her baby when he needed, as though this were the most natural thing in the world, which of course it was.

In 2003 MP Kirstie Marshall was ejected from the Victorian State Parliament (Australia) for breastfeeding her newborn. Ms Marshall said she was not trying to make a statement and did not expect parliamentary rules to be bent for her. "I have since found out that there is a law, or rule, that's actually stated that you can't have a stranger in the House. And as she hasn't been elected to parliament – and I thought that, you know, (Charlotte) being inside me, that was kind of a part of it. That, you know, she's not an individually elected member."
'Charlotte makes a meal of question time.' The Age 27.2.2003

the efficient female

There are other useful human survival strategies, besides the storage of fat and the slowness of growth. Though this is uncertain and may depend on the amount of food available to the individual, there is some evidence that the female metabolic rate is lowered during the first two-thirds of pregnancy, and, though it rises again during the last third, there may be a net saving of energy for the whole pregnancy. This does not mean that women should be underfed while they are pregnant, but that, in comparison with most other mammals, reproduction can continue successfully without women having to devote their time to eating hugely increased quantities of food. Lactation may involve some nutrient-sparing mechanisms, which means that women, again unlike many other mammals, can produce enough milk for their baby's needs without requiring a lot more food. We have populated this planet because our females can reproduce and feed their young with the help of two marvellous strategies: storing excess food in the form of body fat as a supply of energy for the hard times, and adjusting the body's ways of using up the food supply when supporting a new life. Women are like a very economical car that not only has a spare fuel tank, but uses up less fuel per kilometre when it carries an extra passenger.[6]

just like a cow?

When young mammals die it may be because of predators or congenital weakness which might stop them getting their mother's milk (as with the runt who gets pushed out by the siblings). It is

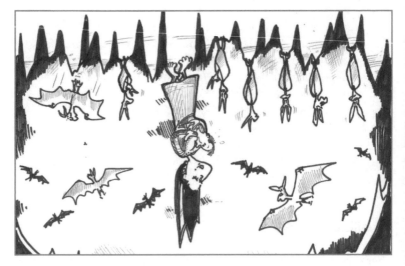

1 'Hanging upside down in caves: the natural way to breastfeed.'
(Cartoon Jack Maypole)

almost unknown for a mammal in her normal environment to produce live young and be unable to produce the milk they need. So why in modern industrialised society is human 'lactation failure' so common? Biologically it is one of nature's star turns, but culturally it has become another human mess. All other mammals suckle their young; monkeys and bats do it, so do the killer whale and the tiger.

One exception is the modern dairy cow who has been bred, fed, and in some cases, treated with synthetic hormones, to produce enormous quantities of milk that could be termed 'unnatural'. Modern calves are removed a few days after birth so that humans can take the milk. Although there is plenty for both calf and humans, modern agricultural organisation does not allow for such compromises. A calf needs between three to ten (at most) litres a day. If left with its dairy cow mother to drink all the milk available (30 to 70 litres), its digestion could not cope and it might die. If it only took the three to ten litres it needed, the poor mother cow would get severe mastitis (inflammation of the udder) and could die.[7]

In the development of dairying over the centuries, selective breeding has favoured placidity, excess milk production and response to intensive feeding with high milk output, but these qualities are irrelevant to the survival of the young, which is the primary purpose of lactation. The human is not at all like a cow, yet join any discussion about breastfeeding and someone will make a comparison between humans and dairy cows: 'You've got to be relaxed and placid to breastfeed'; 'I felt just like a cow'; 'You must eat and drink more to keep up your milk supply, you know what happens to a badly fed cow'. To say that a woman must be like a cow in order to breastfeed is like saying that only Olympic weightlifters can carry a newspaper. Tigers are not placid, yet they suckle their cubs; bats are mammals, but no one suggests that women must hang upside down in caves to be successful breastfeeders. The knowledge of dairy cows has exceeded that of human lactation and has had a misleading influence on the understanding of human mothers and babies.

the use of non-human milk

The human species has only engaged in agriculture and pasturage for 12,000 to 15,000 years, a mere 1% of our time on earth. So for 99% of our existence humans survived without any milk other than breastmilk. Many societies never used animal milk until Europeans persuaded them to do so. Indeed, the majority of adult human beings lack the stomach enzyme, lactase, which is necessary to digest milk. Northern Europeans and some other cattle-rearing groups have the biologically unusual characteristic of producing this digestive enzyme once they are past infancy. Many Asians and Africans or those originating from these regions, suffer pain, wind and diarrhoea when they drink fresh milk. In the past many Chinese considered drinking animal milk as disgusting as drinking a glass of saliva.

Until the invention of refrigeration (and most human beings are still too poor to own fridges) milk was a dangerous food because it is an ideal breeding ground for harmful bacteria. Before the advent of pasteurisation it could (and did) transmit serious diseases such as tuberculosis (TB) and brucellosis. Between 1850 and 1950 bovine TB from drinking infected milk caused over 800,000 deaths in Britain. Up to 1930 when pasteurisation became more common, 30% of TB deaths were caused by milk drinking.[8]

Such problems still occur. The world has been astonished to learn, through the 2008 Chinese melamine-contaminated milk scandal, the extent of lax regulation in the global dairy industry. However milk adulteration is as old as dairying itself and is a recurring problem. Among other adulterants, melamine has been illicitly added to milk and other foods for at least 40 years. This is because melamine is a nitrogen rich substance and the regulators test for the protein content of foods by measuring their nitrogen content.[9]

In the past, except in cool climates, milk had to be drunk immediately (as the Masai do) or made into butter, cheese, yoghurts and other fermented products to be safe. Fresh non-human milk can make a useful contribution to the diet, but it is not essential and for many people it is an inappropriate and even dangerous food. Yet billions of human beings, including most modern Chinese, now believe that cows' milk is essential for the health of infants and young children.

3 how breastfeeding works – and how it was damaged

"Aren't babies clever!"
Ann-Marie Widström, 19931

If they are not prevented from doing so, the majority of babies have the power to stimulate the manufacture of their own food supply and to keep it going in the quantities they need. A baby has to work for her breastmilk by asking for it, signalling when she is hungry, thirsty or needing comfort; and then suckling effectively to maintain milk production. Medical and cultural influences have distorted this process. When allowed to happen, the relationship between a baby and her mother's breast is dynamic and quite different from that with a bottle of artificial milk. A baby is actively involved because it is her suckling that helps establish and keeps her mother's milk-making going. That is why the English word 'suckle' is so appropriate: it means the action of both mother and baby, who are co-workers.

Many people think that lactation only occurs after birth, but several mammals, for example elephants and foxes, are known to lactate without giving birth and suckle the young of other females. In the same way many women, whether they have given birth or not, can stimulate lactation and sometimes sexual partners who enjoy suckling are surprised to find the breasts producing milk.[2] Both childless women, and mothers who stopped breastfeeding years previously, have produced milk, simply by letting a baby suckle their breasts. In the past, and still in some parts of the world, foster mothers, often grandmothers, feed the babies of dead, ill or absent mothers. Concerns about possible HIV transmission (see Chapter 8) have prompted caution about this practice, but in many situations this is the only way to save a baby's life.

In industrialised societies adopting mothers have used various methods to establish lactation. Modern women have used devices (breast pumps or breastfeeding supplementers) or a pharmacological regime. One woman I met shared the breastfeeding of her adopted son with her lactating sister. Her adopted son learned to feed through suckling her sister's breasts *and* her own. Temporarily he got milk from his aunt, but he also gradually stimulated his adoptive mother's breast to produce his full supply.

skin-to-skin changes everything

The fact that humans spend money and time on products to soften their skin shows how much we value that organ. Skin influences human behaviour. Many of the pleasant sensations that come from touching, massage and sex are due to skin-to-skin contact. Yet outdated customs still deprive too many newborns of their first sensual experience of being in the world.

Skin contact between mother and baby has a powerful influence on breastfeeding hormones in the mother and digestive hormones in both of them. Breastfeeding is far more likely to be problem-free and continue for longer if there has been early, uninterrupted skin contact.[3]

At birth a mother instinctively stretches out her arms. If she is standing, squatting or semi-reclining she may reach for her baby and draw her close. If she is lying back her baby may instinctively start crawling up her abdomen. If the mother feels exhausted, the birth attendant can place the baby gently on her abdomen. Back in the 1980s Swedish researchers had the courage to let newborn babies do what they wanted and what talents they showed. Babies know how to crawl to the breast and, through touch, smell and sight, find the areola (that is why it darkens during pregnancy) and nipple. When a baby reaches his target he opens his mouth wide and starts suckling. If undrugged, his reflexes are at a peak just after birth and he knows exactly what to do. It is not a coincidence that gatherer-hunters who spend their lives semi-naked breastfeed without difficulties.[4]

The practice of washing and wrapping a baby is not based on good research evidence but is merely a folk custom converted into medical orthodoxy. People were rightly worried about newborns getting cold. Now we know that newborns are warmest in their mother's arms and more at risk of chilling when in a cot, however well wrapped. Indeed swaddled babies get colder than those who are not.[5] Newborns must stay warm and the place of birth should be a minimum of 25°C (77°F). The newborn can be patted dry of the birth fluids and both he and his mother can be covered. It is now known that a mother's body warms up if her baby is cool or cools down if he is too hot. Bathing removes the vernix, the waxy film on a baby's skin, which is there to protect him from cold and abrasion. Nowadays any well-run maternity unit would not wash babies at birth.

Some newborns (and mothers) need immediate medical attention, but the majority do not. Interventions such as weighing can be postponed until the baby has nuzzled and suckled without

MEN COULD BREASTFEED TOO
"Why is the milk of human kindness made by only half the population? After all, men have nipples and the capacity to use them. Males given certain chemicals lactate with no difficulty. Even a heavy dose of alcohol can do the same as the liver loses its ability to suppress each man's guilty secret, his female hormones. Teenage boys, in a natural desire to see what might be done with their bodies, now and then stimulate their own nipples and (no doubt to their amazement) may eject milk. [. . .]

"A man's pert but useless nipples are his real stamp of inutility. They have no job because of evolution. [. . .] The male's job, if any, is to protect his child as he keeps a weather eye open for what else might turn up. His nipples are just a reminder that he is of common stock with his partner."
Steve Jones, Almost like a whale: the origin of species updated, Transworld Publishers, 2000

interruption; neither mother nor baby should be hurried. Skilled birth attendants interfere as little as possible with skin-to-skin contact and attend to any necessary procedures after the baby has suckled.

A retired midwife was once describing new babies' skins, "There is nothing so beautiful to touch, not even the softest silk." Then she added, "We steal so much from mothers, it is they who should have this joy not us."[6] When skin contact does not happen, we also steal a newborn's rightful contact with the soft skin of his mother's abdomen and breasts.

a born talent

The production of milk works on the supply and demand principle. The more often the baby suckles, the more milk is made. All babies and mothers vary so each couple can find the way that works for them. A healthy, hungry baby is the best milk producer in the world. She stimulates exactly the right amount by suckling when she feels the need. She is superior to the most sophisticated computer programme in the way her appetite is linked to the nutrient and fluid balance of her small body. She can increase or decrease the amount of milk and balance her nutrients according to need; if she is allowed to. Of course, if she is kept apart from her mother's breasts, then she cannot regulate her milk supply. She may signal her needs by turning her head, opening her mouth and sticking out her tongue, making little noises (talking starts far earlier than most people think), but if she is in a hospital nursery or alone in a room then no one will notice her eloquence. If she then has to cry to communicate her hunger, when she gets to her mother's breast she might be too exhausted to suckle effectively. Many people have felt hungry, yet too upset to eat, but they forget that babies are people too. No adult would enjoy a meal in a restaurant where you had to get hysterical to get served. When a waiter is quick to pick up your cues (eye contact, little motions of the hand, turning the body) he or she is carrying out good mothering behaviour – and adults certainly appreciate it.

Mothers need to be close to their babies to pick up these cues. Anthropologist Helen Ball has researched mother/infant night time behaviour. Mothers who share a bed or use a three-sided cot attached to the bed are far more responsive to their babies than those who have a separate cot by the bed. Almost in their sleep, mothers respond, stroke and suckle their babies throughout the night. All the mothers unconsciously sleep in a special position, arm above their babies' heads and knees drawn up, which protects their babies from harm.[7] Breastfeeding was far more successful for the mothers co-sleeping than those who slept apart. Early frequent suckling makes the copious milk production (often described as 'the milk coming in') flow earlier and physical closeness makes this easy.

Quenching a baby's hunger and thirst with other fluids makes suckling difficult. In the same way that most adults hate to be forced to eat when they are full, a baby will be reluctant to breastfeed if she has been given artificial milk or glucose water. She down-regulates the breastmilk supply because her full stomach tells her to stimulate less milk. Her mother's body gets the message that this baby does not need much milk and so reduces production.

Since medical authorities began to supervise breastfeeding, it has been restricted. When babies are fed at prescribed intervals and their time at the breast curtailed, then the wonderful dance that the bodies of a mother and her baby have spent nine months rehearsing cannot be performed. The process gets disrupted and may shut down. That is why so-called 'insufficient milk syndrome' increased as medicalised maternity services became established.

* * *

the patriarchs of breastfeeding

"It is with great pleasure I see at last the preservation of children become the care of men of sense... In my opinion this business has been too fatally left to the management of women, who cannot be supposed to have a proper knowledge to fit them for the task."
Dr William Cadogan, An Essay upon Nursing and the Management of Children from their Birth to Three Years of Age, 1748

How did the practice of restricting breastfeeding get established? One source of the idea of restricting breastfeeding was the influential 18th-century doctor William Cadogan. His 'An Essay upon Nursing and the Management of Children from their Birth to Three Years of Age'[8] was widely read. Cadogan's legacy has done good and harm. He disapproved of tight swaddling clothes. In those days babies were trussed up like well-packaged parcels, and could barely move, let alone kick or play.[9] Cadogan promoted exclusive breastfeeding and condemned pre-lacteal feeds. Wealthy families gave their newborns exotic mixtures of butter, wine or breadcrumbs, while delaying the first breastfeed. Cadogan noted that countrywomen who could not afford these foods or swaddling clothes, had healthier babies than wealthy mothers. He advocated maternal breastfeeding, and persuaded rich women, who usually sent their babies to a wet nurse, to breastfeed their own babies. Cadogan was an observant man who used infant mortality rates to back up his arguments. He made breastfeeding fashionable and this not only saved the lives of newborns, but lowered maternal mortality too. When women exclusively breastfed after birth they were less likely to die. He also improved the care of foundlings, saving many lives through the employment of wet nurses.

The environment of 18th-century London was appallingly unhygienic. Bacteria had not yet been discovered and no one understood how infections spread. Large numbers of infants died of diarrhoea and pneumonia, just as they do today in the poorest regions of the world. Cadogan observed that babies were frequently fed with cows' milk, gruels and 'paps' (mashed mixtures of breadcrumbs or flour, with water or milk) as well as being breastfed and he perceived a cause and effect. His reasoning was sound: a lot of food was contaminated and a source of infection.

Though Cadogan valued breastmilk, he did not distinguish between this and other foods when he decided that 'overfeeding' was the cause of diarrhoea. He therefore advocated only four feeds at regular intervals in 24 hours and forbade night feeding. He did not however suggest limiting the length of a feed. Cadogan claimed that, as a father himself, he had practised all his principles with success. The reader envisages a household with baby after baby thriving on the perfect routine, but if you sneak a look at Cadogan's biography[10] you will find he had just one daughter. Perhaps she happened to be one of those rare babies who stick to a routine and never wake at night. Perhaps her mother was one of those rare women who have plenty of milk despite limited feeding. It is these unusual women who have inadvertently kept the gospel of routine alive, proving the point that restricted, routine breastfeeding can be achieved. I suspect that while Cadogan was attending to his wealthy clients, his wife (or wet nurse) was breastfeeding whenever his daughter wanted and no one told him. Cadogan did not think highly of women and never mentions his wife. He began his essay stating his relief that at last 'men of sense rather than foolish unlearned women' were taking over the supervision of infant care. This taking over of the management of infant feeding by men was significant. An 'unlearned' mother will know about the supply and demand principle. She will feel her milk increasing after a day or night when the baby has been extra hungry and suckling more. No male doctor has experienced this.

Cadogan pioneered a dynasty of well-intentioned but dogmatic men whose ideas influence women's perceptions of their own bodies to this day. Throughout the 19th and 20th centuries, Doctors Budin, Cooney, Pritchard, Truby King and many more, strove with amazing energy and zeal to manage infant feeding the way they thought best. Somehow they ignored, or were frustrated by, the fact that women's bodies had their own way of working. I will return to these men in a later chapter.

the god of routine

As more of the upper classes followed Cadogan's teachings, the ordinary countrywomen, whose babies Cadogan had admired, carried on as they always had, without clocks, books or learning. Over the course of the 19th and 20th centuries ideas about regularity and routine developed to the point of tyranny especially amongst the educated classes who read the books. The source of this religion is complex and wide-rooted. The blossoming of scientific knowledge was in part derived through disciplined exactitude and rigorous observation. Mechanisation and the need for controlled production methods in the growth of industrialised capitalism precipitated the need for timing, measurement, clocks and consistency. The new ideas were applied to humans, and indeed the realization that pulse rates, temperature, blood pressure and respiration had a range of consistent measurements and rhythms endorsed these perceptions of scientific thought. The problems arose when humans were supposed to fit in with arbitrary ideas of what the physical rhythms should be. It was when true scientific observation weakened that most problems occurred.

I come from a generation where the god of routine still ruled: meals, night prayers, bowel movements and baby's crying were all supposed to coincide with the striking of the clock and woe betide the naughty child who experienced hunger pangs, gut cramps or mysticism at the wrong time. The lucky babies were those whose own personal body rhythms happened to coincide with Greenwich Mean Time, but for those who did not fit in, there was a lot of miserable adjustment for both mothers and babies.

In the early 21st century the god of routine is again receiving worshippers. The tragedy is that feeding routines may be necessary (though cruel) for artificially fed babies because baby-led feeding with artificial milks may increase the risk of long-term overweight and obesity. Breastmilk is designed for rapid digestion and frequent feeding. In his early weeks a baby's task is to communicate his individual biorhythms of need to his mother. Fashion persuades parents that they must actively try to control and change their baby's behaviour, despite the fact that his communication skills evolved for his survival. High stress levels result for both baby and parents. Most babies fall into feeding patterns within a few months without any intervention except sensitive responsiveness. In societies who practise this, it is noticeable that families enjoy their babies much more than those who read babycare books, watch clocks and weep.

too much or too little?

Cadogan and others' ideas about the dangers of overfeeding persisted well into the 20th century. As more and more women became subject to orthodox health information, they were instructed to limit feeding time. Extra artificial feeds would be given to 'top up' the baby; thus satiated he would lose his appetite for the breast and the breastmilk supply would go down. Underfeeding was dreaded, but no less than overfeeding. Test weighing of the baby before and after a single breastfeed meant that few mothers were producing the exact quantities that were judged 'correct'.

The advice to restrict feeding certainly did prevent any 'danger' of overfeeding, for the physiological result was that women who fed only at prescribed intervals or removed the baby from each breast after an exact number of minutes, were unknowingly shutting down their milk-making system. Their babies cried, some did not gain weight and these mothers believed that their bodies were innately incapable of producing enough milk for their babies' needs.

To this day 'insufficient milk' is the commonest reason that women give for abandoning breastfeeding. This is more common in societies where free access to the breast is socially deplored. Ironically, an idea that evolved from a fear of a non-existent problem (there has never been any good evidence showing the ill effects of too much breastfeeding) led to the establishment of a real problem.

the good baby

In many societies, a 'good' baby is still judged by the amount of time he sleeps or lies passively alone in a cot. A mother who wants to hold her baby most of the time is judged eccentric and often accused of 'spoiling' him. The separation of a mother and her baby reduces the chances of establishing a harmony between their physiological rhythms. New research tells us[11] that during the 20th century we were misled by medical and nutritional science into trying to make babies gain weight faster by giving them extra foods besides breastmilk. This practice is now implicated in the international obesity epidemic and linked with later chronic diseases.[12]

There are now new preachers of the religion of restriction and routine. Their book sales show that their message fulfils some need in (mostly western) parents, to make their babies conform to an externally prescribed pattern very early. When mothers are allowed and encouraged to be intuitive and responsive to their babies' cues, the pair adapt to each other rapidly and the synergy of two lives can be established happily. A baby's relationship with her mother is the primary experience of love. Does anyone fall in love to a schedule?

soreness and suffering

I have met too many people who consider breastfeeding as an assault course of agonies to be able to ignore the fact that some feel hostile about it. I recall one of my mother's friends who felt the same horror

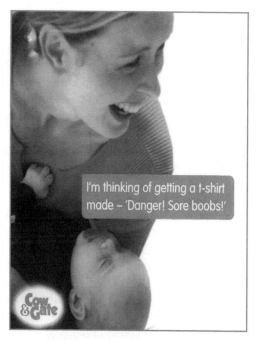

2 Exploiting ignorance: Cow & Gate leaflet 2006

about sex, and I learned that she assumed that sexual intercourse was meant to hurt and be unpleasant; after two children she never let her husband near her again. Nowadays her doctor would be concerned and might refer her to a specialist counsellor. Many women have consulted their doctors about breastfeeding difficulties and been advised to give it up and feed artificially. I leave you, alert reader, to work out your own comparisons with sex.

Misinformation about breastfeeding has been causing pain for years and though I am determined that this is not a 'how to' book, I have to mention sore nipples because they have become an obsession and are shrewdly exploited by the infant formula manufacturers.

The 19th-century discovery of the germ theory of disease was a breakthrough for society, but the resulting overzealous concern with hygiene proved disastrous for breastfeeding. Washing the nipples before and after breastfeeds destroys their protective secretions, increasing the risk of soreness and infection. By the 20th century, books advised scrubbing the nipples with surgical spirit during pregnancy to 'harden them' and massaging with lanolin after the birth to 'soften them'. Some mothers and babies escaped or even survived these persecutions, but not surprisingly more and more found artificial feeding a blessed relief. The suppliers and makers of foods and feeding equipment were eager to provide them with the goods.

Obsessive washing, however, was not the main cause of sore nipples. The disastrous advice to restrict the time the baby spends at the breast persists because the myth survives that suckling itself causes sore nipples. "I advise all mothers to start off by offering five minutes each side every three hours," says a 21st-century best-selling babycare book.[13] How long a baby suckles has nothing to do with nipple damage. Most commonly it is due to the baby being prevented from taking enough of the breast into her mouth and attaching comfortably and effectively. In official international breastfeeding parlance this is called 'good attachment'. Some people call this 'a good latch' and there must be many other explanatory phrases in the world's six hundred languages. Lots of mothers and babies work out attachment between themselves, especially if they have had uninterrupted skin contact and frequent suckling from the start. Confidence plays a huge part and if a woman has seen breastfeeding all her life and assumes it works, then she will have it. When you live in an artificial feeding culture, you miss the unconscious, lifelong lessons of how to hold your baby. Could you enjoy and be skilled at dancing if you had never seen it done and had only read about it in a book?

In societies that hide breastfeeding, poor attachment can happen when a mother does not get skilled help with holding her baby comfortably and close. Sore nipples may be related to other factors – possible candida (thrush) infection, use of creams and balms – but the great majority of breastfeeding problems are due to poor attachment. Some babies are born with a 'tongue-tie' which stops them attaching and suckling effectively. A quick snip by a trained person can resolve this.[14] Many traditional societies recognise and deal with tongue-tie.

Of course suckling may feel strange at first, as any new experience might. Some women may feel a little bit sore, but if the baby is well-attached this decreases quickly. If it gets worse then there is a problem and urgent help is needed. It is just like wearing new shoes: if they fit well, they become more and more comfortable; if they are badly fitted then you will soon get a painful blister. Too many women experience sore, cracked and even bleeding nipples and think this is normal. No wonder word gets round that breastfeeding is dreadful. These women needed skilled help long before they started suffering. To return to the sex analogy, if sexual intercourse is still painful after a week, then there is probably a problem with technique and if the couple cannot work it out between them, they need help.

Everything starts to go wrong if the baby is not well attached. The influence of bottle-feeding makes many people think that 'nipple sucking' is breastfeeding. It is not. If the baby sucks his mother's nipples as he would a bottle teat, it damn well hurts. The milk is not efficiently removed and mastitis (inflammation of the breast) or an abscess may result. That is why so many women say: 'First I got sore nipples, then my milk supply failed so I had to give up.' Of course their milk supply failed. The sore nipples were a sign that the baby's mouth was not in the right place. Not only does a baby's 'nipple sucking' hurt a woman, it stops the message to her brain to keep the system going. Because the milk contains something called 'feedback inhibitor of lactation' or FIL[15], the system eventually shuts down, usually after a lot of misery.

the milk factory

The milking action of a well-attached baby stimulates the right nerves (under and around the areola) which send messages to a mother's brain to keep the milk-making hormones going. Prolactin is the key hormone for producing the milk and oxytocin delivers it to the baby. In a way lactation is the 'normal' state of the body because we need a special hormone (prolactin release inhibiting hormone) to stop us lactating. This is suppressed as soon as the placenta is delivered, allowing the prolactin to rush into a mother's bloodstream. The breast then starts to secrete the early, concentrated milk, called colostrum (some women secrete colostrum during pregnancy) which looks yellowish and is so high in anti-infective properties that it has been called 'the first immunisation'. Thick, treacly colostrum is the perfect consistency for newborns who need time to get the knack of coordinating their swallowing and breathing. A baby's stomach is only the size of his fist and it should not be overfilled. A liquid can pour in too quickly, but a newborn can control the portions of colostrum and practice suckling before the milk starts flowing abundantly.

In some cultures colostrum is thought to be bad or unnecessary and new mothers are told to express and discard it. For example, today in Pakistan most mothers delay breastfeeding to avoid giving colostrum and this is one reason for the high infant mortality rate.[16] In western culture colostrum has, until recently, been viewed with indifference. The focus has often been on 'waiting for the milk to come in' as though colostrum is not milk. Luckily some colostrum lingers in the milk.

Women's experiences vary. Some feel full breasts soon after birth, and even if they do not breastfeed may lactate for weeks. Other women do not feel the sensation of full breasts and some have believed, or were told, that their milk 'never came in'. Because the maintenance of breastfeeding depends on the baby, if he does not suckle, the mother's body sooner or later gets the message that her baby has died and shuts down the mechanisms of milk secretion. FIL tells the body to switch off production when the milk is not removed from the breasts.

Giving full-term, healthy babies anything other than their mothers' breastmilk is a waste of effort and a risk. Glucose and water diminish the appetite and thirst which prompt a baby to suckle effectively. Artificial milk satiates even more and can also prime the baby's body for future allergic reactions, as well as establishing a harmful acid/alkali balance in the gut preventing the growth of the good bacteria which protect against infection.

The evidence for exclusive breastfeeding is now so strong that it is a cornerstone of all mother and child health programmes. Though recommended for many years, its significance was highlighted when researchers discovered the dramatic difference in HIV transmission between exclusive breastfeeding and mixed feeding. Interestingly, in 18th-century England, when Cadogan advocated early, exclusive suckling, more babies survived the first month of life. Despite scientific evidence that (except in rare medical cases) anything other than breastmilk interferes with the establishment of breastfeeding and may do harm, artificial feeds and glucose water are still used in many maternity wards around the world.[17]

The role of the baby in all aspects of breastfeeding has been underestimated, and one scientist described this part aptly as "the baby in the driving seat".[18] Full-term healthy babies are extremely adept at organising their meals to suit themselves and their mothers' bodies – if only other people will let them do it.

As explained above, poor attachment and restricted feeding are the commonest cause of problems and failure. The influence of artificial feeding means that a mother might have played with a doll and a toy bottle when she was a little girl or fed relatives' babies with bottles. If she holds her baby in a position for bottle-feeding, the baby cannot attach well. The baby (too high and not close enough) may suck her nipple instead of suckling her breast and this causes damage. She may need help with positioning her baby so that she can attach well.

when the baby cannot do the work

It is worth adding here that it is possible to produce milk without the baby's stimulus if a mother expresses her milk frequently, either by hand or with a breast pump. These situations arise when a baby cannot suckle, for example if he is born with a cleft palate or is too ill or premature. Such mothers need extra emotional and practical support. If they cannot have skin contact or hold their babies straight away, they need to be able to look at their baby (or at least a photo if they cannot be near all the time) or smell his clothes.[19] Ideally, a mother can undertake the feeding. I saw this happening in Chiang Mai Government Hospital in Thailand where staff taught mothers to tube- or cup-feed their special-care babies. The results were proud and confident mothers who knew that they had contributed to saving their babies' lives and went home having established exclusive breastfeeding.

For many women breastfeeding is not an instinct and has to be learned. Non-human primates, such as chimpanzees, learn about both sex and suckling by observation when they are young. Primates reared in laboratories or zoos have problems with both activities if they have never witnessed them and often cannot mother their young.[20] Humans in most western societies cannot avoid images of sexual activity, but breastfeeding rarely occurs explicitly in films, magazines, television and daily life. Much of the imagery of breastfeeding information has presented it as a medical issue. Images of bottle feeding are all around us, one example being the universal bottle signs outside baby care rooms in shops and airports. In societies where breastfeeding is taken for granted and practised unselfconsciously and openly, women find it easier.[21]

the let-down reflex and the hormone of love

> *"I have given suck and know how tender 'tis to love the babe that milks me."*
> Lady Macbeth in Macbeth, Act 1, Scene 4, William Shakespeare[22]

The hormone oxytocin controls the 'let-down' or 'milk ejection' reflex, triggering a sequence of contractions to squeeze the milk through and out of the breast. As with prolactin, the secretion of oxytocin from the brain is stimulated via the nerves under the areola. Oxytocin is a fascinating hormone: it has a role in sexual arousal, orgasm and childbirth. Eye contact between a mother and her baby increases oxytocin. It is released in both men and women and seems to be crucial in bonding. Mice bred to have no oxytocin have trouble recognising family members. The obstetrician Michel Odent calls oxytocin 'the hormone of love'.[23] In her book The Oxytocin Factor, Kerstin Moberg describes all the amazing things this hormone does to make us sweeter, so much so you feel it could put an end to war.[24] However, one of its effects might work against breastfeeding women. I will save that little fact for Chapter 16.

Many women are aware of the let-down reflex as a tingling sensation of milk pouring through their breasts. They may feel their milk 'letting down' when they hear their baby cry, smell his clothes or even just think about him.

The secretion of oxytocin can be affected by fear or shock, which can trigger the release of another hormone, adrenaline, which may inhibit its circulation. This is a temporary effect. People used to believe that 'nerves' or stress could 'dry up the milk'. Many still do. If stress stopped lactation, the human race would never have evolved because stress has always been an integral part of human existence. The inhibition of the let-down reflex was probably a useful adaptation for survival. Life for our earliest ancestors was dangerous. If an early human was running away from a predatory animal, flowing milk would leave a scent trail, so a reflex to stop flow could be life-saving. When she reached a place of safety, she could put her baby to her breast and restimulate her let-down reflex. Chloe Fisher, who helped mothers and babies in the 1990s Balkan conflict noted that, "Mothers in the maternity ward could hear gunfire and still milk would be dripping from their breasts."[25] If the let-down reflex has been inhibited, then reassurance, a comforting drink or snack, gentle back massage or any other culturally appropriate expression of kindness can redeem it; and we should not forget the most important aid of all, a suckling baby.

In some traditional societies, a woman might believe that a curse or spell is drying up her milk. If the spell is working, then fear has inhibited her let-down reflex. If she believes her milk is threatened, then it may not flow. If she stops feeding, then the milk will truly diminish and the curse is fulfilled. In industrialised societies, the advertising of baby milks and bottles and the doubts of health workers and families provide the modern curses and spells. 'When breastmilk fails . . . ' is the perfect spell to destroy an anxious new mother's confidence. Conversely women whose milk has stopped flowing can have it restored through their faith in a spell or a ceremony.

4 beauty, books and breasts

"I always pass on good advice. It is the only thing to do with it."
Oscar Wilde, An Ideal Husband, 1893

Consider a woman having her first baby in hospital. She may never have seen a baby breastfeeding, let alone closely observe the techniques and rhythms of an entire feed. Her perception of her own breasts may be as sexual objects. She may value them herself in this way and feel some anxiety that breastfeeding may take away their sexiness. For many women, displaying the allure of their bodies might be the one time they feel powerful. Millions of women depend economically and emotionally on a male partner. If a woman gains both social esteem and economic security through her skill in 'keeping her man', then she knows that her body's shape is part of that skill and she has much to lose if she damages that nubile beauty. It is a fact of life that men do abandon women whose youthful bodies have changed, and that abandoned women are poorer. The cosmetics, fashion and cosmetic surgery industries thrive on women's need to maintain a certain, prescribed ideal of physical attractiveness. The promotion of products and processes stimulates insecurities through advertising imagery of impossible and distorted standards of beauty.

Stereotyped ideals of breast shape and size are endorsed by commerce; 'soft-porn' is used in the media to capture attention. By the end of the 20th century cosmetic breast surgery had become almost as socially normal as having a haircut.[1] For the greater part of human existence we went bare-breasted and were accustomed to the great diversity of breast shape. Now instead of feeling proud of their individuality, thousands of women yearn to conform to a ridiculous standard of uniformity. It is not surprising that many women are self-conscious about their breasts. Even in secure, private relationships they may crave reassurance about their breasts' acceptability. Using breasts for feeding a baby may be emotionally confusing if society and personal experience have emphasised their sexual and aesthetic functions. Some women are shy of handling their own breasts. They have been programmed to perceive suckling as a sexual activity performed by adults. (In some societies people roar with laughter when you tell them that grown men behave like babies when they are making love.) A new baby suckling with a powerful animal reflex can be disturbing to a woman who has never seen this happen and has not been prepared for it.

The unfamiliarity of the hospital ward, the busyness of the staff and the presence of strangers, can all inhibit a woman, as do the promotional messages of artificial milk and bottle companies which are still found in thousands of hospitals around the world. People often discuss why so many women do not breastfeed or give up quickly. I believe it is firm evidence of the determination of many women that so many succeed despite giving birth in such an inappropriate environment.

Imagine a young man making his first attempt at sexual penetration. Ask him to set about the project in a special sex centre where there are 'experts' he has never met before, ready to supervise and tell him how it ought to be done. Presume that his partner is as inexperienced as himself, and that he is asked if he is going to 'try and achieve an erection'. When he starts, a busy 'expert', who may never have personally experienced sexual relations, starts telling him how to do it and inspects his body with a critical expression, prodding him and his partner in an insensitive manner. By the bed is an artificial penis, put there, as the young man is told, 'just in case you can't manage it; many young men can't make it. It's not their fault, nature often fails'. Everyone knows how vulnerable the male penis is to psychological stress, and how sensitive sexual partners must be in order to nurture the psyche, as well as the body, of the male. Yet such sensitivity has been conspicuously absent from the experience of most women giving birth in hospital. There are horror stories of health staff snapping at women, pushing the baby on to the breast, then taking her off and distributing the feeding bottles whose very presence is saying, 'You won't do it, you can't do it.' It is another reason why breastfeeding declined as the hospital became the place of birth.

After she leaves hospital, a woman may feel embarrassed while breastfeeding if people disapprove or giggle. Her husband or partner and other family members might express disgust.[2] She may lack faith in her ability to feed. She might feel imprisoned in her home and excluded from normal life if she lives in a society where no one breastfeeds in public. If all this psychological damage occurs and the baby is badly attached and suckling restricted, breastfeeding is bound to fail. These circumstances have been the common experience of too many women.

trying to change old habits

In 1991, UNICEF launched the Baby Friendly Hospital Initiative (BFHI – see Appendix 3) as a strategy to achieve one goal of the 1990 Innocenti Declaration (see Appendix 2); the removal of obstacles to breastfeeding within health facilities. Acknowledging that medical practices and hospital protocols were doing harm was a giant leap forward. Changing matters was more difficult. The BFHI was designed to motivate countries to transform their hospital practices and make the Ten Steps to Successful Breastfeeding (see Appendix 3) the normal standard of care globally. By 2004, 19,000 hospitals in 150 countries had gained 'Baby Friendly' status. Its influence has led other hospitals to abandon some of the damaging practices.

Some Baby Friendly hospitals have let their standards lapse and tolerate old, bad practices. Many governments are in the thrall of the baby food industry. In the early 1990s China led the world in Baby Friendly Hospitals and breastfeeding increased. In 2008, the Chinese contaminated-milk scandal revealed that artificial feeding had become normalised. The BFHI and similar reforms cannot alone prevent the commercial sabotage of breastfeeding or bad advice from others outside the hospital but if fully implemented it can protect mothers and babies from damaging hospital practices.[3]

Some people believe that breastfeeding has returned to industrialised countries, but with some exceptions (eg Norway) while more women attempt to breastfeed, most stop early. Roughly 70% of UK mothers start breastfeeding, yet by six weeks a third, and by six months two thirds, have stopped. Exclusive breastfeeding is only 21% at six weeks and at six months is less than 1%.[4] The picture is similar in the USA.[5]

The baby food companies can maintain good profit margins as long as women hear what a marvellous thing breastfeeding is without getting the support to do it. The decision to feed their babies artificially may be a rational one, when social feedback informs women that breastfeeding is an unhappy experience. A lot of mothers advise their daughters against breastfeeding because they want to protect them from the sense of failure that they themselves endured.

traditional societies and western influences

In most traditional societies babies and mothers have a period of time to establish breastfeeding. Techniques have been learned unconsciously at an early age through observing breastfeeding as an everyday activity.

In gatherer/hunter and peasant societies women's sexual attractiveness is not linked with body shape. Indeed in Papua New Guinea (PNG) there is a dreaded curse that a witch may put on an enemy to make her breasts stay pert and upright like a young girl's forever. A woman's capacity for economic production is a priority; breastfeeding is part of this and consequently enhances her social status instead of being the hidden, private activity it may be in the western world. I must add here that in 2007, the American Society of Plastic Surgeons presented research showing that breastfeeding, even for a long time, does not make breasts lose shape. What does cause 'sagginess' is how fat you are, how many pregnancies, how big your breasts, your age and whether you smoke.[6] This is bad news for PNG women who may be cursed with pert breasts.

I do not want to convey blanket approval for all pre-industrial societies. There are some terrible traditions, female genital mutilation being among the worst. What is notable is that the women who endure this trauma inevitably have more birth problems, yet still go on to breastfeed confidently. This is not always exclusive breastfeeding. Many societies give other substances to babies. We have to differentiate between a woman giving a herbal tea to protect against bad spirits or giving a bottle of formula because she believes she does not have enough milk. Both are to do with irrational belief systems, but the latter does more harm than the former.

People do what others do without question. When I tell friends from my own generation that babies under six months should not have water, they say, 'Oh but I gave my baby water and he grew up healthy.' These breastfeeding mothers gave water not because they doubted their milk supply but because they had been told they must. They did what everyone did. It is the same in traditional societies. My friend Charles who works in rural Guatemala, beamed enthusiastically at a small baby. The villagers feared he had imparted the evil eye and demanded that Charles donate his socks (unwashed), which were boiled in water. The baby was given a few sips of this sock-broth to counteract any ill-effects of Charles' well-meaning smile. Under the WHO criteria of exclusive breastfeeding (see Appendix 7), this anti-evil eye strategy could count as an essential medicine. It is no less harmful or effective than all the chamomile teas, gripe waters, 'water with a hint of rosehip' and all the other nonsense liquids that people give to babies in all societies.

There is enormous diversity of practices. In parts of Morocco, pregnant women are forbidden to be in the same room where a woman is breastfeeding. In rural Guatemala early, exclusive breastfeeding from birth is the norm, yet sweet weak coffee is given at about nine months. In much of Asia colostrum is discarded and pre-lacteal feeds of rice or honey are common. Early feeds are delayed in some groups and not in others. Practices vary according to tribe, clan, family and religion – and yet, despite these adverse practices there are effective support systems which help breastfeeding.

In societies where a woman does hard physical work, she is expected to have a complete rest to recover after childbirth and to establish breastfeeding. There is a common myth that 'Those peasant women squat down in the fields, give birth and then carry on working.' This is nonsense. Most cultural and religious rules make this rest period compulsory, and it is often forty days, just about the time it takes for a mother and her baby to adjust to each other and establish lactation. Relatives and neighbours take on her household and agricultural tasks and care for the new mother, providing a welcome respite from her hard-working life: "I didn't lift a finger for six months when I had my twins; my grandmother did everything for me," an overworked Ghanaian nurse once told me nostalgically.

Urbanisation, migration, family separation and hospital childbirth combine to disrupt such support systems. Without this emotional and practical support, breastfeeding problems develop and failure becomes normal. More and more women lose confidence in their bodies when there is no one close to reassure them. Hospitals, designed originally for the battle-wounded, are noisy places where clattering trolleys, early waking for medical routines and night-lighting disrupt sleep. After birth women need peace, privacy, unhurried emotional support and uninterrupted time with their babies. Staff are often stressed and overworked and their moods may communicate negativity to a new mother. Without special interventions such as a policy overhaul or staff training, breastfeeding help is not a priority. Staff might be reprimanded if they are late with form-filling, but not if they fail to sit with a mother to help her breastfeed in a calm, supportive way.

These western priorities became established in the developing world. When I visited a neo-natal ward in Costa Rica, an enthusiastic young doctor expounded on the hospital's commitment to breastfeeding. As we peered at babies in incubators, a sad young woman was sitting nearby, bottle-feeding her three-day-old baby. I asked the doctor why; he did not know, and asked the woman. "I have no milk," she said. The doctor translated her words without a flicker of reaction, and we sped on to gaze at another technological marvel. It was more important for him to impress us than it was to help this woman. This doctor's benign acceptance of the woman's self-diagnosis confirmed her lack of confidence in her own body. Like many doctors he was probably untrained in the techniques of breastfeeding support. Health workers' experience of breastfeeding failure is often greater than their experience of success. They all know the mantra that breast is best and that milk contains amazing things, which is as useful as knowing that potatoes are edible and nutritious, without ever learning how to cook them.

Many health workers acknowledge that they learned more from their own babies, other mothers and the breastfeeding support groups than from their training. Faith in the process is conspicuously lacking and this mistrust is communicated to mothers. When health workers ask a woman, 'Are you going to try and breastfeed?'[7] they imply the likelihood of failure. Do driving instructors start off with the assumption that most of their clients will never drive a car?

I once discussed breastfeeding by childless women of adopted babies with a paediatric nutritionist. He confidently stated that this procedure was impossible, because the breast 'had to be primed with the post-natal hormone influx', and that this would be 'difficult to manage pharmacologically'. One woman who breastfed her adopted babies (without any drugs) lived in the same town where this doctor worked, but these facts did not fit in with his understanding of the way women's bodies work and he could not accept them.

Health workers often need more breastfeeding support than mothers. Derrick Jelliffe and his wife Patrice set up a relactation unit in Uganda. Mothers were well fed and rested, and suckled their babies frequently in order to restimulate lactation after they had misguidedly abandoned it for artificial-feeding. They were also given a small dose of chlorpromazine, a tranquillising drug which has the side-effect of inducing lactation. This project was carried out years ago and it is now known that chlorpromazine should not be given to breastfeeding mothers. The Jelliffes knew that relactation could happen without medication, but the main purpose of the drug was to inspire confidence in the health workers. They could not believe that relactation could happen without western medical aids, and their faith in pharmaceuticals communicated itself to the mothers, thus aiding the process. We have to have placebos for health staff administered via the patient![8]

Faith alone does not make breastfeeding easy in a society ignorant of ordinary techniques, but where breastfeeding is still normal, the fact that a woman takes it for granted that she can breastfeed has a potent effect on her success. Relactation is now a well-recognised and well-managed procedure, and is particularly important in disaster situations where an artificially fed baby is at great risk of death. In less dire situations, the ignorance of lactation is still so widespread that thousands still believe that once a woman stops breastfeeding she can never restart.[9]

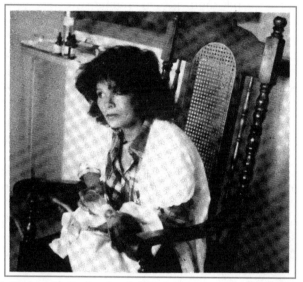

3 Woman bottle feeding her three day old baby because she believed she had no milk. (Photo Gabrielle Palmer 1987)

old habits die hard

Babies need to breastfeed when their bodies tell them to. This may be quite seldom or quite frequently depending on the individual baby, but on the whole frequent feeding works better. After birth there is a time of 'calibration' when the mother's and baby's responsiveness to each other sets the mother's body to produce the right amount of milk for her baby or babies. Breastmilk changes over the hours, weeks and months, according to a baby's needs; and it changes during a breastfeed.

To my amazement and horror many mothers are still told to change breasts after a set time (for instance two minutes a side) in the belief that this 'protects' the nipples. The result is that a baby might take in two helpings of what some people call 'fore-milk', which though full of important nutrients and enzymes, does not slake a baby's hunger because it may not include any fat-rich 'hindmilk'. It is like having a meal with two soups and no main course; you feel full but unsatisfied. The baby stays hungry and may have pain, wind and colic because he has not had a nutrient-balanced meal. The concept of 'fore' and 'hind' milk can do harm because it can make some women solemnly try to control the balance of their feeds. When babies feed frequently in the gatherer-hunter style they may actually take in more of the vital fats than the controlled, spaced feeds of industrialised societies. Babies, like adults, are all different: some feed quickly and others slowly, some from one breast at each feed and others from both. The key is to learn from the baby. Babies fall off the breast spontaneously with sleepy satisfaction when they have taken what they need. Indeed this is a sign that the baby has been well attached. Babies can translate the nutrient needs of their tiny bodies into their suckling behaviours, but medical rules based on mistaken theories have sabotaged their skills.

Today, in spite of 'baby-led feeding' being recommended, it is still rare in industrialised society. I have heard midwives suggest that mothers 'demand feed every two hours'. Health workers ask mothers how often a healthy, full-term baby has fed during a 24-hour period. This pressures a woman into making a responsive, spontaneous act into a monitored, self-conscious task. Does she count how often she kisses and hugs her partner or older children or chats to colleagues or friends? Michael Latham, Professor of Nutrition at Cornell University, described real 'demand' feeding when he said, "Asking a woman in rural Africa how often she breastfeeds is like asking someone with an itchy rash how often they scratch."[10]

sinister female fluids

The profound mistrust of breastfeeding is complex, but a primitive male fear of the polluting quality of women comes into the argument. Many cultures have beliefs in the power and pollution of female fluids. Zulu tradition claims that manhood may be lost if breastmilk falls on a man's skin. In Mozambique a friend assured me that women deliberately killed men by having intercourse when they were bleeding from their vaginas. Some European Christian churches still have cleansing ceremonies which coincide with the end of the lochia, the blood loss after childbirth. A Christian priest told me that he believed it was an irrational horror of menstruation that was behind the resistance to the ordination of women priests.

After childbirth women are both bleeding from their vaginas and secreting milk from their breasts and modern theories of disease have been used to endorse ancient primitive emotions. I would have dismissed these theories as obscure nonsense if I had not been confronted with many expressions betraying their revulsion. Many men twitch at the mention of menstrual blood. When I first explored this subject I thought it was a matter of male disgust of women, but I have since learned that many women are alarmed by their own secretions. As many have pointed out to me, when nurses and midwives used to play a joke on young doctors by putting expressed breastmilk in their coffee, telling them only after they had drunk it and then laughing at their disgust, it was not just the men who were horrified.

In 1980s Mozambique, though child mortality rates were high, it took the late President Machel's personal intervention to persuade Portuguese doctors that mothers should stay with their babies in paediatric wards. The excuse for keeping them out was 'hygiene', yet mortality rates fell when mothers were allowed to stay with their babies to breastfeed and care for them. Separation of mothers and babies has been a persistent practice in many countries, despite evidence that it is harmful both physically and emotionally for the baby and mother. There is not a single scientific study to show that separated babies have fewer infections than those left with their mothers, indeed the contrary has been shown.[11] Why should the health worker bottle-feeding the baby be less of a carrier of disease than the mother who has been protecting the baby in her body for months?

The discovery of HIV and the fact that it could be found in breastmilk led to a resurgence of these fears of female fluids. The very expression, 'mother to child transmission' (MTCT) implied that only women transmitted the virus. As one HIV worker expressed it, "It is as though a woman is seen as a vector." The child's father may have introduced the infection either before or after conception.

Male ambivalence towards female bodies seemed to be behind some early 20th-century doctors' doubts and fears about breastfeeding. Dr Koplick, a leading paediatrician of his time, wrote in 1903, "The thumb may be used to exert pressure on the breast, thus aiding the flow of milk. In this way the infant is prevented from drawing the nipple too far into the mouth."[12] The implication is that the fearful nipple could do harm if it went 'too far', when in fact this advice is a recipe for nipple damage and inadequate milk production. To this day women may be told to 'hold the nipple and breast between the fingers so that the baby can breathe'. Did no one notice that babies have nostrils at the sides of their noses? Babies do not suffocate at the breast, but it is a recurring male fantasy – in the 1986 James Bond film The Living Daylights a man is killed by being crushed to death between a woman's breasts.

Influenced by the ideas of Dr Koplick and others, thousands of women have fearfully breastfed in this way, sincerely believing that their baby could choke if they did not 'control' the procedure. The idea that the means of sustaining your baby's life could actually kill her must have scared many mothers.

the mistakes sanctified in print

Since I wrote the first edition of this book over twenty years ago, information about breastfeeding has improved. However, in books and magazines and on the internet, there is still much bad advice, often sitting poisonously amidst a nest of lovely pro-breastfeeding statements.

I delve into a selection of popular parenting books from my local library and to my dismay find the following example:

"The major (and often only) cause of breastfeeding problems is improper latch-on. I prevent this in mums I work with, because I meet with them four to six weeks before their due date. I explain to them how their breasts work and show them how to place two little round elastoplasts[13] on their breasts, 25mm above and 25mm below the nipple, which is precisely where they'll be holding their breasts when nursing. This gets them used to placing their fingers properly."[14]

How have trillions of women managed to breastfeed without a pre-birth supply of elastoplasts (ouch) and tape measures to get the precise millimetres? How sad that the poor author understands the importance of good attachment, but gives advice that prevents it. Such 'proper' placing of the fingers has caused a lot of trouble.

I then buy the current range of pregnancy and parenting magazines and am spoilt for choice in finding text which subtly undermines breastfeeding. One magazine feature titled Secrets of Breastfeeding Success plus a step-by-step guide begins:

"If you can, put your baby to your breast as soon as she's born. Research shows skin-to-skin contact makes breastfeeding easier. Keeping calm will help your milk flow better. If you feel tense, stop and take some deep breaths. Try to lie down 15 minutes before the next feed."[15]

Imagine reading these words when pregnant with your first baby. It implies that breastfeeding is difficult, that you are likely to feel tense and that you will know the exact time of your baby's next feed. It implies that milk flow is all to do with mood-control, which is nonsense.

Then, in boxed text below, is the heading, 'SHIELD YOURSELF FOR SUCCESS' followed by the statement: "A correctly fitted breast shield is essential for successful expressing, so Medela has this advice on how to check your shield is OK." As I read this, it dawns on me that this is 'advertorial' promoting Medela products, and sure enough a page-footer indicates this. The information is not all bad, but the overall impression is that breastfeeding is difficult, exhausting and that an array of expensive equipment and specialist knowledge is needed to do it. The visual information is damaging with the big opening breastfeeding picture for this article showing a badly attached 'nipple sucking' baby with his lower lip turned in. The magazine carries other advertisements for bottles, milks and baby foods.[16]

I now turn to the internet and easily access a milk company website. Amidst snippets about breastfeeding, the Cow & Gate site tells me that 'it is hard to tell how much milk your baby is getting'. There is an entire section entitled: 'Is my baby getting enough milk?' There then follows a list of signs some of which have serious clinical implications, such as jaundice or dehydration. Where it should say, 'Contact a health worker immediately', the advice begins: "If you are worried about whether your baby is getting enough milk, try feeding them more regularly." Does this mean to a stricter schedule or more frequently? It is unclear.[17]

I recall some African friends falling about with laughter when I told them that women read books to learn how to breastfeed. Many women in industrialised countries do seem to crave instructions. It is a measure of their lack of confidence. Much information is still inadequate, undermining or just plain wrong.

Despite much improvement, some books for health workers are still appalling. A nutrition book aimed at US nurses reinforces damaging myths and gives no useful information. It states, "Mothers need to be reminded to have the newborn 'latch on' to the entire areola not just the nipple." Areola size varies widely and for the women whose areolas spread 20cm (almost 8ins) back from their nipple, their babies need mouths like carps to achieve such a miracle. Without any explanation of how to help a mother and her baby it continues:

> "Otherwise the milk is not expressed successfully and the baby becomes frustrated and cries. All of this produces an interaction of anxiety between the newborn and the mother, frequently resulting in poor nutritional intake. Mothers who do not have adequate support and education may discontinue breastfeeding because of the poor quality of the interaction."

Well, they are certainly not going to get support if the poor nurse got her education from this book. The very next paragraph states: "Commercially prepared formula is recommended for infants during the first 6 to 12 months."

The authors also imply that a mother's food intake influences breastfeeding success and that timing is important. Top of two lists of questions to ask the mother are: "What is your routine pattern of food intake?" and "How many minutes are you feeding the baby with each breast?" The correct answer to both questions is of course 'Mind your own business!' Any mother who does know the answers needs lots of support to escape the damage of this book's misinformation.[18]

This book was published in the USA in 2001 after a decade of good breastfeeding support information disseminated by official bodies such as WHO, UNICEF, the American Academy of Pediatrics (AAP), the International Lactation Consultants' Association (ILCA) and many other breastfeeding support organisations. Publication time lag does not excuse; in the same year other US paediatric textbooks provided accurate and useful breastfeeding information. I note that a second edition of the nutrition book for US nurses has been published. In this mothers are encouraged to "allow the baby to nurse 5 to 10 minutes at each breast and schedule feeding every 3 to 4 hours".[19]

Improvement in information has taken place all over the world, thanks to devoted research scientists, health workers and campaigners who have spent decades unravelling the misinformation that has been disseminated for over a century throughout health systems, in company materials and medical textbooks. Out-of-date textbooks not only sit on health training school shelves but are even sent as charitable donations by the well-meaning.

the vanishing knowledge

Ordinary women tend to know about breastfeeding. In many less-developed societies, the idea of being unable to breastfeed does not exist. When anthropologist Leslie Conton asked Usino women in Papua New Guinea (PNG) about breastfeeding they were amazed: "Why does she ask us all this? All women know how to breastfeed!" and they laughed at the thought that she might not know how to feed an infant.[20] As Conton points out, most adult skills were learned by observation and practice, rather than verbal instruction, so the idea of formulating verbal descriptions of the breastfeeding process was strange. Even if the 19th-century doctors had discussed techniques with ordinary women, the women might not have been good at describing actions they had never analysed. Much of our knowledge of infant feeding comes from cultures undergoing rapid development where a crisis already exists, so that most groups are already being damaged by contact. It is therefore vital to grasp the vanishing knowledge from those rare societies which are still relatively undamaged. When I trained as a breastfeeding counsellor, I was taught that one could avert milk leaking by holding the heel of the hand to the breast for at least one minute, and I solemnly absorbed and disseminated this 'new fact'. This knowledge already exists in many places: in Africa I have noticed women unconsciously performing this action just as I might obliviously scratch my ear.

PNG is a poignant example of the vulnerability of traditional societies to outside influences. In the 1970s a rapid increase in malnutrition and death due to bottle-feeding was stopped through legislation banning the open sale of feeding bottles. Twenty years later, implementation of the law had lapsed and advertising via satellite television went uncontrolled.

5 a taste of infant feeding

> *"A millionaire's baby who is not breastfed*
> *is less healthy than an exclusively breastfed baby*
> *whose mother is in the poorest social group."*
> Professor J Stewart Forsyth, Ninewells Hospital
> and Medical School, Dundee, Scotland, 2006

Most of us are irrational about risk.[1] We leap into our cars without a second thought but pray when we get on a plane, yet flying is far safer than travelling in a car. When it comes to health we all know a smoking, drinking old person who disproves public health messages. My own mother was a marvellous example. Born in 1912, artificially fed from birth with sweetened condensed milk (SCM) without vitamins A and D, she grew up in a damp house with an outside lavatory. My granny was an unhygienic and terrible cook; she skimped on food to buy other necessities. My mother smoked until she was 84 (luckily for her children she went off cigarettes when pregnant) and in her later years drank far more alcohol than was good for her. She had a negative approach to life. All these factors are strongly associated with ill-health and premature death. My mother never had a serious illness, produced four healthy children and lived to be 91. Just because I witnessed her remarkable resilience does not make me able to claim that SCM as a breastmilk substitute, poor diet and hygiene, smoking, alcohol and a negative outlook are the recipe for a long healthy life. In 1912 almost 83,000 babies died.* Throughout the 20th century millions of smokers suffered illness and early death. My mother was unusual and lucky.

In industrialised countries, despite strong evidence, public health messages do not emphasise the risks of not breastfeeding. This coyness seems not only due to a desire to spare the feelings of parents, but also the delicate emotions of the artificial milk companies. When the US Office on Women's Health sponsored an advertising campaign showing the risks of artificial feeding, pressure from the manufacturers led the US Federal Administration (ie the US Government) to crush the campaign.[2]

*An IMR of 95/1000: cf 2006 IMR England and Wales 5/1000

46

breast is not best[3]

Messages about the 'benefits' of breastfeeding imply that artificial feeding is normal and safe, and that breastfeeding is a bonus. It is not like that. Artificial feeding is risky. This basic fact upsets people who feel insulted if they or their mothers did not breastfeed but most women do not 'choose' how they feed their babies: they do what their culture and society expects. Humans are herd animals and we tend to do what everyone else does. Family attitudes, friends' reported experiences and advertising can be far more powerful influences than a woman's own 'choice'. Millions who have 'tried' to breastfeed gave up because general ignorance, hospital and health workers' practices, all interwoven with cleverly targeted product promotion, sabotaged normal infant feeding . . . breastfeeding. The Chinese parents who fed their babies the contaminated Sanlu milk, did so because it had become normal in China to abandon breastfeeding early. Many Chinese mothers did not get the right support to establish and sustain breastfeeding so they believed their bodies could not produce breastmilk, or they gave up after a few months because they thought that was just fine. When they returned to work, no one had told them how to maintain breastfeeding. Global press reaction echoed modern Chinese parents' assumptions, that not breastfeeding is normal.[4]

I do not have the space to include all the effects of being artificially fed. Also most infants are neither exclusively breastfed or exclusively artificially fed. This has proved a headache for researchers who often have to adjust their feeding definitions (see Appendix 7) to the existing infant feeding practices of the societies they are investigating.

The following is just a 'taster' of the evidence of the effects of how a baby is fed. Perhaps the most conservative and cautious summary is within the policy statement of the American Academy of Pediatrics (AAP) who refer to the benefits of human milk alongside saying that breastfeeding should be "the normative model". AAP's policy emphasises the fact that human milk feeding decreases disease but avoids saying 'artificial feeding increases the incidence and severity of a wide range of short and long-term diseases'.[5] This is not just a game of language. The old mantra 'breast is best' is a cliché. Would the thousands of Chinese parents have bought any artificial milk if health workers and the media had consistently explained that artificial feeding increased the risk of a baby getting ill even if the artificial milk was of the highest quality? And if there had not been widespread advertising by all the infant feeding product manufacturers? It is not just contaminated milk that makes babies sick. In every country, rich or poor, thousands of babies are treated for illness every day because they are given foods and fluids other than breastmilk. Paediatric wards are not full of exclusively breastfed babies.

Even in the USA, where artificial feeding is assumed to be safe, it has been calculated that 720 babies between the age of one and 12 months, die each year because they are not breastfed.[6] Besides the well-known likelihood of diarrhoea and respiratory infections (the commonest causes of infant illness and death), not being breastfed increases the risk of meningitis, ear, urinary tract and blood infections. An artificially fed baby is more likely to suffer sudden infant death (SIDS, also called cot/crib death), diabetes, certain childhood cancers, overweight and obesity, high blood cholesterol and asthma.[7] Immunisation may not work so well because 'take up' (ie antibody response) of vaccines is poorer in a child deprived of the immunological effects of breastfeeding.[8] If you were breastfed you may carry living cells from your mother in you for your whole life and in a way be 'closer' to your siblings. That is why before the invention of special drugs to stop rejection, kidney transplants were more successful if the donor and recipient were breastfed siblings.[9] Being artificially fed may prevent a child from achieving his full potential intelligence.[10] If a baby is not breastfed and has a medical procedure like a heel prick test, he will suffer more pain.[11] His jaw and teeth development may be impaired, requiring costly dental treatment.[12]

Artificial feeding hurts women too. Not breastfeeding her baby straight after giving birth may increase a woman's risk of continued heavy bleeding.[13] Not breastfeeding leads to the early return of her menstrual periods which can lead to iron deficiency anaemia (IDA). Breastfeeding is especially protective for women who normally have heavy periods.[14] Women who artificially feed risk becoming pregnant again; closely spaced pregnancies damage the health and endanger the lives of both mothers and children.[15] The longer a woman breastfeeds, the lower her risk of breast[16] and ovarian cancer,[17] bone disease and hip fractures in later life.[18] Not breastfeeding can increase a woman's risk of type 2 diabetes,[19] rheumatoid arthritis[20] and gall bladder disease.[21]

Progress in medical care and health services has been a great boon for those who have access to them, but it has disguised the risks of artificial feeding. During the last half of the 20th century antibiotics dramatically reduced deaths from infections. Due to overuse and misuse, we are now entering an era of antibiotic resistance. Reports from both low and middle-income countries show that 70% of hospital-acquired infections in newborns resisted WHO's recommended treatment.[22] Early exclusive breastfeeding could prevent many such infections and save lives. More than a third of deaths in children under five happen during the first month of life (about four million babies). Breastfeeding within the first hour would save 22% of these babies.[23] That means 880,000 babies could be saved simply by not removing them from their mothers, and by supporting early suckling.

the clever food

The following is not an exhaustive account of breastmilk's amazing properties. I merely want to highlight a few facts. Despite a long record of mishaps (see Appendix 6) manufacturers of artificial milks claim to match the known nutrients in breastmilk. The subject they avoid is 'nutrient bioavailability' (ie how much is actually taken up by the body) because whatever new ingredient they add to an artificial milk they cannot ensure that the baby's body will utilise it. The nutrients in breastmilk are so well-absorbed that there is very little waste. After the first treacly, copious stool called meconium, many babies have frequent slightly-soiled nappies. Once exclusive breastfeeding is well-established, some delightful babies only produce a soiled nappy every few days.

The low proportions of some nutrients are as important as the abundance of others. It is difficult for a baby's immature kidneys to filter out the waste from excess proteins and minerals. It is because cows' milk is too rich in these nutrients that it has to be diluted and modified when used for human babies. Early overload of these nutrients as well as excess calories[24] may have long-term ill-effects.[25] Breastmilk comes with its own regulating substances which not only raise the bioavailability of some nutrients, but lower it when it is dangerous.

For example, breastmilk carries digestive enzymes which compensate for the fact that babies cannot produce their own enzymes in the first few weeks. Bile-salt stimulated lipase (BSSL) is a lovely breastmilk enzyme. It comes along in the milk, minding its own business and doing nothing much in the first part of the baby's gut. Then it meets bile salts from the baby's liver and bursts into action, breaking down the fats so they can be transported to build the baby's brain and nervous system. Apparently only a few special mammals produce milk with both the enzyme and the substrate. Humans share

VITAMIN D

Vitamin D is a hormone triggered by sunlight on the skin. Deficiency (VDD) stops bones absorbing calcium and causes rickets, the soft-bone disease which leads to malformations such as bandy legs. VDD in a pregnant woman can cause low birth weight, neonatal convulsions and heart problems in her baby. VDD was not a problem for our ancestors because they lived semi-naked in sunny regions.[26] When some early humans migrated to regions north of 50° latitude (much of Canada, Northern Europe and Russia) they had to get vitamin D during the sunny months for body-stores to last the winter. In spring, summer and autumn, five to 15 minutes outside in the daytime provides enough vitamin D for pale people. Dark-skinned people need more time or more skin exposed so citizens of Asian and African origin are more vulnerable to VDD. Babies need to be naked in sunlight (or artificial UVL) for 30 minutes a week, or two hours if clothed but bare-headed. Rickets is rare in sunny countries unless a baby is kept covered or indoors.

Historically a disease of poverty wherever factory work, bad housing and polluted air deprived people of sunlight, rickets has re-emerged. Shopping malls, computers and TV, enclosed transport and fear of other humans keep families indoors. Fewer people hang out washing, shop in the open air, walk to work or sit with their babies in the sunshine. Fear of skin cancer makes health professionals over-anxious about sun-exposure. Protection from sunburn is important but some take this to extremes. A balanced approach is needed. Food is a poor source except for fish livers. Most dietary vitamin D comes from artificially fortified foods such as fat-based spreads (UK) and milk (USA and Canada). Excess can be toxic and in the 1950s over-enriched baby foods caused serious infant illness. Concerns about over-dose have faded, but the UK's upper limit is half of the USA's recommended dose. Some health authorities suggest vitamin D supplements for breastfed babies only but babies fed on infant formula (vitamin D fortified) have developed VDD. In pregnancy vitamin D is crucial (a child's bone mineral content at nine years is related to his mother's pregnant status) but supplementing a lactating mother makes no difference to her breastmilk. The autumn-born baby of a mother with enough vitamin D will have sufficient stores to last until spring. In northern countries, supplementation may be necessary for pregnant women who avoid the sun and for some autumn/winter born babies. Individual assessment prevents the risk of excess amounts.[27]

this talent with gorillas, dogs, cats, ferrets and seals. In contrast a breastmilk protein called lactoferrin, binds with iron to prevent too much being utilised. Excess iron encourages the growth of harmful bacteria in the gut.[28] Iron is an important but dangerous nutrient. Too much or too little makes us ill. Recent research has found that babies who are born with sufficient iron stores and are fed iron-fortified artificial milk have poorer neurodevelopment.[29]

Breastmilk has similar proportions of nutrients, immunological and growth factors the world over. A mother's undernutrition has little effect on her milk, but there may be lower concentrations of vitamin A, iodine and B vitamins if her diet is deficient. In the past,

---

VITAMIN K

Vitamin K is needed for blood clotting and deficiency is associated with a rare condition called haemorrhagic disease of the newborn (HDN) which can cause brain damage and death. (In the absence of intervention HDN occurs in between four to 70 cases per 100,000 births, ie between 0.004 to 0.07% of the population.) Vitamin K is found in dark-green leafy vegetables, cucumber, cheese, yoghurt and certain oils (olive, rapeseed, soya). It is also made by bacteria which live in the gut. If a mother has enough vitamin K in her diet during pregnancy, her baby is born with enough body stores until his own personal germ farm has got going. A woman will naturally push out some faeces as she gives birth and if her baby arrives in the common way with his face downwards, he will ingest a few useful micrograms of faeces which quickly colonise his gut with vitamin K-producing bacteria. If his mother has a C-section or her bowels were emptied with an enema before birth, this beneficial contamination will be prevented. Some medical textbooks point to exclusive breastfeeding as a risk for vitamin K deficiency. There are two aspects to this. Firstly, the biochemical markers which indicate low vitamin K in a baby (who has not received the synthetic dose) decrease as breastfeeding becomes established. Scientists see this as a self-correcting phenomenon and point out that most babies with apparently low levels of vitamin K never get ill. The problem is that there is no way of identifying the very few who might get HDN. The second point is that supplementing pregnant and lactating mothers benefits both mother and child and may increase breastmilk concentrations by 200%. Vitamin K is now administered routinely to babies (but not to mothers) in many countries, either by injection or an oral dose.[30]

babies of poor women subsisting on over-polished rice developed infantile beri-beri due to vitamin B1 (thiamine) deficiency. Improved rice processing had conquered this disease but in the 21st century it has been reported from refugee camps. Iodine deficiency is readily remedied by salt iodization and iodized oil doses for women and children. Political apathy is a cause of its persistence in deficient areas.[31]

Vitamin D is naturally low in breastmilk because humans evolved to get it from sunlight not food. Vitamin K may be low if a mother's diet is deficient. (See boxes for information on vitamins D and K.) In poor regions vitamin A deficiency is common. Scientists can actually judge a woman's vitamin A status from her breastmilk better than from a blood test. Severe vitamin A deficiency causes blindness. It also impairs the immune system, increasing the risk of death from measles, diarrhoea and respiratory infections in infants and young children. Giving a mother a large vitamin A dose soon after birth maximises the vitamin A in her breastmilk and protects both herself and her child from infections and death. In wealthier regions, most people have plenty of vitamin A in their diets, so supplementation can be toxic and it is forbidden for pregnant women because excess amounts can cause birth defects.[32]

Despite marginal diets the nutrient quality of breastmilk is remarkably adequate for the majority of women.

the robustness of lactation

The world over, even undernourished women can produce enough milk to support their babies' growth and development.[33] If you consider that all women are designed to feed twins, then you realise that feeding one baby is unlikely to tax the body's capacity. As K-strategists (see page 12) the human female evolved to survive reproduction and stay healthy enough to reproduce again after a period of recovery. Biologically the contraceptive effect of breastfeeding (see Chapter 10) is part of that recovery. It seems that breastfeeding has a beneficial role in protecting women's health.

Extra food makes little difference to breastmilk output. It is the baby's behaviour (and free access to her mother's breasts) that controls the amount of milk. Food supplementation can even do harm. When scientists gave Gambian mothers high energy biscuits to see if this increased their breastmilk, it made no difference to milk supply but did decrease the infertility effect of breastfeeding, thus increasing the danger of closely-spaced births.[34]

During the Second World War in Singapore, Dr Cicely Williams was interned in the Sime Road concentration camp together with other British women, 20 of whom were pregnant: 20 babies were born in the camp, 20 were exclusively breastfed and 20 survived and grew up healthy.
Personal communication Cicely Williams 1984.
See also: Baumslag N. J Hum Lact 2005; 21:6-7

When nutritionists worked out the theoretical energy needs of lactation, they arrived at a figure of an extra 500 calories (2,100 kilojoules) a day. This amounts to an extra helping of normal daily food such as rice, dahl and vegetables, a peanut butter sandwich or a small bowl of shelled nuts.[35] Chances are that if you are a breastfeeding woman reading this book and live in North America, Europe or Australasia you need no extra food because most of us (I include myself) eat more than we need and have a body fat store to provide this energy. However in poor regions many women do not get enough food to lay down fat stores. Even then they still lactate successfully. These women need extra food to protect them from malnutrition which puts them at risk of illness. Diet before and during pregnancy does make a difference to whether a baby is born healthy, but lactation is astonishingly robust and persists in the worst conditions as evidence from prison camps and women suffering from anorexia nervosa shows.[36]

Just because our bodies work so brilliantly does not mean I am advocating less food for women. On the contrary, pregnant women need priority for good food. How well or poorly girls are fed from birth influences their own and their children's long term health, but lactation works well despite disadvantage and may even break the cycle of intergenerational disadvantage. Women can feel proud of this physical resilience.[37] It is like being good at running marathons.

Over the years breastmilk has been criticized for being too rich, too weak, too little or too much, and doubt is widespread. A common media image of breastfeeding has been of a hungry mother in a famine rather than of the millions of ordinary women who breastfeed without fuss. Reporters have referred to babies 'sucking on empty breasts' when they have no evidence to prove this statement. A withered breast reflects a mother's weight loss, not her state of lactation. If you went on a crash diet and walked hundreds of kilometres in the heat, you would have sagging breasts. But you could still produce milk to keep your baby alive.

more than a food

Breastmilk is much more than a food: its secretion is part of a process which affects the mother and the baby both immunologically and hormonally. Immunologist Lars Hanson views not being breastfed as a state of immunodeficiency.[38] A baby's immune system is not fully developed at birth and she relies on her mother's antibodies which were transferred to her in the womb. These 'passive antibodies' linger for many months and help the artificially fed child survive. Breastfeeding provides an intermediate immunology system while the baby's own immune system is developing. Pathogens are destroyed or weakened by the anti-infective factors in breastmilk. As the placental antibodies gradually disappear a baby develops her own. During this crossover phase, breastfeeding makes the disease-challenge less of a risk. Interestingly, the thymus gland (which controls the development of the immune response) of an exclusively breastfed baby is double the size of the thymus of an artificially fed baby.[39] This is because breastmilk contains a vast range of substances which transmit messages to the baby's body tissue to signal it to develop in a particular way. The power of breastfeeding can be illustrated by the fact the thymus size is actually related to the number of breastfeeds a day.[40]

The difficult conditions in which most of the world's babies live makes this protection essential for health and life, but even in the rich world it is important. Of course breastfed babies can get ill, but they stand a much better chance than their artificially fed sisters and brothers. A mother's breast is like an efficient pharmacist: it produces general disease preventing substances for everyday use and then makes up specific medicines to order as need arises.

Babies and mothers are challenged by the same pathogens. Disease is diagnosed by the mother's body before anyone else notices. A mother, like everyone, meets pathogens and manufactures her own specific antibodies. But unlike men and non-lactating women she transfers these to her breast through her body's immunological network. Breastfed babies' illnesses are usually less severe and less life-threatening. For example they are less likely to die from measles which still kills children where immunisation programmes are inadequate. Where immunisation programmes do function breastfeeding improves the effectiveness.[41] The antibodies in breastmilk are also thought to protect the breast itself from disease as well as the baby.

In certain circumstances breastmilk can also transmit disease, most notably HIV, but even then specific anti-infective factors are at work which protect most babies from infection.[42] The world is full of disease-causing organisms and yet even in the worst conditions, not every baby dies. Miraculously the majority live, thanks to this amazing system of disease protection.

faster, bigger, fatter: how should babies grow?

The fascinating properties of breastmilk are too numerous to describe here. They include anti-inflammatories, substances which influence our lifetime's immune system, growth factors and hormones which trigger responses to nutrients. Until recently, health workers and scientists worried about breastfed babies' growth because it did not conform to the growth curve of the international reference standards. Astonishingly, these were based on the US National Child Health Survey (NCHS) standards yet were adopted by WHO and the majority of governments. They were established by measuring mainly white, artificially-fed babies, mostly from one region in mid-USA, between the 1920s and 1970s. Eventually, WHO acknowledged the bad science behind these standards and launched research to discover the biological basis of optimal human growth. This was based on the careful observation of exclusively breastfed infants in six very different countries. WHO now state that: "Arguably, the current obesity epidemic in many developed countries would have been detectable earlier if a prescriptive international standard had been available 20 years ago."[43]

Nutritionists now realise that obesity starts in infancy, or even before. Infants who gain weight too rapidly are likely to develop into overweight or obese adults. Even though they can appear gloriously plump, it is rare for an exclusively breastfed baby to become overweight. Babies who are artificially fed or mixed fed with extra artificial milk and high energy solid foods are at risk of childhood overweight and obesity.[44]

Of course if a baby stops growing he should be checked for illness. Too often a slowing of weight gain is attributed to a mother having insufficient breastmilk when there may be other reasons. Breastfeeding is often 'blamed' for a problem which it is helping to solve.[45] Insufficent breastmilk is a sign that both mother and baby need help to diagnose and resolve the problem. Most breastfeeding difficulties can be resolved through improving attachment. A baby who is not stimulating enough breastmilk is usually a sick baby. It used to be assumed that weight loss preceded infection but a breastfed baby who feels unwell may not suckle effectively and as a result loses weight. Supplemental milks, cereals, water, juices and infant 'teas' may have triggered the illness. Giving a baby anything other than breastmilk before six months increases the risk of infection, allergy and even death. Whatever the supplement, it is nutritionally inferior to breastmilk; it fills a baby's stomach, decreases appetite at the breast and thus reduces the breastmilk supply.[46]

ROSE PETAL'S STORY

Rose Petal was born at 37 weeks' gestation with a severely malformed gut. Surgeons carried out intricate surgery but her bowel would not function and she developed jaundice and septicaemia. After discussing all options her parents decided on palliative care at home. Her mother had been advised to stop breastfeeding because her baby was expected to die within two weeks. Rose Petal proved unable to digest and absorb infant formula and was losing weight. A friend offered to supply some of her breastmilk which was fed to Rose Petal along with other local mothers' milk, offered after an appeal. After three months she stopped losing weight and even started gaining a little. Her mother tried unsuccessfully to relactate. Then collecting enough breastmilk locally got more difficult. Rose Petal's parents turned to the milk-banks and Gillian Weaver of The United Kingdom Association for Milk Banking (UKAMB) coordinated a supply of breastmilk by collecting surpluses from different milk banks. Rose Petal's grandparents helped with the coordination. With Gillian's input and help the country-wide milk banks took it in turns to supply Rose Petal. The Red Cross provided a volunteer driver to collect and deliver the milk. Rose Petal began to improve and grow a little. She subsisted on breastmilk and rehydration fluids which proved essential for her electrolyte balance. She continued with these and carefully selected foods for three years. She had ups and downs but her very survival disproved all expectations. Nine years later Rose Petal's parents still feel profound gratitude that donated breastmilk kept their daughter alive at a time when hope had been lost.

This account is adapted from 'A Case for Donor Milk Banking – Rose Petal' by Gillian Weaver, UKAMB News, April 2002; and with help from Rose Petal's mother.

premature and low birth weight babies

Many people associate the care of premature and low birth weight (LBW) babies[47] with incubators. These were invented by the 19th century French doctor, Pierre Budin. Inspired by methods for rearing newly hatched chicks, he designed glass-sided 'hatcheries' to keep babies warm but also so that mothers could see their babies. Budin knew that mothers lost heart and were more likely to abandon their infants if they could not touch or see them. He commented, "The life of the little one has been saved, it is true but at the cost of the mother." Budin encouraged as much contact as possible. Regrettably his pupil, Dr Martin Cooney, lacked such sensitivity. He spent his life commercialising his "human hatcheries", exhibiting them at trade fairs and exhibitions. German doctors 'gave' him premature babies who were not expected to live and in 1896, 3000 visitors viewed his infant exhibits at the Berlin World Exposition. Throughout the next four decades, Cooney displayed 'his' infants in Europe (eg at Covent Garden in London) and in the USA. In 1940, infant hatcheries were still on display at Coney Island amusement resort near New York.

Unlike Budin, Cooney forbade mothers to be involved in their infants' care. He restricted visits on the pretext that they caused infection. Cooney's methods, which included scrupulous hygiene and one nurse per baby, became the prototype for the care of premature and LBW babies in US hospitals. In the 1920s and 1930s mothers were

4 The custom of forbidding mothers contact with their newborns spread all over the world. This is a notice in Benghazi Hospital, Libya.
The British had left their stamp on the Libyan medical schools; other Libyan doctors had trained in Ireland. (Photo Gabrielle Palmer 1994)

encouraged to provide breastmilk but discouraged from contact with their babies. We can still find Martin Cooney's legacy today when health systems lack provision for mothers to stay close to their vulnerable babies.[48]

There are many different reasons for a baby to be born too small or too early. Among some of the known causes is a mother's own long-term poor health and nutrition, and the stresses during her life. This is why poorer mothers are likely to have smaller and more vulnerable babies. Babies who suffer growth retardation in the womb, even if they reach full-term, are at risk of illness and death. Other babies might be growing well and an event such as a mother's infection, or a sudden shock such as a car accident, might trigger an early labour. As a generalisation the early baby who has been growing well in the womb has a better chance than the growth-retarded baby.

Human milk is vital for these babies. Premature breastmilk is different in composition to full term milk, and adapted to the baby's need. Extremely premature or tiny babies may not be able to suckle and swallow, but almost all mothers can express their milk and this can be a life-saver. Such mothers need lots of support. Logistical and financial help to stay near their babies should be a priority. If a mother has died or is too ill to express, donated human milk can be used. Very early babies may need supplementary nutrients. Human milk fortifiers are commercially produced and in some hospitals are added routinely to mothers' expressed breastmilk. This can be a risk because the milk of mothers of preterm babies has variable protein levels and excess can cause harm. Some mineral supplementation may be needed for very low birthweight babies but for most, mothers (if given the right support) can meet their babies' needs and make a big difference to survival and long-term health.[49]

During the 1980s, breastmilk for premature babies was disparaged by some doctors. Research, mainly funded by the infant feeding product industry, was published that claimed that babies who had been fed on 'special' pre-term formulas grew better than those on breastmilk. This news spread round the world. On a closer look, it turned out that the supposedly breastmilk-fed babies were mostly fed 'drip milk' which donor mothers were advised to collect from the second breast while suckling her baby on the first. Drip milk tended to be lower in fat and therefore did not provide enough energy. Nowadays guidance for donor breastmilk expression is properly regulated with scrutiny of the nutrient balance. These studies also ignored the issue of adequate support and information for the mothers of the LBW babies. Later crucial differences came to light: bone density was better in the breastmilk-fed babies, and among the artificially-fed babies there were high rates of necrotising enterocolitis (NEC).

A mother's own milk is always better for her baby than donated breastmilk, but this is still better than artificial milk. Awareness of HIV has led to testing of breastmilk donors and routine pasteurisation of all donated milk. This has contributed to improved standards for supervision of human milk banks around the world.

kangaroo mother babycare

"Kangaroo mother care is a basic right of the newborn and should be an integral part of the management of low birth weight and full-term infants in all settings at all levels of care in all countries."
The Bogota Declaration 1998

Animals cuddling and feeding their babies draw the biggest crowds in zoos and wildlife parks. We love seeing mammals exhibiting mothering behaviour and cry 'aaah' when sea otters float on their backs with their pups, or joeys peek out of a kangaroo's pouch. We feel alarmed when captive apes ignore their young and intuitively know it is harmful, yet such maternal neglect became routine for the tiniest humans born in 20th-century hospitals. If modern standards for well-run zoos were applied to human society it would have to be closed down.

In 1979, in the main maternity hospital in Bogotá, Columbia, Drs Edgar Rey and Hector Martinez were short-staffed, ill-equipped and overwhelmed by the high infection and death rates of LBW babies. Separated from their ailing infants in incubators, and unable to bond, many mothers abandoned their babies. In desperation, the two doctors initiated an entirely different approach. Tiny, premature babies, wearing only a nappy, were tucked in between their mothers' breasts, held in place by clothing. Babies had continuous skin contact, and access to the breast, and slept, woke and fed in this warm, secure environment. If they needed to be tube-fed or given oxygen, this was all managed without moving the little one from his cosy nest. This method was called 'kangaroo mother care' (KMC) because it mimicked the joey in the pouch of a mother kangaroo. Babies not only survived, they thrived; mothers bonded and families were overjoyed. In the hospital, staff morale blossomed and costs fell. Rates of infection, death and abandonment dropped dramatically. In contrast to conventional care, babies' oxygen levels, heart rates, breathing and temperatures remained stable so that mothers and babies (some of the babies weighing less than 2kg, 4.2lb) were able to go home a few days after birth, where KMC continued. If a mother needed to shower, another family member held the baby in the same way, but otherwise the baby stayed tucked between his mother's breasts 24 hours a day.[50]

Kangaroo mother baby care is one of the great leaps forward of the 20th century. Wonderful interactions take place with KMC. If a baby gets too cool, his mother's breasts warm up; if he gets too hot, they cool down. Vulnerable babies sometimes stop breathing (apnoea), but with KMC this is rare. They sleep better, feed better and hardly cry at all. Mothers produce the right amount of breastmilk, probably because the skin contact stimulates their bodies to do so. A baby who cannot yet coordinate his suckling can be tube or cup-fed expressed breastmilk while staying close to his mother's breast. With KMC he progresses more quickly than incubated babies to normal breastfeeding.

Nils Bergman, a South African paediatrician, feels passionately about KMC and sees it as the biological norm. Compared with other mammals, even full-term human babies are born immature and need to stay close to their mothers during the sensitive period after birth. The unstable heart rates, irregular breathing and purposeless movements of a newborn alone in an incubator or crib may be signs of separation terror. Bergman believes that when a baby is left alone to cry and eventually stops, this silence is an act of desperation. Solitary babies are in danger and crying is evolution's method of alerting a mother that her baby needs her urgently. If ignored a newborn mammal's instinctive survival strategy is to feign death through silence to evade predators. This is a painful thought in a society where leaving a baby to cry until he 'settles' is normal. We cannot prove whether Bergman is right or wrong because experiments can never be done, but the fact that 'kangaroo care' babies do so well, despite their initial vulnerability, tells a lot about the 'normal' treatment of all newborns, whether healthy or LBW.[51]

KMC is more common now than thirty years ago, but it is still not the norm. KMC does not exclude the use of technology; all LBW babies need to be stabilised immediately after birth. If they cannot breathe they need to be ventilated with a sophisticated machine, although this may be unavailable or malfunctioning in poor countries.

A

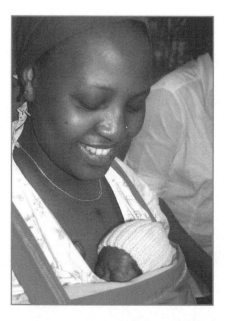

5 Mother and her baby in KMC Unit in Kalafong Hospital, Pretoria, South Africa. (Photo by Dr Elise van Rooyen with permission of the mother 2008.)

review of KMC evidence found significant reductions in hospital-acquired infection, severe illness, later respiratory infection and non-exclusive breastfeeding at discharge. The babies gained more weight per day and mothers had a greater sense of competence. There were no differences in infant mortality assessed after 41 weeks' gestational age (ie the baby had reached the normal age to be born) of babies cared for either with KMC or conventional care.[52]

This review rejected many research studies with methods below the high standards demanded for academic scrutiny. There were too few 'randomised' trials. One particular problem was 'blinding': ensuring that the researchers did not know in which group (high tech or KMC) the babies belonged. Researchers may guess which babies are which, especially if they are themselves staff involved in KMC care, and this limits the impartiality. What this review did not mention was that the practices of 'conventional care' for LBW babies have not been based on impartial research. Isolating babies in temperature-controlled glass boxes evolved out of Martin Cooney's profit-led 'infant hatcheries', not well controlled research. No one did that sort of research in the early 20th century. LBW care was based on medical opinion not scientific proof. Michel Odent once said, "We do not

A MOTHER'S INITIATIVE

"I was born in 1947 in a private nursing home in Colombo, Ceylon [now Sri Lanka]. The medical records have been lost, but my mother told me that I was premature, weighed 1.1kg and could not suck at all. I was told that no one gave me a dog's chance. My mother took me home in a shoe box lined with cotton wool and gave me what would now be called 'kangaroo care'. She created a 'wick' out of cotton wool, squeezed her breastmilk onto it and let it seep into my mouth. This did the trick. I rapidly gained weight and learned to suckle. I was breastfed, together with other foods, for four years."

This is Dr BJC 'Chris' Perera's account of his mother's initiative. He went on to be a successful paediatrician, rising to the top of his profession at an exceptionally early age. He did research, published and became the Founder President of the Sri Lanka College of Paediatricians. He practises both as a clinician and academic. Chris was a seeded national tennis player. He has no high blood pressure, diabetes or other diseases of affluence and still plays competitive tennis. He has been in the vanguard of breastfeeding protection in Sri Lanka.

know whether premature babies do what they do because they are premature or because of the way they are treated in hospitals".[53] The results of KMC show that babies do behave very differently according to how they are cared for.

In 2004 I had the privilege of visiting the 25-bed KMC Unit at Kalafong Hospital in Pretoria, South Africa. It was a complete contrast to the usual incubator-packed rooms, where tiny humans isolated in transparent boxes lie in a world of machines and tubes. Women were attending to normal tasks, talking on their mobile phones, making a drink, going to the bathroom. The most noticeable thing was the calm atmosphere and the women's faces. In contrast to the tense mothers I have seen sitting by incubators, they were relaxed, even joyful. Many wore special wrap-around blouses in gorgeously patterned African cloth which the unit had designed and were producing. On each mother's chest, slightly above the line of her blouse a tiny head would be emerging, either sleeping serenely or gazing with uncanny alertness. When a mother looked down to check, her smile was a ray of light on her baby.

The hard facts were just as inspiring as the emotional atmosphere. During the 18 months after KMC was introduced, 466 infants of whom 81% weighed less than 1,751g were admitted with their mothers. One

infant died and 32 returned to the high-care neo-na~~
mothers were breastfeeding when they went home wit~~
of some HIV-infected mothers who had made a d~~
breastfeed. The average stay was 13 days, three less th~~
was introduced.

Dr Elise van Rooyen who runs this unit is one of many South Africans dedicated to KMC. It is planned that KMC should become the normal care for all LBW babies in South Africa, and there are already some spectacular results. In Sebokeng Hospital in Vereeniging, 122 babies weighing less than 1,800g died in 2000 and 120 died in 2001. After KMC was introduced in 2002, just one baby died.[54]

We know that high-tech care, especially when combined with breastmilk feeding, saves the live of thousands of LBW babies throughout the industrialised world. We also know that many babies born too small or too early survive with medical or social problems.[55]

Most people do not have the choices that affluent people take for granted. As Professor Malan of the University of Capetown says, "In affluence, KMC is a precious gift. In financial constraints, it is a useful addition to infant care. In poverty, it may be the only means of survival."[56]

the importance of other foods: 'complementary feeding'

The WHO and UNICEF guidance on infant feeding avoids the word 'weaning'. It causes confusion both in English and other languages. To some 'weaning' means 'coming off' the breast and/or bottle, to others it means the introduction of solid foods to a breastfed or artificially fed baby's diet. Ask a roomful of people what 'weaning' means and each assumes they all have the same understanding. They do not. The official term for stopping breastfeeding is 'cessation of breastfeeding' and for starting other foods, 'complementary feeding'. They are both a bit clumsy but they are clear.

Most foods are nutritionally inferior to breastmilk, lessen the baby's appetite for the breast and therefore reduce breastmilk supply. Most babies under six months have not developed the muscular coordination to chew and swallow solid foods, which is why parents liquidise foods, make up sloppy cereal feeds or buy expensive little jars of purée and spoon them into their babies' mouths. Parents may get upset when their baby rejects their unnecessary offerings. Feeding cereals and solid foods early is not just a waste of time, money and effort, it does harm. Babies get more infections, more allergies and are

.e likely to die if they get complementary foods before six months.[57] Scientists knew this for years before WHO made it official policy. This delay had less to do with scientific doubt than with behind-the-scenes pressure from the baby food industry who did not want to change labels. WHO policy to delay solid foods could mean a loss of millions of dollars' worth of sales, so lots of lobbying went on. Still today, doctors close to the baby food industry are trying to prove that early cereals are essential for young babies. WHO guidelines have been adopted in many countries, but companies are still selling products with incorrect labels all over the world.

The six month guidance is a public health message and individual babies vary. If a baby is a week away from his first half year and grabs food off your plate, chews and swallows it easily, then he is probably ready to eat solid foods, but many babies are coaxed to eat food they do not need. Other children may not even need to start till later. One healthy child in Australia was growing well on exclusive breastfeeding at fifteen months. Scientist Peter Hartmann was asked after a lecture whether he had looked at this child's iron status. He replied, "No, I couldn't catch him".[58] I know several thriving breastfeeding babies uninterested in solid foods as they neared their first year. They are now healthy adults.

Most babies at about six months start showing developmental skills such as sitting unaided, grasping objects and putting them in their mouths, and chewing, all of which indicate readiness to try other foods.[59] Our nearest relatives, chimpanzees, depend on breastmilk alone for about three years and then spend another two to three years on breastmilk and other foods, until a mother finally refuses her breast. Her baby may protest with displays of temper. The chimpanzee mother deals with these tantrums with sensitivity and firmness.[60] Anthropologist Kathy Dettwyler has considered a range of physiological and other signs and judges that between two and a half and seven years of breastfeeding is probably the 'natural' period for the human primate.[61]

Breastfeeding continues to provide most of a child's nutrients after six months and around half in the second year, but there is an increasing need for extra iron and zinc[62] mostly available in animal foods. Absorption of iron in plant foods is not so high. The mixture of foods is important: for example, drinking tea with food (giving tea to babies is common in some regions) inhibits the absorption of iron; eating fresh fruit and vegetables enhances it. Human beings flourished for thousands of years before they started cultivating and eating cereals which are poor sources of iron. Some scientists consider that settled agriculture led to stunting in our ancestors. 'Boxgrove man' who lived in southern England around 300,000 years ago and was over 1.8m (6ft) tall would have grown on a diet of animals rich in iron and zinc.[63] Scientists have speculated that our ancestor infants crawled about freely and ate iron-rich soil.[64] They probably also ate insects which are rich sources of minerals and other nutrients.

Iron-deficiency anaemia is a serious global problem of malnutrition in young children. It is in part due to a mother's deficiency during pregnancy and to non-exclusive breastfeeding before six months.[65] However a significant cause is early clamping of the umbilical cord after birth which became the norm during the 20th century. Waiting for two minutes, or until the cord has stopped pulsating, before clamping, enables blood transfer from the placenta to the baby. This will make a big difference to a child's long-term iron stores and is especially important for babies born to mothers with low iron themselves.[66] How many mothers rich or poor have control over the timing of cord-clamping? In rich countries, there has been a trend to harvest cord-blood for stem-cells. Harvesting 100mls of blood from a newborn is equivalent to taking over a litre (2.5 pints) from an adult.[67] Such theft can cause immediate problems and also jeopardise his long-term nutrition and health.

But it is not just at birth that we steal nutrients from small children. We live in a distorted society where those who do not need large quantities of animal foods eat excessive amounts and those who need them do not get enough. Poverty restricts the choice of foods for millions of humans while others consume far more animal products than they need. If most male adults halved their meat consumption and most toddlers doubled theirs, both groups might be healthier. Both at household and at global level the most nutritious food often goes to the most powerful. Family foods can be the ideal for a growing baby if these are varied and nutritious, but for thousands of families they are not. In the shanty towns of Southern Africa, a mother may only have maize meal, sugar and tea in her store box; anything extra is too costly. Continued breastfeeding will provide some well-absorbed iron, but gradually her baby needs more and if she does not get a mixed and varied diet with some meat, fish, vegetables and fruits, a baby may become anaemic.

Influential nutritionists are keen on providing fortified foods through the 'market'. The Global Alliance for Improved Nutrition (GAIN) is a 'public-private partnership' which claims to reach 160 million people and aims to provide fortified foods for a billion. If you look on the GAIN website you can be forgiven for thinking that all the world's nutrition problems are about to end.[68] But caution is needed. Search on and you will find that the giant food company Danone is on the board of GAIN*. Danone is the second biggest (after Nestlé) artificial milk and baby food manufacturer in the world. This was not stated on the GAIN website. Danone owns baby food company Blédina and Numico (which owns Nutricia, Cow & Gate and Milupa). They all violate the WHO Code, thus undermining infant nutrition and the Convention on the Rights of Child. The conflict of interest is breathtaking.

Fortification of some basic foodstuffs with specific nutrients can be a helpful strategy. However there is a trend to promote the use of commercialised complementary foods. These can be useful, but there is a danger. For example, Ready to Use Therapeutic Foods (RUTF) have saved the lives of children with severe, acute malnutrition. But RUTF use has sometimes led to decreased breastfeeding and it has often been the lack of exclusive breastfeeding which has led to the malnutrition in the first place.[69] And often it was the promotion of a commercial baby food which led to the non-exclusive breastfeeding.

I have met hundreds of parents who bring their children up on breastfeeding and family foods and they thrive. These families can afford plenty of food and know what is good. I must also add that I know vegetarian families whose children have grown up tall, healthy and intelligent and have never eaten a scrap of meat or fish in their lives. You can get iron from non-animal foods but you need to ensure bioavailability by judicious combination.

Ignorance about older babies' needs is common in all countries, but it affects poor children most. Children need priority for the most nutritious parts of the family meal, but often the best bits go to adults. When food is short either within the household or in the community at large, the child often misses out.

There is another type of malnutrition: childhood obesity. This is increasing in poor as well as rich countries. Overweight and obesity is associated with the early introduction of solid foods.[70] Tastes and eating habits are formed early in life. The companies involved in GAIN are among those who profit from selling high fat, high sugar processed foods which are associated with overweight and obesity.

* September 2008.

artificial milk for babies

In the 1860s, a German chemist, Justus von Liebig* (1803–1873), often called 'the father of modern nutrition', invented the 'perfect infant food'. It was made of wheat flour, cows' milk, malt flour and bicarbonate of potash. Though patented, commercialised and delivered in liquid form, it did not sell well. A powdered form was then developed with some of the cows' milk replaced with pea flour. To von Liebig's annoyance, some doctors claimed it was indigestible and did not match human milk, but one of his devotees argued:

"If we were to say that this preparation does not agree with newborn babies, such a statement could not be supported on theoretical grounds, since in the food they get the very same ingredients as in mother's milk. As therefore this milk agrees with them I cannot understand why they should be unable to digest Liebig's Food."[71]

Artificial milk has been a hit and miss affair, relying on experimentation on babies. Its composition has been as much influenced by nutritional fashion as by facts, as both the Syntex story in Chapter 15 and the 'novel oils' account below, illustrate. Artificial milk is an entirely different substance from human milk, containing no living cells and not adapting to each baby's individual and changing needs. I compare breastmilk with cows' milk, the commonest basis of breastmilk substitutes, not because it is the most appropriate substance – chimpanzees' or horses' milk might be better – but because it has been the most available and therefore the most used.** As a marketing report states: "The choice of ingredient used to supply the proteins to infant formulae will depend on two main factors, the price and the carbohydrate used in the formula." It then explains that the carbohydrate maltodextrin (which sounds so delightfully scientific) is derived from maize with potatoes as a secondary source.[72] As you read on, you may be amazed to realise that a product presented as 'closest to mother's milk' might actually include potatoes, fungi and beans, depending on the price of course.

By the 1960s, due to both nutritional fashion and economic

---

* von Liebig was a brilliant chemist who did all sorts of clever things, including inventing the stock cube.
** In 1998, a zoologist from London Zoo contacted Baby Milk Action (IBFAN UK) to ask where he could find human milk for a baby elephant because he judged it to be closest to elephant milk.

expediency, artificial milk manufacturers tended to replace most or all of the butterfat in cows' milk. Coconut, palm and other vegetable oils were used because they were cheap as was beef tallow, a waste product from the meat industry. So was groundnut oil which might trigger peanut allergy or contain traces of cancer-causing aflatoxins. Agro-chemicals are used in most large-scale oil crop production and the refining processes may remove nutrients. Vegetable oils cannot replace breastmilk fats which help the brain and nervous system to develop, so marine oils came into favour, but there was the risk of environmental pollutants and the marketing impediment that mothers (and some babies) disliked the fishy taste.

Since 2002 some companies have been trying to imitate certain important fats in breastmilk (please do not be put off by their long names), notably long-chain polyunsaturated fatty acids (LCPAs) called arachidonic acid (shortened to either AA or ARA) and docasahexanoic acid (DHA) which are crucial for brain, nerve and eye development. They are one reason for breastfed babies' better brains, eyes and general development. You might think how kind the companies are who add these products to artificial milks. However, Charlotte Vallaeys and the team at the Cornucopia Institute (CI) have gathered some disturbing facts. The Martek Biosciences Corporation make the imitation AA and DHA (called 'novel oils' with the patent names DHASCO and ARASCO) from laboratory-grown fermented algae and fungus using the hydrocarbon hexane in the process. Scientific studies have shown no extra benefit to infants. The CI reports that:

> "The FDA have not affirmed the safety of Martek's algal DHA and fungal ARA oils added to infant formula. In a written statement, FDA officials noted: 'Some studies have reported unexpected deaths among infants who consumed formula supplemented with LCPAs. The unexpected deaths were attributed to SIDS, sepsis or necrotizing enterocolitis. Also some studies have reported adverse events and other morbidities including diarrhoea, flatulence, jaundice, and apnea in infants fed LCPAs' ..."

These 'novel oils' are used in so-called 'organic' products. Apparently the FDA has no legal power to stop the addition of such ingredients and does not give approval for novel ingredients in infant formula. The FDA can only raise questions when a company requests for an ingredient to be given the status of "Generally recognised as safe" or "GRAS". The FDA has told the manufacturers that they must perform rigorous in-market surveillance. Meanwhile the artificial milks containing these novel oils are aggressively advertised as having a beneficial effect on infant brain and eye development. But then as a Martek investment promotion explained in 1996: "Even if [the DHA/ARA blend] has no benefit, we think it would be widely incorporated into formulas, as a marketing tool and to allow companies to promote their formula as 'closest to human milk.'"[73]

The European Food Safety Authority (EFSA) has to deal with thousands of companies submitting applications for health claims. Martek claimed about a follow-on milk that: "DHA and ARA support neural development of the brain and eyes." EFSA said that Martek failed to demonstrate causality and were denied permission to use this claim.[74]

beans, beans, beans

Soya beans are also used as a basis of artificial baby milks, not because different foods were analysed to find the best for babies, but because the soya industry sought profitable outlets.

Like any pulse, soya beans can be a useful food in a mixed diet, but it would be unwise to subsist on them alone. Yet quite a few babies do. The soya industry expanded in the 1950s and 60s during the years of protein obsession mainly to supply animal feed products. Soya contains substances which inhibit nutrient-absorption and cause nasty side effects, so it is limited in animal feeds to avoid growth and fertility problems.

The continuing use of soya-based infant formula (SIF) is alarming. For over twenty years scientists have recommended that it should be available only on a doctor's prescription but it is still sold on the open market. In the USA, SIF makes up 20 to 25% of infant formula sales, in the UK around 3%. UK government scientists stated in 1999 that "the use of SIF should be discouraged through professional and parental education as more suitable alternatives are available." In 2003 they stated "there is cause for concern about the use of SIF. Additionally, there is neither substantive medical need, nor health benefit arising from [its] use." The UK Chief Medical Officer has stated that non-breastfed babies with allergies or lactose intolerance should be fed with hydrolysed cows' milk-based infant formulas. The only reason for allowing SIF on the UK market is to placate vegan parents who do not breastfeed. Health officials from Australia, New Zealand, Canada, Ireland, Switzerland and Israel have all issued warnings against the use of soya-based artificial milks for babies.

Soya contains phytoestrogens, naturally occurring plant chemicals similar to the human hormone oestrogen. These may influence the timing of puberty and menstruation, fertility, thyroid function and cancer-risk. Soya contains much higher levels of aluminium, fluoride and manganese (all potentially harmful to brain development) than breastmilk or cows' milk. Soya and SIF contain phytic acid which binds to calcium, iron and zinc making these essential minerals less available to the body. SIF is sweetened with sucrose (ordinary sugar) or corn syrup which cause more tooth decay than lactose (milk sugar). SIF is often used because of cows' milk allergy, but it can be just as allergenic as cows' milk. A SIF-fed baby is more likely to become allergic to soya in foods later on. Genetically modified (GM) beans may be used in SIF production unless the company states otherwise. In 2005, Nestlé's website verybestbaby.com was still promoting its soya-based formula as "complete nutrition for babies 0 to 12 months" and suggested its use if "you want a vegetarian-based diet for your baby". A baffling statement because vegetarians (unlike vegans) drink cows' milk.

Nestlé actually produce hydrolysed cow's milk protein formulas which scientists say are safer for the non-breastfed baby who is at risk of cows' milk allergy. Dr Tracie Sheean of the US Food and Drug Administration's National Center for Toxicological Research stated that infants fed SIFs have been placed at risk in "a large, uncontrolled and basically unmonitored human infant experiment".[75]

a safe alternative to breastmilk?

The artificial milks for babies which have come to be called infant formulas are manufactured to internationally agreed standards. As they lack all the enzymes, anti-infective properties and growth factors, they cannot really be compared with breastmilk. However they are assumed to be safer than the unmodified animal milks and cereal gruels used in the past. What does surprise many people is that powdered infant formula (PIF) contains disease-causing microbes or pathogens. In 2002 outbreaks of serious infection and one death amongst babies in a US hospital intensive care nursery were traced to Enterobacter sakazakii within powdered infant formula.[76] The particular product was withdrawn and the US FDA banned the use of all PIF in hospital nurseries.[77] Belgian babies had also become seriously ill and two had died from the same cause.[78] The US FDA regulations had stated that a certain amount of 'colony forming units' (that is, germs that can multiply) were acceptable. PIF was not guaranteed nor required to be free of pathogenic organisms.

In 2004, a WHO/FAO Workshop discussed the illness and death caused by Enterobacter sakazakii and Salmonella. Both pathogens survive the heat processes of production. Other 'toxigenic' pathogens, (germs that trigger defensive toxins which harm or kill the baby) "such as Clostridium botulinum, Staphylococcus aureus and other Enterobacter species" can be found in PIF. The workshop noted that "the true magnitude of the problem is unknown due to *lack of surveillance* [my emphasis]". Among 10 key recommendations, the workshop called for regular alerts to the fact that PIF is not sterile and may cause serious illness, and that manufacturers should be "encouraged" to reduce pathogens in products.[79]

All my working life, the discussion of infection in artificially fed babies had focused on faulty preparation by mothers and carers. The whole 'baby milk issue' started because 'we', the clean, educated mothers could artificially feed correctly and 'they', the dirty, uneducated mothers could not. We will never know how many thousands of babies have died from pathogens in the tin because the process was masked (or exacerbated) by feeding with unhygienic water, bottles and teats. It was only after the Belgian babies died that I read enough to learn that Enterobacter sakazakii had been associated with neonatal deaths since 1958.[80] Enterobacter sakazakii causes a life-threatening meningitis and survivors may be brain damaged. No exclusively breastfed baby is known to have been infected with Enterobacter sakazakii. WHO/FAO Guidelines issued in 2006 emphasised that PIF must only be reconstituted with boiled water that is cooled to no less than 70°C (158°F). Manufacturers' instructions should be reviewed. More than a year later, a Baby Milk Action survey of company telephone 'carelines' found that most companies had not changed their instructions.[81]

the food code: the codex alimentarius commission

The basic standards of quality for our food are set by the Codex Alimentarius Commission, commonly called 'Codex'.* Codex 'belongs' to FAO and WHO and convenes international meetings to discuss important matters like food labelling, the levels of permitted toxins in foods, and whether we can call 'non-dairy creamer' 'milk' or

---

* The Latin word 'codex' means 'account book' or 'ledger'; it also means tree-trunk and was used colloquially to mean 'blockhead'.

'whitener'. Governments can set higher standards than Codex, but they risk charges of barriers to trade by the World Trade Organisation (WTO) and have to prove that the higher standard is necessary. For example the EU and the USA have argued about the import/export of milk from cows treated with bovine somatotrophin hormone (BSH) or chlorine-disinfected chicken. The EU has to prove to WTO that doubts about BSH and chlorine-washed meat are scientifically valid. Governments take the Codex standards seriously because they become the model for legislation and regulation and the benchmark for such disputes.

When Codex discusses standards for artificial milks for babies they get lobbied by bodies such as the International Dairy Federation (IDF) and the governments in their thrall, and sometimes by NGOs such as IBFAN. For example, in 2005 the Codex committee wanted to set an upper limit for vitamins because high levels are dangerous. The IDF lobbied against this because lower levels require a shorter shelf life, which raises distribution costs. Vitamins deteriorate during storage. Babies given the 'freshest' products might get dangerously high doses; babies getting the long-stored products might get dangerously low doses.[82]

The shelf-life issue is problematic. A Codex scientific working party investigated the safety of additives for preservation in infant formulas. The scientists reported that "few additives have been investigated in relation to their effects on very young children. It is therefore prudent that foods intended for infants under 12 weeks should contain no additives at all." In other words, all infant formulas should be made up from fresh ingredients everyday and refrigerated as any fresh product because, "It is likely that the detoxicating mechanisms, the permeability of certain tissues, and other protective mechanisms of the infant aged up to 12 weeks may not have developed to a point where they are able to cope with substances that present no problem to the adult."[83] So the very products which are so blithely promoted as "closest to breastmilk" contain substances, not included in the labelled ingredients, which have no proof of safety.

When Justus von Liebig invented his "perfect substitute for mother's milk" he matched it to the substances he could analyse. The situation is the same today; we can only describe what is known and there is still so much to learn. The list of both design and production errors is scandalously long (see Appendix 6) and these are only the recorded cases. Each new development highlights the flaws in the previous product which was always presented as 'closest to human

THE LIFE SAVER

Every year 10 million children under five, most in poor countries, die from infections of the chest and gut. Babies under six months who are not breastfed are five times more likely to die from pneumonia and seven times more from diarrhoea. In Brazil, artificially fed babies were 17 times more likely to need hospital admission for pneumonia than breastfed babies. There is a dose-related effect. Non exclusive breastfeeding doubles the risk of death. Exclusive breastfeeding has a very low risk of infection or death. A breastfed baby who gets water, juices or herbal teas has a slightly higher risk. If he gets other milks such as infant formula or cereal foods, the risk is much greater.

A baby who gets no breastmilk at all has the highest risk of infection and death. When researchers looked at all the possible means of preventing infant and young child death they found that improving breastfeeding practices could prevent more deaths than any other single strategy; even more than such key benefits as the provision of safe water, sanitation, immunisation and medical services.[89]

milk'. In the later 20th century, one company, GenPharm, patented a process to use milk from transgenic cows containing the human milk proteins lactoferrin and lysozyme.[84] GenPharm had a collaborative agreement with Bristol-Myers Squibb to "market a nutritionally enriched infant formula worldwide". The drive to get cows and goats to produce 'human milk', or at least products within human milk, continues with the alleged motive of scientists who "hope these findings will one day lead to milk that protects infants and children against diarrhoeal illnesses, which each year kill more than two million children worldwide."[85] One can marvel that animal scientists seem unaware that women already produce what expensive research is seeking. Obviously the profit motive drives these commercial laboratories but it is astonishing when internationally renowned doctors show the same ignorance. The winner of the 1998 Nobel Prize for Medicine, Dr Ferid Murad, declared: "Diarrhoea is the biggest killer of babies, but no one will find a cure because there is no market in Africa."[86]

Since 2008, the world's consciousness has been raised by the Chinese Sanlu milk scandal, but the contaminant, melamine, has been found in 22 other brands including those of the market leader Nestlé.

Even in the absence of corruption, any artificial milk might change because of an ingredient's price rise, a new cattle treatment, an accidental factory contamination or because the quality control inspector is off sick. As the discovery of widespread melamine contamination reveals, many governments have simply neglected and underfunded food inspection, naively (or cynically) leaving companies to monitor their own practices. The long journey from nutritionists' theories to babies' stomachs means the possibility of error is endless. The bottles, teats and feeding paraphernalia may include such risky substances as bisphenyl A and phthalates which may contaminate the baby's feed.[88] Farm, factory, laboratory, packaging, transport, storage and kitchen are all managed by human beings who have only a lifetime to learn their tasks. Nature has had millions of years.

environmental pollution

Environmental pollution affects the feeding of all children.

The pollutants that most threaten our health and lives are known collectively as Persistent Organic Pollutants or POPs. There are twelve particularly nasty ones called the 'Dirty Dozen'.[90] Most are chlorine-based compounds (organochlorines) such as PCBs and dioxins. They come from PVC plastics, electrical equipment, pesticides, herbicides, the paper industry, timber treatments and other products which have proliferated since the 1940s. Their harmful effects on human health and life outweigh their benefits.

Just in case some readers feel confused, because the word 'organic' is associated with healthy foods grown without chemicals, let me explain. Chemicals are called 'organic' because they contain a carbon atom, carbon being the building block of life. 'Inorganic' (ie not containing carbon) chemical pollutants include the heavy metals such as lead and mercury, which are highly toxic. There are also toxic chemicals which include both a heavy metal and carbon in their molecule structure, such as organic mercury compounds.

POPs are designed to last a long time in the product; for example in the insulation around electrical wires. The harm begins either during the manufacturing process, or when these products eventually break down and are absorbed into soil, water, air and food. POPs are highly toxic; they can damage sperm, causing male infertility, or miscarriage, birth defects and childhood cancers. After industrial accidents, such as the 1976 chemical-factory explosion in Seveso, Italy, there are more malformed and stillborn babies. POPs leach into our environment through waste incineration, seepage and contamination from industrial processes. We all have POPs in our bodies, mostly from food, especially dairy, fish and meat. POPs accumulate up the food chain and are stored in the body fat of both men and women.[91]

As humans are top of the food chain, these pollutants are found in breastmilk. During the past three decades, some environmental campaigners have issued press releases highlighting the pollutants in breastmilk. The campaigners' goal to shock the powerful to stop contaminating industrial processes has led to mothers abandoning breastfeeding. Industrialists have worried more about the fall in profits if forced to clean up.

The benefits of breastfeeding still outweigh the risks of artificial feeding. POPs certainly do harm in the womb. Pre-natal exposure can damage a baby's nervous system, developing brain, immune and endocrine (hormone) system and lead to developmental problems and learning difficulties. Study after study shows that breastfeeding counteracts the damaging effects of pre-natal exposure.[92] Even in extreme circumstances this is true. Evidence from Vietnam, where the organochlorine defoliant 'Agent Orange' was used as a weapon of war, showed an association between heavily-sprayed areas and birth defects. However, breastfeeding was beneficial.[93] Research shows that artificially fed infants exposed to high levels of POPs before birth, have more adverse effects than those who are breastfed. No one is sure why this happens and research would be difficult. As scientist Maryse Arendt so cogently points out, there is no control group for comparison, because no human beings are free of environmental pollution.[94]

The little spark of light in this gloomy account of our contaminated world is that by 2004 most countries had signed up to the 2001 Stockholm Convention on POPs. The cheering news is that in the countries where there has been effective legislation, POP levels in humans have decreased. Where there has been no legislation it has not. So it can be done. The depressing news is that while parts of the rich world clean up their own mess and get more smug, more manufacturers 'invest' in the poor world because they are attracted by the lower production costs of lax pollution control. We in the richer countries thus get products at a cheaper price; but what is that price?

There is another angle to this story. WHO and the UN Environmental Programme (UNEP) are carrying out a Global Coordinated Survey of POPS in Human Milk.[95] They are doing this because "human milk is the ideal matrix to generally monitor levels of persistent pollutants in the environment." Scientists could investigate blood, semen or body fat, but they frankly say that human milk is better because you get information about two people, the mother and the infant, for the price of one. The Survey Guidelines state that the researchers and interviewers must be well-informed about breastfeeding. There are strict ethical rules and every woman must give fully informed consent. Each woman will complete a questionnaire with many details of her life and donate her expressed breastmilk for sampling. She will be an unusual woman if she is not somewhat alarmed by the survey's subject matter. Women who are already fretting about breastfeeding could have their anxiety levels raised, and even those who have never had a moment's doubt might think, 'If they are looking for poisons in my breastmilk, will my baby be harmed?'

But fair enough, just as the armed forces are expected to take risks, so too must women endure some pain if they are to have the honour of helping to save humankind. When I read the Survey Guidelines, I came across this sentence: "Those completing the questionnaire may be offered a small gift for their time. This item should be of nominal value and ideally promoting breastfeeding by the mother – for example, a small pillow for supporting the baby during breastfeeding." How much patronizing can a woman endure? She gives her time, private information and her breastmilk. She endures some stress because the informed consent reminds her that her baby might be harmed. She is then given a 'small pillow to promote breastfeeding'. Can pillows promote breastfeeding? If she is the sort of woman who uses pillows for breastfeeding, it is likely she can afford her own. If she is not, then the researchers are introducing the mistaken idea that she needs a manufactured 'aid' to breastfeed. And as for promoting breastfeeding, if she has agreed to donate her breastmilk, does she need any promotion? Women need protection and support for breastfeeding but many are sick of being urged to breastfeed. There is nothing more annoying than being told to perform a task that you were just about to do anyway.

Despite the current evidence that breastmilk is not yet so polluted as to reduce its amazing powers, there is no room for complacency.[96] Women can try to minimise individual risk before conception, during pregnancy and while breastfeeding. If possible they should avoid polluted food. Fish is one of most nutritious foods we can eat, but some may be contaminated with POPs and heavy metals. Fish meal is commonly used for animal feed so pollutants in fish can concentrate in meat, dairy products and eggs. Women should never 'crash diet' because this may release contaminants stored in body fat into their bloodstreams. For adults who eat a typical 'western' diet[97] reducing their intake of meat and dairy products, even during pregnancy, is likely to improve health. Increasing the range and intake of fruit, nuts and vegetables can provide the micronutrients promoted in animal products and reduce both animal fat and pollution levels in the diet.

The most important action for every one of us, is to do whatever we can to halt the production and careless disposal of these poisons, otherwise our grandchildren may not have the chance to bear healthy babies. If breastmilk becomes too contaminated to use, our chances of bearing healthy children, or even being able to reproduce at all, will be in jeopardy.

Artificial feeding carries pollutants which are not listed on product labels. Cows' milk and milk products are responsible for half our daily exposure to POPS.[98] Although cows' milk fat is often replaced with other oils, there can be no guarantee that these are contaminant-free. Water can also be a risk. In the 1980s in the USA, carcinogenic chemicals found in two Abbott-Ross formulas were traced to a polluted well. 'Blue-baby' syndrome, when deoxygenated blood circulates, has affected artificially fed babies where water contained high nitrate levels from agricultural fertilizers.[99] However water engineers worry most about POP residues. In the UK, bore holes were closed because of permanent POP contamination, but as the legal cases were settled out of court this information was never publicly documented. You only find a substance if you have a specific test for it and it would be impossible to search for every pollutant, especially those present in minute (but dangerous) quantities. One chemical engineer tried out a new test on his own tap water and discovered a POP (tetrachloroethylene) in it. His incidental curiosity revealed that a whole town had been drinking dangerously contaminated water for years. Bottled waters (whose packaging and distribution cause pollution) may be too high in minerals to be safe for babies and they may also contain pathogenic microorganisms which are more likely to increase in a bottle than in tap water.[100]

One pollutant, bisphenol-A, is used in the manufacture of polycarbonate plastics used for feeding bottles for infants. It can leach into milk, has a high affinity for fats and is associated with cancer and diabetes. Canada has banned its use in feeding bottles. Glass feeding bottles or ordinary household china cups are safer than plastics.

Another group of pollutants, phthalates, are used to make plastic more flexible and are found in bottle teats, bottles and even in infant formula.[101]

The heavy metals, lead and mercury can damage the central nervous system and brain development. Mercury pollution mostly comes from fish and dental fillings. Industrial pollution and car exhaust fumes are the main sources of lead. Lead was added to petrol for 70 years, despite available, alternative technologies, not because it was the best strategy but the cheapest. General Motors and other companies sponsored phoney research to maintain its use. Though anti leaded-fuel campaigners had worked hard, unleaded petrol was put on the market for other reasons: "We stopped lead in gasoline in the US, not because it was bad for children's brains but because we wanted it for our catalytic converters."[102] The lead-using technology is still being sold to developing countries and unleaded fuel remains the privilege of the rich world. Lead is the number one pollutant of children in poor countries. It comes from car exhaust, old paint and dust. Children ingest it in food, lick it from their hands and breathe in car fumes. 'Soft' water (ie low in calcium salts) absorbs lead from old pipes. An exhaustive review of mercury and lead ingestion and breastfeeding concludes that "Habitual diets consumed by lactating mothers pose no health hazard to breastfed infants. Instead, cows' milk-based formulas pose a greater risk of infant exposure to neurotoxic substances."[103]

The most abundant metal on earth, aluminium (not a heavy metal) is easily absorbed into babies' bodies and has been associated with brain damage. It is found in water and in high levels in milk from cows grazing in areas under acid rain. Soya beans avidly take up aluminium from the soil. Premature babies have suffered permanent kidney and brain damage from aluminium in their feeds.[104]

Radioactive contamination is worse for artificially fed infants. Following the 1986 Chernobyl nuclear reactor accident, evidence from Italy and Austria showed that breastmilk contained 1/300th the amount of radioactive iodine and caesium found in cows' milk. Sweden had comparable results in the most affected areas.[105] Strontium 90, resulting from the nuclear testing of the 20th century, was ten times lower in breastmilk than in cows' milk. Also radiation levels in breastmilk are much lower than in a woman's own body.[106]

Radioactively contaminated milks were exported from Europe to poor countries after the Chernobyl disaster. At that time Poland had appealed for aid donations of artificial milk because of fear of contamination of their own cows' and human milk. Some months later, consignments of Polish powdered milk turned up in Bangladesh. There were also reports from Egypt, Nepal, Ghana, India, Mexico, the Philippines and Sri Lanka of imported milks containing unacceptably high levels of radioactive contamination. For the same reason, Brazil returned large quantities of milk to manufacturers in Ireland. Subsequently the Gambia was flooded with mysteriously underpriced milks made in Ireland. Thailand banned the sale of several European branded radioactively-contaminated milks whereupon an EC official warned Thai officials that European aid would be cut if they did not lower their stringent safety standards.[107]

6 it's not just the milk that counts

*"I would rather have cows' milk from a breast
than breastmilk from a bottle."*
Carole Livingstone (1942–2003), poet and teacher

The friend who said the words above was born in the USA in the 1940s when early physical contact was discouraged. Artificially fed from birth and rarely cuddled, she felt a lifelong deprivation of a mother's warmth. Luckily the theories about restricted mother/infant contact are now discredited. Nevertheless it has become increasingly common to feed babies expressed breastmilk (EBM). Expressing can take as long as suckling, but if it is done outside an employer's time, the pursuit of profit will not be interrupted. EBM is a useful back-up when it is impossible for a mother and baby to be together, but too often distorted priorities and a lack of organisational imagination, rather than necessity, keeps them apart.

It was 'discovered' in the 1940s that babies in orphanages who received all their supposed nutritional requirements, did not grow because they were not cuddled. Everyone needs to be stroked and touched and the benefits of skin contact do not just affect mothers and babies. Lonely people may visit the hairdresser more than necessary to get the physical contact they need. They might keep pets so as to stroke another live creature, and people buy teddy bears for babies. It is a sad symbol of our modern culture that we buy excessive numbers of soft toys for our babies. Parents who believe they must leave their baby to cry and sleep alone from an early age, will tuck numerous cuddly toy animals into their baby's cot, as though they unconsciously know their baby is deprived and needs comfort.

It is now known that babies' brains develop according to how much they are loved. Neuroscientists have used sophisticated technology to observe the workings of babies' brains. Their discoveries have shown that the quality of parents' and carers' affection and responsiveness shapes development. The parts of the brain which influence social and emotional relationships do not develop automatically but in response to the way a baby is cared for. As Sue Gerhardt describes: "Love facilitates a massive burst of connections in this part of the brain between six and 12 months.

Neglect at this time can greatly reduce the development of the pre-frontal cortex."[1] This is the area which shapes our social and emotional selves. Many abandoned and deprived babies, from the notorious Romanian children's homes of the 1980s Ceausescu regime, were found to have gaps in these crucial areas of their brains and as a result many who survived physically were irretrievably damaged emotionally. Adoptive parents often found it difficult to bond with and love a child who was intrinsically incapable of interacting emotionally with another human being.

Some women who have breastfed their own children have held a fostered or adopted baby against their naked breast when they artificially feed. With bottle-feeding, the milk may go down rather quickly and not with the stop-start rhythms of breastfeeding. The baby may feel full before his oral and touching needs are satisfied and need a dummy or a thumb to suck. It is remarkable how rare thumb or object sucking is in societies where unrestricted access to the breast is the norm. It has become socially acceptable for a baby to suck anything, be it bottle, dummy, soft toy, blanket or the nearest adult finger, while the ideal object, a breast, is denied. Some babies are less secure in the presence of strangers and that is when they need the breast most, yet in industrialised society this is the time mothers are most discouraged from giving it. Even an empty breast can provide solace and in some cultures men may offer their nipple to comfort a crying baby whose mother is absent.[2] Breastfeeding is an inadequate word because it is not merely putting food in a stomach, it is also our first experience of love and it works both ways. Where Baby Friendly Hospital practices have been established it has been noted that fewer mothers abandon their babies than before.[3]

Sometimes breastfeeding has been so damaged that it can spoil a mother's relationship with her baby because of the tension that unhappy feeding can induce. In her book A Life's Work writer Rachel Cusk evocatively describes her sense of misery and isolation as she struggles, after a ghastly birth, to breastfeed. She conveys the insensitivity and ignorance of those who are supposed to support and help her. She is deprived of the heady joy of motherhood because no one is taking care of her.[4] Her story is far too common. Of course mothers who artificially feed their babies love them, but a bit of plastic and silicon does not convey to the baby the primal contact that a soft, warm breast can. Nor can bottle-feeding convey to the woman the warm sensual feelings that can be experienced through suckling a baby.

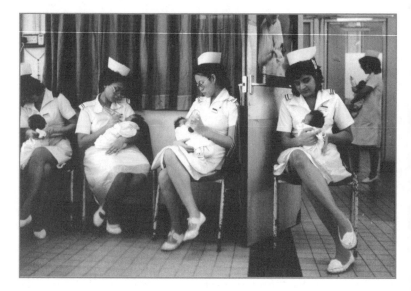

6 Nurses bottle-feeding newborns in a Singapore maternity ward.
(Photo Raghu Rai 1980s)

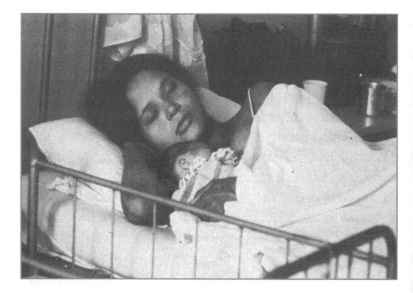

7 Woman sleeping with her newborn baby in a hospital bed.
(Photo courtesy of UNICEF 1980s)
Who is bonding with whom?

bonding

"The two people who need each other at this time,
more than they ever will at any other in their lives, are separated."
Ashley Montague, Touching: the human significance of skin,
Harper & Row, 1986 (1st edition 1971)

The concept and importance of bonding came to public attention through the work of Klaus and Kennel in the 1970s.[5] Observation of animals revealed the fact that infants were rejected if the mother could not nuzzle them within a certain time. Researchers who separated primate mothers and infants experimentally, observed that the loss of contact was devastating and the ill effects could last through generations.

As I explained in Chapter 3, skin-to-skin contact after the birth affects the hormone levels and behaviour of both mother and baby. One observational film vividly illustrates the power of spontaneous mother/baby interaction. As the birth attendant gently places the baby on his mother's abdomen, he gradually crawls towards her breast, smelling, nuzzling, mouthing and exploring with tiny hands. At first the mother just holds her baby, but after about half an hour, oxytocin is coursing through her body, prompting her to stroke and talk to her baby, who also makes communicative noises. As this happens, the mother's nipples slowly change shape. Eventually after around an hour of 'talking' and touching between mother and baby, the baby gapes his mouth and suckles his mother's breast with superb skill.[6]

It is a measure of the universal sabotage of these natural talents that the BFHI was needed (see Appendix 3), in the attempt to halt the 'normal' practice of removing babies, leaving mothers bereft and confused. Because hospital staff routinely separated mothers and babies it became harder for women to feel comfortable with their newborns making them more inhibited about breastfeeding. We can also surmise that like other primates, these effects might be passed onto the next generation. Nowadays the maternity ward supervision of bonding has been made into a uniform, time-measured ritual. Though uninterrupted skin-contact for as long as the mother wants is the ideal, any closeness is better than the cold callousness of nurseries full of bawling newborns where there has been immeasurable and unnecessary suffering. Even with supportive practices every mother reacts differently, and some take longer than others to fall in love with their babies. If an infant or mother is seriously ill, bonding may take longer, but fortunately there seems to be human scope for emotional healing and love can survive setbacks.

If you compare the breastfeeding couple with the relationship which preoccupies modern western culture, the romantic attraction of two adults, 'bonding' is presumed to occur with the first kiss or meaningful physical contact. It is taken for granted that couples need to cuddle and that this strengthens the emotional bond – yet still in too many circumstances mothers are supposed to love their babies while unrestricted physical contact is discouraged.

A baby's crying is biologically designed to motivate us to stop it. A breast is the best comforter, yet in western society it has been viewed merely as a conveyor of 'feeds'. Actual physical cruelty to babies is often triggered by an infant's ceaseless crying and many parents have felt an impulse to hurt their child when they cannot stop this noise. There is now some evidence that breastfeeding can protect against child abuse and neglect.[7] The German word for breastfeeding, 'Stillen', means to quieten and soothe as well as to give the breast. This function is just as important as conveying nutrients to a stomach. A breastfeeding mother is being caressed and loved by her baby so it may be easier to love him or her, as babies are more contented when close to a human body. Of course there are breastfed babies who continue to cry, but this seems to be a greater problem in western society.

My own (British) culture has viewed physical contact with alarm, though attitudes are now changing. For example in the UK, the USA and some others, it is still unacceptable for heterosexual men to hold hands, even though it is common in many countries. Touching strengthens the bonds of friendship and it is sad when custom inhibits actions such as stroking and holding hands which can defuse aggression and misunderstanding. Jane Goodall's work with chimpanzees has shown how effective these actions can be, enabling the chimps to transcend their fear of one another.[8] Television, film and computer visuals reflect our values when they show sexual contact and aggressive conflict as common images, but rarely show non-sexual physical contact (except violence), such as suckling.

Modern western society appears to be confused about the borderline between physical closeness and genitally-focused sexuality. Breastfeeding is on the borderline of these feelings and if our taboos are in turmoil, this may explain some of the rejection of breastfeeding.

harshness still survives

In 2007 British viewers of a TV programme called Bringing up Baby were astonished to hear a nanny urge a mother to leave her small twins to cry and to put them in a pram outside in the chilly British weather. The babies had needed special care after birth and were just ten days old. Their mother lacked confidence in her breastfeeding. The nanny encouraged her to feed artificially and insisted that the babies sleep in a separate room, in contradiction to UK public health policy. Sleeping alone in the first six months doubles the risk of cot death (SIDS).[9] The nanny instructed the mother not to look her infant in the eye while she was bottle-feeding otherwise he would 'think he was boss'. Supposedly this regime of cruelty was based on the teachings of schedule-obsessed Frederick Truby King (see Chapter 10), but even he did not urge avoiding eye-contact which can have serious, adverse emotional consequences. The programme led the National Society for the Prevention of Cruelty to Children (NSPCC) to issue a statement that these methods were "outdated and potentially harmful".[10]

bottle-feeding and bottled-feelings

I know that stating these facts can be painful or even enraging to some women who have not breastfed their children, but the continued denial of the risks of not breastfeeding and the value of breastmilk, supposedly to spare women's feelings, is a patronising deception. The whine about 'not making mothers feel guilty' is such a cop-out. If someone told me I had been driving my car dangerously for years, of course I would be upset, but I do not think I should be denied that information just to spare my feelings. I drove my own children in a car without safety seats in the days before they were used. I cannot say, 'well my children are alive so it must be safe'. I am just grateful my children are alive and that they are better-informed about child safety so they can protect their children. So too with breastfeeding. No woman need feel guilty for 'failing' to breastfeed, though she has the right to feel angry or sad for being denied support and information when she needed it.

I did not bring up my first baby in the way I now believe is best. I tried to suckle him to a routine. I let him cry, I stopped breastfeeding too early. He has survived physically and I hope emotionally. Luckily tough human babies can survive a lot of mistakes, but the more vulnerable ones cannot and it would be better not to have to put so many babies to the test.

One argument put forward in favour of artificial-feeding has been that the father can feed the baby. Advertisers use this idea to sell infant feeding products. However, though a minority of fathers do bring up babies, the great majority do not. It is ironic that as the approval of breastfeeding grew in industrialised countries more fathers expressed interest in getting involved in feeding. The reality is that few fathers actually do take the whole responsibility of infant care and most artificial feeding is still done by mothers. I certainly applaud the greater involvement of fathers and wish that all societies did more to support the skills and responsibilities of fatherhood. However I often wonder whose emotional needs we are discussing. Some men are jealous of breastfeeding babies and mothers; it is something that men cannot do and they can feel excluded. As there is evidence that men can lactate, maybe there is hope for them yet![11] Babies need a lot of care besides breastfeeding: bottoms and noses have to be wiped, nappies changed; bathing, cuddling and massage are all important, and there are many years of providing other food, helping with dressing, reading stories and playing games. Lots of fathers and babies have warm, close relationships without the symbolic bottle binding them together. New parents often forget that babies have a habit of hanging about the house for 20 or more years, so there is plenty of scope for paternal bliss. If fathers did everything for their children except breastfeed they would be the main childcarers.

breast pumps

Each year in the USA around six million breast pumps are sold.[12] As only three million US women start breastfeeding, does this mean that every woman needs a brand new pump for each breast after every birth? I get the impression of a vast, whirring milking-shed. These statistics are disturbing, especially when selling and renting breast pumps may be more financially rewarding than spending time helping breastfeeding mothers. Where is the baby when a mother is using a machine to take milk out of her breasts? And what has happened to a woman's hands that she needs a machine to remove her milk? Do women buy more than one pump because there is no impartial information to guide them to buy the right one first time, or do pumps wear out before the next baby is born? In wealthy Norway some hospitals still use 50-year-old pumps because they work so

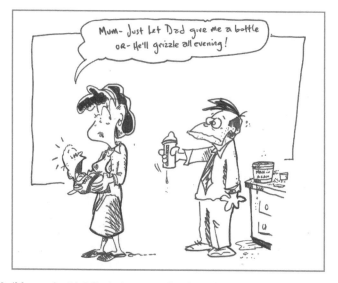

8 'Mum – just let Dad give me a bottle or he'll grizzle all evening!'
(Cartoon Jack Maypole)

much better than the new ones, so pumps can be made to last.[13] Do hospitals stockpile vast numbers? And what are the ecological implications of all the discarded pumps? Do they go into landfill? Do the plastic parts contain pollutants and do they decay safely?

Women express their breastmilk for lots of different reasons. It is a requirement of the BFHI accreditation that all breastfeeding women be taught hand expression. A baby might be preterm, sick and unable to suckle. A healthy mother and baby might be adjusting to each other and feeding a little expressed milk might help them through an early difficulty. A woman might feel uncomfortably full and her new baby might find it easier to attach if her breast is softened. She might want to squeeze some milk into her baby's mouth to entice her to suckle. A woman might want to donate her milk or store it for later use. Then there are emergencies, sudden illness or surgery, work away from the baby and so on. In the past a baby might have been wet nursed in these circumstances; or fed a breastmilk substitute, as many still are. In the USA women who use pumps are less likely to stop breastfeeding early, so increasing pump use could signal that breastmilk is valued more than it used to be. I want to ask whether all those women who use pumps were ever taught how to hand express, saw other women doing it or felt they had a choice of technique.

In some countries, pumping has become the default method of

expression, and hand expression has become an afterthought. It would be safer if it were the other way round. Just as the medical marketing word 'infant formula' has entered ordinary (and legal) vocabulary, so the word 'pump' has gradually replaced 'express'. For the majority world, pumps carry the same risk as feeding bottles and teats; most women and many health facilities do not have the means or the conditions to use them safely. Pathogens cling to equipment and though breastmilk antibodies might help combat this risk, it would be safer to avoid complicated tubes and parts. In South Africa, policy guidelines suggest limiting the use of pumps. They are expensive and if shared could cross-infect, not only with the usual hospital sourced pathogens such as Staphylococcus, but also cytomegalovirus (CMV), hepatitis B and HIV.

Pumps (both electric and manual) are not without risk in rich countries. The USFDA recorded 37 adverse events in nine years. These included tissue damage, infection, pain and soreness and contamination of the pump. Medical investigators claim that there is underreporting to the USFDA and consider surveillance systems inadequate.[14] One US lactation consultant visited a South African neonatal unit and was impressed with women's skills and confidence with hand expression. She noted their lack of inhibition and how adept they were at eliciting the let-down reflex. They came from a culture where breast exposure, public breastfeeding and ease with handling their own breasts was normal.[15]

What suits individual women varies. I know a British mother of three who breastfed for around six years and returned to work soon after each birth. No one had told her what to do. She told me "I couldn't be bothered with a pump, hand expression is so much faster and easier." I have met other women who said the exact opposite. No one can say which works better. A review of the limited research found that no single study had asked mothers if they had achieved their goals for expressing milk. Moreover eight out of ten evaluation studies of pumps had been paid for by the manufacturers. Few studies had analysed the women's support systems and circumstances. The conclusion was that mothers needed to feel valued and supported whatever method they used.[16] When research midwife, Sandra Lang, worked with mothers of low birth weight (LBW) babies, she found that women who wanted to use pumps expressed best with pumps and those who preferred hand expression produced best by hand. Sandra suggests (as do others) that hand-expressed milk might have a higher fat content than pumped milk.[17] This may be important: small

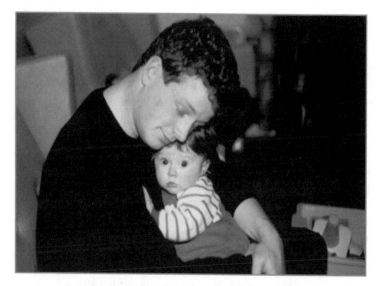

9 'There's plenty of scope for paternal bliss'.
Stephen Clark with his son Lewis. (Photo Jacquie Clark)

babies do not need large quantities of breastmilk, but nutrient balance is crucial. For example, fat proportions may be influenced by the style of expression.

I am not against pumps; they seem to be helpful for mothers of very LBW babies. I certainly believe it is up to each woman to decide what she wants to do. But many women are not given an informed choice. It is an uncanny coincidence that pumps, which are heavily promoted and advertised, have become the default method of expression. There has been no well-designed research to discover whether hand-expressed and pumped breastmilk is different. And of course a baby might elicit breastmilk with a different balance of nutrients and other factors from either pumped or hand-expressed milk. Almost all investigation into breastmilk has used pumped milk. A great deal of research-funding and sponsorship of events is financed by pump companies. Though I am convinced of the sincerity of the scientists involved, there is a financial motive for ignoring the possible benefits of hand expression. There is also the question of impartiality about different brands of pump. Some scientists present lecture slides with a pump company logo in the corner, allowing their academic kudos to promote a single brand. Several pump companies also manufacture bottles and teats and aggressively market them in defiance of the WHO Code.

the culture of separation

Western culture seems to have a drive to separate mothers and babies. The goal of independence starts at birth and mothers who want to stay with their infants most of the time are viewed as 'possessive' or eccentric. Many mothers internalise this value and yearn for time away from their babies quite soon after birth. On a brief visit to Japan I noticed a completely different attitude to motherhood amongst a wide range of women. Apparently this is because when a baby is born in Japan, he or she is seen as a separate being and the goal of care is to bring this separate creature into the family fold and stay close.[18]

One aspect of the issues of separation and closeness is that we have to confront the fact of the physical and sexual abuse of small children. Although not exclusively their crime, men are the principle abusers. There is also the occasional case of baby snatching, often by mentally ill women. When infants spend their early life close to a mother's body, they are much better protected than those left alone in cots and prams.

7 your generous donations could do more harm than good

"After all, breastfeeding mothers are the most sustainable, local, efficient, life-saving emergency response."
Marie McGrath, nutritionist and aid worker
The Guardian 30 May 2007

feeding babies in disasters

Those wasted babies that are filmed and photographed during disasters are often only alive because of the breastmilk that they have managed to take in. The life-saving value of breastfeeding is never better demonstrated than during disasters, or as aid agency jargon now calls them: 'complex humanitarian emergencies' or CHEs.[1]

Towards the end of the 20th century, aid agencies were reporting 428 disasters per year; by the 21st century there was an average of 707 disasters each year. There are an estimated 26 million human beings living in, or trying to move from, devastation or temporary shelter in their own countries. There are a further 11.4 million refugees far from their own lands.[2] They have been through war, rape, drought, famine, flood, earthquake, or some combination of these events. People may lose every scrap of substance in their lives: a bit of land, their home, their animals, seeds, a precious identification document or a dearly won qualification certificate. They lose agricultural or artisan's tools and the small stock of useful items that people build up over the years: a sewing machine, buckets, a hoe or water container. And they lose their loved ones, especially the sick, the young and the old who succumb to disease more quickly during any disruption of ordinary life. Most disasters occur in poor regions and most refugees are given asylum by poor countries. Disaster can hurt the better-off too, as when the 2004 Asian tsunami struck tourists and the 2005 Hurricane Katrina affected both rich and poor, but the aftermath is always worse for the poor than the rich, as both these events showed.

In any emergency, breastfeeding can and must continue. It saves the lives of infants and young children, and of their mothers through reducing the risk of pregnancy. Babies are at great risk of death if they are not breastfed. During the 1998 war in Guinea-Bissau, children who had stopped breastfeeding were six times more likely to die. Those breastfeeding had no higher mortality than during peace time.[3] Women maintain adequate growth in their babies even when they themselves are undernourished. During the West Darfur famine in the Sudan in 1984 and 1985, the infant mortality rate did not increase, whereas child deaths quadrupled and adults deaths doubled. This protection for babies was attributed to exclusive breastfeeding. Moreover, the mothers' mortality rates were lower than the overall adult death rate.[4] These facts contrast tragically with the 1991 plight of Kurdish refugees whose babies died because their mothers believed they could not breastfeed. Some ill-informed aid workers supplied bottles and powdered infant formula, thus contributing to the death rates.[5]

Occasionally, when there is no wet nurse available, artificial feeding is needed. Just how seldom can be illustrated by the fact that when around a million refugees crossed the Rwanda/Zaire border in July 1994, there were just six babies in need of temporary substitute feeding. One orphan was being wet nursed by a pregnant woman who then had to stop by the roadside to give birth. Health workers from an aid agency first gave the baby some boiled water and then purchased infant formula from a local store which they carefully made up and fed to him in a clean cup. In these conditions bottle feeding is far too risky. With all six babies, the health workers' aim was to find foster mothers willing to breastfeed because they knew that continued artificial feeding risked death.[6] It is an inspiring fact that in the midst of the horrors of conflict and flight, there are always acts of selfless generosity. Women willing to suckle a needy child are not hard to find but local cultural attitudes and the risk of HIV transmission have to be considered.

Where mothers are accustomed to artificial feeding, protecting infant nutrition can be more difficult. The 2006 conflict between Israel and Hezbollah in Lebanon led to 900,000 people being displaced (ie having to leave their homes and be refugees in their own country) including 50,000 infants. Mixed feeding was the norm and many mothers believed they could not breastfeed in such stressful circumstances. These problems were exacerbated by inappropriate distribution of artificial milks though it was obvious that conditions were not conducive to safe artificial feeding. In the chaos that characterises disasters some aid workers did not even follow their agencies' guidelines (some are excellent). As in the world at large, many, including high-ranking field staff, were ignorant and poorly trained about infant feeding, even those from the key agencies (such as UNICEF) responsible for coordination. Many staff did not know how to support the mothers and babies, who needed skilled assessment, targeted help and follow-up, not infant formula chucked off the back of a truck.[7]

A striking characteristic of much-publicised emergencies is the zeal with which well-meaning people send things. The mere mention of human suffering compels people to have a spring clean and amass quantities of old clothes, kitchenware and unwanted canned food. Fuel and time is squandered dragging this round the world. The intentions are good, the results appalling. Competent aid agencies rarely use this stuff. Companies also have their spring cleans and unsellable drugs and baby foods get dumped. Few people check sell-by dates in an emergency.

Imagine having your house blown away, one of your children killed and the whole family going down with diarrhoea. You pull together a makeshift shelter and start helping your neighbours with theirs, when their son tells you there has been an aid delivery. You rush to claim and struggle home with your share only to discover a load of cumbersome and unsuitable goods. Your need is for well-organised emergency services to support you with basic water, food and health care. Instead, you have to waste precious energy sorting through miscellaneous cans and packets with unreadable labels, and strange garments.

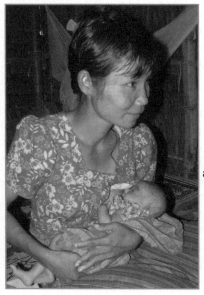

10 Baby Sa Bei aged seven weeks born just after the 2008 Myanmar cyclone. Her mother abandoned her in order to find her other four children and husband. San San Min is fostering Sa Bei and with intermittent help from breastfeeding counsellors has succeeded in stimulating her breastmilk to feed Sa Bei.
(Photo Nina Berry)

A 2006 TV news report[8] showed two chirpy Englishwomen gathering a vanload of cast-off children's footwear in the UK and driving all the way to the site of the recent Pakistan earthquake. The shoes were tipped out in a heap and children scrabbled through them. Whilst the commentary applauded the young Englishwomen, the camera shot lingered over a trainer with a split and unwearable sole. This gift would damage both the recipient's feet and the local economy. Local shoemakers and traders, struggling to get their businesses back to normal after the earthquake, would endure more hunger because of this harmful generosity. A cash transfer would have enabled people to buy any shoes they needed. If you are caught up in a disaster your immediate need is for money, guidance and skilled helpers who have contacts with the powerful. You need new underwear and clean, warm bedding, not Aunty Mildred's old evening-dress; you need cooking containers that can function on open fires or kerosene stoves. You need food that you can eat, something familiar, not scary and strange. You need appropriate drugs. You need local goods in quantities that can be fairly distributed to all. Money means that trading can get going again as quickly as possible.[9]

However, although all this useless stuff gets in the way and impedes the aid workers, it does not directly kill people. Artificial milk, baby foods and bottles do. They kill babies and small children by transmitting infections because it is very difficult to use such products hygienically in emergency conditions.

Despite consistent evidence about the harm they do, commercial baby food products still get distributed in areas where they are deadly and it is not just misguided charity. A disaster can be a wonderful marketing opportunity. During the Balkan Wars of the 1990s, donations of infant feeding products poured in to the devastated regions of Former Yugoslavia. In 1994, advertisements appeared on TV in Scotland. Sponsored by Nutricia's* Cow & Gate brand, they presented an appeal "on behalf of the children of Bosnia who need your help right now". The voice of Jeremy Irons hit just the right note of urgency and gravitas as the camera homed in on a woman breastfeeding her baby. A concerned female voice asked, "How must that mother feel, knowing that her baby is aching with hunger?" Then the camera panned to another breastfeeding woman as the voice said, "How must this mother cope, knowing she's helpless to protect her daughter from illness and infection?" The viewers then saw boxes

* Nutricia has since been bought by Danone.

unloaded, a bundle of old-fashioned feeding bottles, milk being poured and then a close-up of a baby lying on her side with a propped bottle. The advertisement was for an aid agency, Feed the Children, who claimed to have sent thousands of tons of 'life-saving baby packs' each containing '30 items to keep a baby alive and healthy'. There was a phone number for people to make donations. When members of the public called, it was suggested that as well as donating money, they could purchase Cow & Gate infant feeding products and send them to the agency for transport to Bosnia.[10]

Thankfully for the children of Bosnia, this advertisement was seen by some alert Scottish midwives. They sent copies to people who could do something to stop these misguided efforts. The UK IBFAN group Baby Milk Action contacted Feed the Children and established a dialogue. Paediatrician Professor Andrew Tomkins from London's Institute of Child Health debated on BBC World Service radio with the agency's director, who it turned out was quite unaware that he was creating risks. A bright young nurse in his employ quickly caught on, and educated herself and her colleagues about the realities of infant feeding in emergencies. The agency changed its name, and stopped sending artificial milk and bottles.

Was the whole sorry episode due to ignorance? In part, yes; but if Nutricia/Cow & Gate could afford to hire Jeremy Irons, make the advertisement and pay for air time, they could afford to do the basic research and check the facts and the international guidelines. If they had any concern for Bosnian children's survival and health they could have asked UNICEF or WHO for a rapid assessment of need and conditions. If there was a real need for artificial milk (which their own filming of breastfeeding mothers contradicted) they could have earmarked the exact quantities and quickly printed labels in the appropriate languages. They could certainly have warned the public against sending any product labelled in English. In keeping with WHO resolutions, they should also have ensured that any baby who was already artificially fed (and whose mother was unwilling to relactate) would be individually assessed and would receive the donated product together with the necessary support of water, fuel, equipment and follow-up health surveillance, for as long as was necessary. All this information was available and Nutricia/Cow & Gate were not short of funds or staff to seek it out.

By the end of the 1990s an investigation found that a significant proportion of aid in Macedonia had been unsolicited. NATO countries loaded up their planes with products and merely documented tonnage. Out of 3,500 tonnes an estimated 40% was baby food, the quantities depending on stocks donated not on estimated need. Agencies were uncoordinated and there was no monitoring to ensure that World Food Programme (WFP) guidelines, advising against the general distribution of powdered milk, were respected. Only after a nutritionist from UN High Commission for Refugees (UNHCR) arrived in the region did an improvement in the coordination and monitoring of infant feeding get established.[11]

In 1999 during the Kosovo crisis, when almost 700,000 people fled their homes, some NGOs sent in food parcels with infant feeding items and out-of-date UHT milk. It cost other agencies such as UNICEF an estimated US$500,000 to gather up and destroy inappropriate foods, including 27 tonnes of breastmilk substitutes. In camp conditions, bottle feeding is lethal, yet an unsolicited donation of 60,000 baby bottles and teats had been accepted into a UN warehouse. They were stored for several months and then destroyed, wasting money, time and energy. One agency tried to resolve some of the problems by re-labelling donated infant formula with local language labels, but they could not keep up with the flood of products.[12]

And what did the people of the Balkans really need? Just some simple support with breastfeeding. This mostly involved re-training the doctors, nurses and midwives who still thought that babies should be separated at birth and bottle-fed with any fluid available. Chloe Fisher, midwife and breastfeeding expert went to help. She found mothers delivering in makeshift barracks where health staff still tried to find a separate room for the babies. She found newborns being fed Intralipid* because of the assumption that babies must be fed something white in a bottle soon after birth: another 'generous' gift from a spring clean of surplus stock. Chloe and others made a difference. Breastfeeding rates soared and there are many healthy young people in that region today whose mothers exclusively breastfed because of that war. It is one good thing that came out of that terrible time.[13]

So did the world learn from the Bosnia experience? On 26 December 2004, an earthquake off Indonesia triggered a massive tidal wave, the tsunami. A tidal wave of goodwill did some damage too and Sri Lanka was a victim of both. A press picture released by one national aid agency showed a glamorous young aid worker demonstrating the

---

* Intralipid ® is a brand name of a fat emulsion used for intravenous feeding.
  It is based on soya bean oil and egg phospholipids. It is not designed for infants.

use of infant formula to Sri Lankan mothers, some of whom were calmly breastfeeding their babies while they watched the bottle-feeding lesson. This was not the only agency to do this, but it was guileless enough to issue the press photo.[14]

Sri Lanka is a remarkable country. Still fundamentally poor, with an average per capita annual income of just US$1,300, it has a good public health system. Its under-five mortality ranking is better than the Bahamas, which are more than ten times richer. At just 11/1,000, its infant death rate is half that of Saudi Arabia. Breastfeeding is the norm and three-quarters of babies are still suckling at two years. Sri Lankan paediatricians value and understand breastfeeding. What is more, despite endemic internal conflict, the country has adequate infrastructure and emergency services. With financial support they were able to deal with the destruction of the tsunami themselves. The young aid worker innocently promoting products in her attempt to help was not just risking the immediate sickness or death of infants just after a disaster, but was undermining years of good breastfeeding policies implemented by skilled health workers and women's support groups.

8 hiv and breastfeeding

"We all knew that not breastfeeding in Africa could kill, but somehow we expected HIV-infected mothers to be different. We were wrong."
Dr Nigel Rollins, Professor of Maternal and Child Health,
University of KwaZulu-Natal, South Africa 2007

It is April 2000 and in a BBC TV programme a well-known journalist is describing the effects of HIV on a South African woman, Maqquma:

"For Maqquma, feeding her family is the immediate concern. There's one meal a day here. But if she dies from AIDS, it's the older children who'll have to become parents to the younger ones. They will join a generation of orphans in remote villages across South Africa. It isn't just the food that's in short supply, so too is the most basic health care and information. Maqquma breastfeeds her baby. If the child isn't already HIV-positive, this is a common method of transmission."

The journalist turns to Greta, a social worker and asks: "Does Maqquma know about the danger of breastfeeding her baby when she's HIV-positive?" Greta translates his question and Maqquma's face crumples with shock as she replies. Greta translates her answer: "She says she doesn't know. She didn't know anything."[1]

How did Maqquma feel, hearing this shattering information from strangers with a film-camera? And how else could she feed her baby? The journalist talks confidently, but actually he has no idea whether Maqquma will infect her baby or not. He does not know the levels of virus or antibodies in her blood; or whether she is exclusively breastfeeding. He seems not to know that, despite the risk of transmission, the majority of HIV-infected women who breastfeed have not infected their children. Despite covering the poorest areas of the world, the journalist appears unaware that the alternatives to breastfeeding can be lethal. If the woman had been bottle-feeding her child in front of the camera, would he have delivered the news that her baby would be likely to die? Is he aware that if Maqquma had artificially fed from birth, her baby would have had a greater risk of dying from diarrhoea or pneumonia, than from contracting HIV? The journalist was not alone. His assumptions echoed the general

Of the 38.6 million people living with HIV, 17.3 million are women of whom 76% live in sub-Saharan Africa (SSA). The majority are unaware of their status. More than three-quarters of all AIDS deaths occur in SSA. Globally, 2.3 million children under fifteen are living with HIV. In SSA alone, there will probably be 16 million orphans by 2010. Overall in the world, AIDS accounts for 3% of under-five mortality, in South Africa it accounts for 40%. Scaling up prevention strategies in 125 low- and middle-income countries would avert an estimated 28 million new infections.
Sources UNAIDS, WHO, UNICEF 2007

confusion about HIV and infant feeding.

Research by far-thinking scientists has now uncovered some important truths which may make life a little bit easier for the most powerless women.[2] However in 2000 the policy makers were still arguing. The attempt during the 1990s to protect babies from HIV-infection resulted in some near disastrous policies. Breastfeeding was almost destroyed in the regions where it was most vital for survival. In late 2000, an African doctor working with UNAIDS told me: "The biggest problem for HIV in Africa is breastfeeding, we must do everything we can to stop breastfeeding promotion in Africa."[3] Yet earlier that year WHO had published a review which proved how vital breastfeeding was for early survival, especially in the areas where HIV was most prevalent.[4] Somehow this man had forgotten the realities of the continent of his birth and ignored the scientific evidence. It was as though in regard to HIV/AIDS he had more fear of breastfeeding than of unsafe sex, needle-sharing and unscreened blood transfusions.

The HIV and infant feeding policies of the 1990s inadvertently created an experiment which caused more infant death and proved that for most communities, breastfeeding was essential.[5]

the risk of transmission

HIV is transmitted through blood, semen, vaginal fluids and breastmilk. It cannot be cured, but modern anti-retroviral drugs (ARVs) help to keep the virus in check and slow the progression to AIDS, the condition when the immune system stops working and opportunistic infections attack the body. With the right care HIV-infected people can stay healthy for years. Without treatment for HIV-infected mothers, scientists estimate that 5 to 10% of babies contract

HIV in the womb; 10 to 15% during birth and 5 to 20% through breastfeeding. To get this into perspective, think of a town where there are 100 pregnant women living with HIV. Out of these, 7 of their babies may contract HIV before birth and 15 during birth. If these women breastfeed for two years, then another 15 babies might get infected. Sixty-three babies will be HIV-free. This means that the majority of untreated HIV-infected mothers give birth and breastfeed without transmitting the infection. When you consider that some of those babies might take in around 500 litres of breastmilk which is carrying the virus, something special must be happening. Exclusive breastfeeding dramatically reduces the risk of transmitting HIV.

In the rich world, mother to child transmission (MTCT) has fallen from 25% to less than 2% because of anti-retroviral drugs, Caesarean-section births (C-sections), exclusive artificial-feeding, excellent healthcare and effective support. The last two are essential because the first three measures all pose other health risks for mother and child.

Any child who is not breastfed will need more medical treatment, wherever they live, but in much of the world this is simply not available. Many poor women do not go to health facilities during pregnancy because they are too far away or too expensive. After a scandalous tussle over pricing by the drug companies,[6] ARVs are now available for women who can access health services, if they are functioning. A package of drug treatment called 'highly active anti-retroviral therapy'(HAART) reduces MTCT, but it is unavailable to many. In 2007 less than a third of women were getting the drugs they needed. There are not enough staff to cope with everyday health problems (more people die of malaria than AIDS) let alone carry out C-sections and administer drugs and other care for all HIV-infected women – over 13,000 health workers who trained in sub-Saharan African (SSA) countries now practise in Australia, Britain, Canada and the USA. A quarter of doctors and one in 20 nurses trained in Africa work in a rich country.[7]

If a woman has high levels of the virus in her blood and breastmilk and low levels of CD4 cells (the white cells which combat infection) then she is more likely to infect her child. Most poor women do not have access to sophisticated monitoring services to know their CD4 and viral load status. If a woman contracts HIV for the first time while she is breastfeeding, then she is more likely to infect her child. The longer she breastfeeds, the more risk there is of transmission. This is not, as far as is known, because the risk gets greater but because the more often you are exposed to a risk, the greater the probability if its happening. Just as the more often you travel by car, the more chance you have of being in a car accident. An HIV-infected woman is eventually likely to develop AIDS, especially if she does not have ARVs. A mother suffering from AIDS is more likely to transmit HIV to her child.

meetings, meetings, meetings

In 1992, the UN experts did what UN experts have to do: they met at WHO in Geneva and formulated a policy.[8] Aware that breastfeeding was vital for child survival, they also knew that rich babies could survive artificial feeding. They wanted to say: 'If you are HIV-infected but are educated, financially secure, have clean water, electricity and consistent supplies of infant formula, then you can artificially feed whether you live in London, Lagos or Recife. If you are HIV-infected, uneducated, poor and live in a shanty town, a crumbling tower block or a mud hut, and have erratic fuel supplies then you have no choice but to continue breastfeeding.' They avoided geographical boundaries because they knew that some HIV-infected mothers were living in luxury in Africa and others in appalling conditions in Europe or North America. Of course this was all dressed up in the necessary UN-speak. They used the diplomatic term 'settings' – as in 'settings where there is high prevalence of infectious diseases' – to mean places of squalor, poverty and ignorance. The decision makers were confronting the world as it is, but considered it too delicate and offensive to state baldly the harsh realities of our complicated and unjust society.

The policy was misinterpreted to mean that there was one rule for industrialised nations and another for the 'developing' world: a double standard. This was too much for the poor countries' leaders, who believed they were being told to let their people die, so the policy makers had to go back to the drawing board.

The next policy, launched in 1998, changed direction and attempted to give every HIV-infected woman in the world the 'choice' to decide how to feed her child.[9] They presented all the possible options. A woman would have a discussion with a counsellor who would help her decide whether to breastfeed or replacement feed. According to her circumstances she could choose either to breastfeed, to find a wet nurse free of HIV, to use commercial infant formula, or to use home-made formula if she had a cow or a goat and could learn to dilute the milk, and add sugar and a vitamin/mineral mix if available. Or she could use donated milk from a human milk bank if one existed. Or she could express her own breastmilk and heat-treat it at home. Having been helped to decide according to her individual circumstances, a woman must then be supported to carry out her 'choice'. The problem was: where were all these health workers well trained in counselling? Many were filling the gaps in health service staffing in Europe or North America.

who chooses?

If the privileged and educated from the rich world were confused by all these choices, imagine the bafflement of poor, uneducated HIV-infected women and the health workers expected to guide them. Many African or Asian women had no concept of 'choice'. Depending on local custom, most women had to accept what their husband, brother, parents or in-laws told them to do. If the family expected a woman to breastfeed then she had to do so. If they insisted she give infant formula or traditional porridge or herbal teas, then she did. "When I got home my sister said the baby must drink starch water, the thing with salt and sugar", a mother of a four-month-old told researchers in South Africa.

Also, women were used to health workers telling them what to do and health workers were used to being bossy. Both found it hard to cope with the process of choice. The only verb in Zulu to describe how a health worker interacts with anyone is translated as 'to tell'.[10] Health workers had their own prejudices and many were poorly trained. If HIV could be transmitted through breastfeeding, then many believed the risk to be 100% and they would advise a woman not to.

The UN policy makers knew that presenting the use of infant formula as a choice could cause problems. Already some governments, for instance, in Thailand, were providing free ARVs and infant formula for HIV-infected mothers but supplies sometimes ran out. Poorer governments could not afford to copy the Thai experiment. There were also fears that the infant formula companies would exploit the situation and provide temporary free supplies in order to expand markets in impoverished countries.

There were some HIV/AIDS experts who wanted to forbid all HIV-infected women from breastfeeding. In industrialised countries some HIV-infected women who wanted to breastfeed were threatened with removal of their babies, driving some parents 'underground' when they most needed support.[11] You cannot police every second of intimate life. Yet some health and social workers, who would never

SARAH'S STORY

Sara is a lawyer. She discovered she was HIV-infected during routine antenatal screening. She was advised to have a C-section and not to breastfeed. She could accept the first edict but found the second difficult. Resident in the UK but originally from overseas, she was close to her extended family who would be eagerly involved in every detail of her new baby's life. If she did not breastfeed they would guess her HIV status and be aghast. They might even reject her and her baby. The neonatologist, obstetrician, virologist and midwifery manager met to discuss her case and agreed that she should be supported to breastfeed. This decision reflected UK national policy[13] and also the UN guidelines.[14] Sara planned to breastfeed exclusively for two or three months and then change rapidly to exclusive artificial feeding. Her virus levels would be monitored and she would continue with her ARV regime. Sara's breastfeeding was supported by one dedicated midwife with help from the infant feeding specialist. Both had made her aware of the importance of good attachment and frequent effective feeding to keep her breasts healthy and minimise the risk of transmission. If there was the slightest problem they would use donor milk from a human milk bank.

Sara bore a healthy daughter who breastfed beautifully from the start. On the evening of the third day, the midwifery manager arrived alone at her bedside. She informed Sara that if she continued to breastfeed, this might be a 'child protection matter', an implicit threat to take Sara's baby from her into social care. It was as though the group decision had never taken place. Sara immediately began artificially feeding her baby. If the other staff had been consulted they could have helped Sara to express and pasteurise her breastmilk using the single-bottle pasteuriser in the unit. Starting artificial feeding at such an early stage after some breastfeeding could have increased the risk of HIV transmission to Sara's baby.

consider checking condom-use in the bedroom, or removing a partner who refused to practise safe sex, believed they had the right and duty to check every second of a mother-and-baby relationship. It touched on the overwhelming philosophical question of who is responsible for the baby.

UNICEF had already been criticised for being too committed to breastfeeding and accused of neglecting the issue of mother-to-child HIV transmission.[12] It was clear that the UN health agencies could not recommend replacement feeding without finding a way to make it possible. The plan was to set up Prevention of Mother-to-Child Transmission (PMTCT) programmes in eleven pilot countries and learn from the experience. Since its formation, UNICEF has been viewed as the agency which distributed 'stuff'. It provided vaccines, education packages and . . . milk. Having taken years to shed its old milk-provider image, UNICEF was back where it started and the problems came back too.

hard lessons

To avoid promotion of a brand or company, UNICEF commissioned a generic infant formula, manufactured by a company that did not violate the International Code of Marketing of Breastmilk Substitutes.[15] Its label conformed to Code requirements and the graphics showed safer cup feeding rather than bottle-feeding. Some governments requested the free formula, but others such as Botswana and South Africa decided to buy their own on the open market. There were difficulties from the start. The generic infant formula arrived late and there were storage and distribution hitches. The labels (in French, English and Spanish) had to be translated into local languages and people bickered about who should do this. It was also difficult to monitor use.

Wherever infant formula is distributed free, there are problems. A baby must have sustained supplies. Anyone who has lived in a poor country knows that fragile infrastructures cause hitches in distribution systems. Bad roads, power cuts and bureaucratic blockages slow up deliveries. There is also 'leakage'. Pilfering exists everywhere and infant formula has high market value. In the USA, US$7 billion worth of infant formula is stolen and resold each year, sometimes with the expiry date changed.[16] In countries such as Kenya where infant formula costs 84% of the minimum urban wage, its black market value is high. If you are poor you have cash flow problems all the time, so free hand-out products get traded. Selling the free infant formula may just stave off family hunger, eviction or some pressing debt. When women run out of formula, they either reduce the number of feeds or over-dilute them or give sugar water or fruit drinks. Some mothers go back to breastfeeding and mixed feed, the worst option for MTCT.

'Choice' flew out of the window. In several countries, health staff simply told HIV-infected mothers to formula feed; they were negative towards women who wanted to breastfeed. Mothers often felt forced to choose a particular option.[17] Staff were lax about giving adequate feed preparation instructions and neglected to ask women about their home conditions. In Rwanda only 8% had adequate sanitation and just 41% adequate water, yet staff pressed women to use infant formula. Untreated water must be boiled for ten minutes and the charcoal stoves commonly used in Africa take 10-15 minutes to reach boiling point. Giving a baby six to eight feeds a day takes prohibitive amounts of fuel and time. Night feeding is a problem when you do not have electric light. Even in relatively prosperous Botswana, only 27% of HIV-infected women had a fridge and even then many mothers stored the prepared feeds at room temperature.[18, 19]

Some breastfeeding advocates became dejected and confused. Funding for breastfeeding promotion efforts dwindled and in much of Africa the energy drained from BFHIs. Few could grasp that, if a mother did replacement feed, it was vital that the closeness intrinsic to the principles of 'The Ten Steps' be maintained. The BFHI was designed to protect and promote exclusive breastfeeding, but its provisions always included the acceptance of medically indicated replacement feeding. When this occurs, it is vital to meet the emotional needs of mother and baby through constant contact.

spillover

The greatest worry about the provision of free infant formula was that it would lead to 'spillover', the term describing the effect on the general population of artificial feeding by HIV-infected mothers. If health workers were seen to endorse it for some, then the message would get across that it was safe for all. And it did. Because of the stigma of HIV/AIDS some women wanted to keep their HIV status secret, often from their close family. They would tell their families and neighbours that they 'were sore', 'had not got enough milk' or their milk had 'dried up', reviving the myths that breastfeeding could be inadequate or unreliable, and any difficulties incurable.

good intentions: the example of botswana

With its low population (less than 2 million), good infrastructure and successful economy Botswana had been called the Switzerland of Africa. Using its diamond wealth wisely, the government invested in education and public health. There were reliable water supplies and high levels of literacy. Between 1970 and 1990, immunisation increased, child malnutrition fell steadily and the infant death rate more than halved. Protection of traditional breastfeeding was part of their health success.

Then HIV/AIDS struck and this spectacular progress went into reverse. By 2003 over 37% of its citizens were HIV-infected, one of the highest rates in the world. Nevertheless experts were optimistic: if any country could be the flagship for successful HIV policies, then Botswana was the one. The government dramatically increased expenditure. UN agencies, NGOs and philanthropists (Bill Gates donated millions) provided finance and support. The national HIV/AIDS strategy was rolled out including the national Prevention of Mother to Child Transmission (PMTCT) Programme which provided ARVs and free infant formula for twelve months. All HIV-infected women were advised to artificially feed and 89% decided to do so.[20] The Botswana Ministry of Health was doing exactly what the HIV/AIDS experts advised.

Then disaster arrived. Between November 2005 and February 2006 there were unusually heavy rains and flooding. Infant diarrhoea broke out, hospitals were overwhelmed and death rates soared. In the first quarter of 2005, there had been 9,166 cases of infant diarrhoea and 21 deaths of children under five in all 22 health districts. For the same quarter in 2006, in just 12 health districts, 22,500 babies had diarrhoea and 470 died. The US Centre for Disease Control (CDC) analysed the reasons. The children were mostly around nine months old, almost all under two, and 93% were not breastfeeding. Many developed acute malnutrition, including the severe form called kwashiorkor, during or after the diarrhoea. The main risk factors for death were not being breastfed or having kwashiorkor (itself associated with not breastfeeding). Whether the family was poor, had clean water, lived in town or countryside or what germ had triggered the diarrhoea had no bearing on the risk of death. Deprivation of breastfeeding was the killer. The bitterest fact was that the babies whose mothers were HIV-free had died from lack of breastfeeding because artificial feeding had become 'normal' again through the Ministry of Health policy. The worst fears about spillover had come horribly true.

During 2003 Nestlé had distributed promotional leaflets in Botswana. One was for New Pelargon infant formula and claimed that "Diarrhoea and its side-effects are counteracted".[21]

The researchers into Botswana's tragedy were well aware of the crucial effect of not being breastfed on child survival. In other parts of the world, some appeared oblivious to the ill-effects of artificial feeding.

how could they not know?

Researchers in Haiti followed up 106 babies born to HIV-infected mothers for fifteen months. They provided free infant formula, drug treatment for HIV, comprehensive medical care and lots of extra support to ensure the artificial feeds were hygienically prepared. There was no breastfeeding. Twenty-two babies died, most before six months of age. That is an infant mortality rate (IMR) of 207/1000, which is over three times Haiti's national IMR of 60/1000. "Despite perinatal HIV treatment, mortality in children born to HIV-infected mothers remained high. Bacteremia, particularly with Staphylococcus aureus, is a partial explanation for excess illness." The researchers did not appear to consider the absence of breastmilk as a factor in infection; nor that Staphylococcus aureus is one of the intrinsic pathogens found in powdered infant formula. Astonishingly, these researchers concluded that there could be no nutritional cause for the babies' infections 'because of the provision of infant formula'. One has to ask: how can a medical team reach the dizzy heights of career progress (research is prestigious) and not a single member be aware that breastmilk contains factors which destroy Staphylococcus aureus, and that those very bacteria are among the intrinsic contaminants in infant formula?[22]

a randomised clinical trial

The gold standard of research method is the randomised trial whereby you select people to reflect the population at large and allocate different treatments and see what happens. Such research eliminates bias and is intended to show up the true causes of a problem or effect. For example you might test a new drug by randomly selecting people with certain characteristics and giving half of them a placebo (an inert substance) and the other half the drug. Trials can be 'blinded': when the researcher but not the subject knows who is getting the real drug. They can also be 'double blinded' when neither researcher nor subject knows who is getting the drug. Obviously you could not have a blind trial with infant feeding method, and random allocation would be unethical because you cannot tell women to do something that might risk their babies' deaths – though I have to tell you that I heard the suggestion made in the early days of the HIV/AIDS pandemic.

In the 1990s researchers believed they had found an ethical way. They asked HIV-infected pregnant women in Kenya to take part in the study and whether they were willing to be randomised to feeding method. If they said yes, they were randomly allocated either to formula feed or to breastfeed and their babies were observed for two years.[23]

The results were distressing. The breastfed babies had a much higher rate of HIV infection transmission, but large numbers of the formula-fed babies died of other infections, especially in the first two months. So the mortality rate at two years was more or less the same. Nevertheless people got very excited about this study because it seemed to show that formula feeding prevented MTCT.

But there were flaws in the research. Even though they had invited over 2,000 women to take part, most refused and a mere 18% of the invited women participated. One of the researchers said, "All these women were quite indifferent as to how they fed their babies."[24] What an unusual group of women. They did not reflect the wider population as the 82% refusal rate indicated. Then there was the question of the real feeding method. Breastfeeding was not exclusive. As anyone in Kenya can tell you, at that time almost all babies were given other milks and maize porridge well before six months. To complicate matters further, some of the women allocated to formula feeding did a bit of breastfeeding too. These women lived in adequate conditions with running water and sanitation, and they were educated. The research project provided constant supplies of free infant formula and health care for both mothers and babies (but did not provide ARV drugs). They were therefore not at all typical of most African women. Despite this, many people in the HIV/AIDS field saw these research results as the green light for widespread artificial feeding by HIV-infected mothers in Africa.

exclusive breastfeeding

In 2000 another UN policy meeting took place and the whole issue of exclusive breastfeeding was discussed. This was because some daring and caring research had been published.

In the late 1990s some scientists in Durban South Africa were trying to discover whether vitamin A supplements to HIV-infected pregnant women could reduce MTCT (they did not.) The women received counselling to help them decide whether to breastfeed or artificially feed. Unlike many other researchers into MTCT, these individuals really understood breastfeeding and they explained the general benefits of exclusive breastfeeding to the mothers. The global rate of exclusive breastfeeding was around 38% but in sub-Saharan Africa it was about 30%. In South Africa it was as low as 7%. Most babies were fed a mixture of breastfeeding, other milks and/or maize porridge, but because these women had received sensitive and helpful counselling, some of them exclusively breastfed for just a few months. Their babies had the same rates of HIV transmission as those who were formula fed. The babies fed a mixture of breastfeeding and other fluids and foods had the highest HIV rates.

For those in despair about the increasingly muddled implementation of the UN policy, these results were a beacon of light in a dark landscape. However, in research you cannot prove a point if some results are merely a spin-off finding which had nothing to do with the original quest. The scientists had been looking for an effect of Vitamin A and discovered the exclusive breastfeeding data. More research had to be done and it was initiated. However the concept of exclusive breastfeeding protecting against MTCT was plausible enough to influence the policy makers.

the ugly but useful acronym: 'afass'

This time a new approach was devised to help local decision-making. The experts knew that the current 'choice' policy was not working, so in 2000 they devised new criteria which went thus: "When replacement feeding is acceptable, feasible, affordable, sustainable and safe, avoidance of breastfeeding by HIV-infected mothers is recommended. Otherwise exclusive breastfeeding is recommended during the first months of life." This became known as the 'AFASS' criteria: acceptable, feasible, affordable, sustainable and safe.[25]

More research was carried out and it showed that mixed breastfeeding doubled the risk of transmission in the first six months and that early exclusive breastfeeding was protective. Replacement-fed babies were twice as likely to die in the first three months of life.[26]

I know I should not show favouritism towards particular individuals working in the impossibly difficult field of HIV/AIDS, but I have to burst out and say that those South African researchers who dared to question the anti-breastfeeding policies deserve prizes for disentangling the facts out of the bias, emotion and ignorance. They were not the only ones, but they had a special strength. They worked in Africa and they saw with their own eyes the conditions in which women were expected to prepare 'safe' artificial feeds. They knew that asking a woman not to breastfeed was far too difficult. They also thought about the biological facts, seized on an intelligent hunch and ran with it.

It is not easy to establish exclusive breastfeeding in a world where

---

HOW EXCLUSIVE BREASTFEEDING PROTECTS

Scientists do not yet fully understand how or why exclusive breastfeeding protects but they have some plausible ideas.

a) A baby's gut is programmed to receive breastmilk and nothing else during the first months of life. The gut walls have a mucosal barrier which allows nutrients, growth and anti-infective factors through, but keeps out pathogens and allergens. Any fluids or foods (other than breastmilk) can damage the gut wall and allow pathogens and allergens to get through. So if a mother is HIV-infected, then some of the virus in her milk may cross through ruptures in her baby's gut wall.

b) Exclusively breastfed babies' guts contain different microbes from artificially fed or mixed-fed babies. One in particular, 'lactobacillus bifidus', creates an acid environment which inhibits the growth of pathogens. Mixed feeding encourages the growth of other microbes and undermines this protective effect. Giving solid foods dramatically disturbs the balance of gut microbes, many of which are pathogenic.

c) Exclusive breastfeeding keeps a mother's breasts healthier. Mothers who get sore, cracked or bleeding nipples, mastitis or an abscess (all inter-related) are more likely to transmit HIV. Poor attachment and restricted breastfeeding prevent the effective removal of milk and can lead to these conditions. When a baby is given other fluids or foods, he is likely to remove less milk. Good attachment protects the nipples so there is no risk of blood getting into the baby. Exclusive breastfeeding necessitates frequent milk removal and prevents mastitis and breast tissue damage.

d) Breastmilk is brimming with anti-infective factors. HIV-infected women have no less than non-infected women. HIV-infected women's breastmilk contains specific anti-HIV factors. Breastmilk composition may differ with exclusive breastfeeding and have more disease protection.

mixed feeding is normal, but it is possible as researchers have shown. Women change their practices when they are given knowledge and support. What seems to escape the attention of many policy makers is that women rarely make decisions alone. Few women leap up after the birth to prepare a bottle of infant formula or sugar water for their newborns. It is health workers or relatives who tell women what to do. During the early months, mothers all over the world hear the question: 'Do you think he's getting enough?' And company promotion works its spells on everyone.

Community-based promotion of exclusive breastfeeding can work wonders. Counsellors do not need to be health workers, they just need high quality training, good supervision and support.[27]

reality, clarity and sanity

In 2006, the experts met again and fresh air blew through the room. WHO issued a Consensus Statement on the prevention of HIV in pregnant women, mothers and infants. It made clear that decisions depended on a woman's individual circumstances, taking into account the local situation, the state of the health services and what support was available.[28]

If AFASS conditions existed, then avoidance of any breastfeeding was the surest way to avoid MTCT, but they were well aware that the majority of women could not meet these criteria. The new guidance went thus: "Exclusive breastfeeding is recommended for HIV-infected women for the first six months of life unless replacement feeding is AFASS for them and their infants before that time."

They recommended exclusive breastfeeding for six months unless AFASS conditions changed. And if after that time, replacement feeding was still not AFASS, then they advised continuing breastfeeding together with complementary foods. Women should only stop breastfeeding when a nutritionally adequate and safe diet without breastmilk could be provided. In a poor country such as Mozambique, finding enough nutritious, local food to replace breastmilk after six months could double the cost of feeding a child, something few households could afford. In some areas enough of the right food is just not available.[29]

In rich countries, the AFASS criteria are often ignored and women are given no option. Women like Sara (see page 103) suffer because their own informed decisions are disrupted by insensitive practitioners. Today, improved drugs, testing and viral monitoring mean that the risk of MTCT transmission through breastfeeding is very low. The other health staff could see that replacement feeding was neither acceptable nor feasible in Sara's circumstances.

We also have to think of those 2% of babies in rich countries who are born HIV-infected, despite good health services. The WHO Consensus Statement states that if babies are known to be already infected, then their mothers are strongly encouraged to continue breastfeeding. If mothers are supported to breastfeed these babies have a better chance of more life. Most HIV-infected babies die, but some have survived and are reaching adulthood. UN policy recommends that these babies be breastfed. In the iThemba Lethu orphanage in South Africa, HIV-infected babies who were malnourished and sick started to thrive when fed donated breastmilk. This inspired paediatrician and researcher Anna Coutsoudis to set up the first milk bank in Africa, a venture most people had thought impossible.[30]

The 2006 WHO Consensus Statement urged a revitalisation of breastfeeding protection, promotion and support and the implementation of The Global Strategy for Infant and Young Child Feeding (see Appendix 1).

The last decade of the 20th century provided a painful experiment in re-learning that artificial feeding kills babies. There is more hope now that some inspired and inspiring people have patiently looked at the reality of life for most women.

9 life, death and birth

"My mother's life made me a man."
John Masefield, poet 1878–1967

risk

If breastfeeding is so wonderful, how do so many survive artificial feeding? Firstly we have to remember that adaptation is part of evolution and the fact that humans are omnivores is a great advantage. A survivor is just that and many animals get by in less than ideal conditions. Natural selection favours those who adapt to adversity. Survival involves a wide range of factors and, though a priority, food is only one. Genetics, living conditions, a mother's lifelong nutrition[1], a father's and even grandparents' life experiences[2], birth weight, birth spacing, medical care and a host of known and unknown factors all play a part. It is the increasing control of some of these factors, as well as better management of artificial feeding, that contributed to the 20th-century falls in infant mortality in the industrialised world. An exclusively breastfed child can die, just as an artificially fed child can survive, because of a range of risk factors, but this does not mean the risks are equal. There is an account of a 17th-century man orphaned at two weeks old, who was reared on beer and lived to be 70, yet no one could say that feeding an infant beer is a low risk strategy.[3] This man was clearly rather unusual, as are the babies today who survive without breastfeeding. Most of them live in the protectively organised environment of industrialised society or, like the infant beer drinker, are exceptional.[4] What has happened in the rich world is that, while removing the ideal food and feeding method, there has been progress in the elimination of other immediate risks. It is important to remember that it is still only a minority of the world's population that can be artificially fed from birth without getting ill or dying.[5]

In the artificial-feeding cultures of industrialised countries there is an assumption that infant infections are normal, but death is not expected; parents do not expect to lose a child to illness. There is a tremendous back-up system for these babies. There is clean water, sanitation, waste disposal, dry housing and hygiene awareness as well as health surveillance, immunisation, and rapid, effective treatment in the case of illness. Antibiotics have had a dramatic effect on reducing deaths from infection. An artificially-fed child in Paris, London or Sydney may develop an ear or respiratory infection or diarrhoea, but rapid access to transport and good medical facilities provide speedy diagnosis and treatment. As I mentioned in Chapter 5 antibiotic resistance is becoming a serious, global problem. A British Medical Journal article states that "existing antibiotics are losing their effect at an alarming pace" and should be considered a non-renewable resource. Misuse and overuse have contributed to this problem.[6]

Even with the huge benefit of breastfeeding, a baby with malaria in a rural African village may die if untreated.[7] His mother might walk for a whole day to take him to the nearest clinic. If it is planting or harvest time she cannot chance two days' absence from her tasks because the community's food supply for the coming year might be jeopardised. Without telephones, transport, decent roads or well-staffed health services there is no safety net for such emergencies.

Because people who live in richer regions are often unclear why artificial feeding is so dangerous in poorer regions it is important to spell out in detail what normal conditions of life are like for the majority of human beings.

normal life

Water: About one-sixth of the world's population, over a billion people, lack access to safe water. A piped water supply in your home is one of the most effective protections against disease, but just 6% of rural African households have this. For the rest, women fetch water from wells, rivers, lakes or ponds. These might be eight or more kilometres away. Water-fetching takes between fifteen minutes and over an hour, depending on the distance. There are often queues (some women start out in the night to avoid them), and in East Africa waiting time has tripled in the last four decades. Water containers usually hold around 20 litres which weigh 20 kilograms*, the same as the baggage allowance on most airlines. Imagine carrying that on your head for over an hour every day. Similar problems of access to water exist in parts of Asia and Latin America. An average person in a poor country uses just 10 litres of water a day; in a rich country the figure is 200 litres. Flushing a toilet uses about 15-26 litres a day.

Some urban areas are better served. In towns about 70% have piped water in the home compared with 25% of rural households, but even in the cities, it is hard to practise basic hygiene if you are poor.

* Just over 5 US gallons, which weigh approximately 44lbs.

Normal conditions

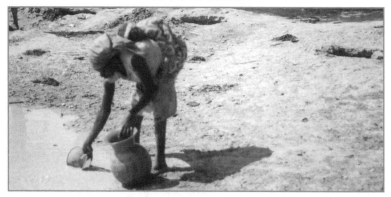

11 Collecting water, Niger. (Photo Sandy Cairncross)

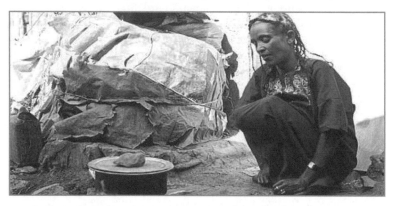

12 Cooking the family meal, Ethiopia. (Photo Venetia Dearden, Courtesy of Save the Children, UK)

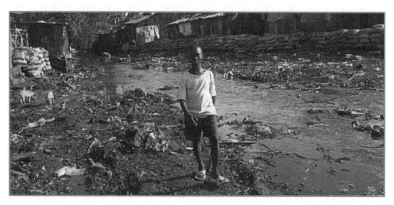

13 A river may serve as an open sewer, Sierra Leone. (Photo Anna Kari, Courtesy of Save the Children, UK)

Every home in an elite suburb of Jakarta may have a luxury bathroom or two, but in the slums a family will be lucky if there is a water tap in their street. The urban poor often have to buy water from vendors and therefore limit amounts. In Indonesia, 70% of the population (220 million) rely on water from potentially contaminated sources.[8]

Containers in the home are easily contaminated. Water needs boiling to kill the microorganisms in it but there is another problem. Because powdered infant formula contains intrinsic pathogens it must be made up with boiled water cooled to no less than 70°C (158°F) no more than half an hour before each feed. The charcoal fires commonly used in Africa take 10 to 15 minutes to reach boiling point. Cow dung fires in South Asia may take even longer. Preparing six to eight feeds a day takes prohibitive amounts of fuel and time. And, then, how do you cool a feed quickly if there is no running cold water? Everything stays hot in tropical climates, and the more slowly the feed cools the more pathogens can multiply. In hot climates refrigeration would help, but when most incomes barely achieve subsistence levels, only a minority can afford fridges.[9] Unreliable fuel supplies mean that even those that exist do not always function.

Most people think first of safe water for drinking and cooking, but water's role in hygiene is crucial for survival. The inevitable and invisible contamination of your hands through wiping your bottom is part of normal life and most societies have traditional hygiene practices after defecation and before food preparation. But if you have a very limited water supply (and no soap), it is very difficult to prevent oral-faecal contamination. Most of the common diarrhoeal diseases are spread this way. Many readers will have been on hiking trips in remote areas where they had to let their own standards fall. For millions of people, every day is like a hard hiking trip. You may be able to boil the water for the baby's feed, but can you scrub and dry your hands thoroughly for six or eight baby feeds a day when you only have a few litres for the whole family?

Sanitation: Over a third of the world's population, 2.5 billion people, lack adequate sanitation. Exposed human waste is a major cause of disease. The construction of public sewerage systems and household plumbing contributed significantly to the health improvements of the countries that are rich today. Despite this knowledge, one in three human beings has no access to any type of lavatory or latrine. Disposal of waste, sewage treatment and vermin extermination are taken for granted in western society. If you live in a city squatter slum (as about a billion people do), your lavatory may be the street and your home a breeding ground for insects. You share your living quarters with far more people than the average North American or European does. Three toilets and one shower between 250 households is common in many cities of sub-Saharan Africa. Open sewers are normal in poor countries. If well-maintained and free-flowing, they are better than no sewer at all, but many become informal rubbish tips and get blocked, creating a paradise for rats, mosquitoes and other vectors of disease.[10] Consequently everyone, especially a baby, is exposed to more infections. With his mother's milk brimful of anti-infective factors, combating the pathogens in their common environment, a slum baby can do remarkably well when exclusively breastfed, but deprive him of this protection and the inevitable infections can lead to death.

Fuel: Fuel is essential to boil the water for artificial feeds and sterilisation of utensils. Even in wealthy regions, fuel costs erode the household budget, but poor people spend a much higher proportion of earnings on fuel. Whether it is wood, charcoal, dung, kerosene, or liquid bottled gas, fuel is expensive, using up half the income of many families. In Jakarta, where a daily wage may be the equivalent of US$1 a day, the kerosene to boil 20 liters of water costs about US$0.25. Artificial feeding requires small quantities of freshly boiled water for each feed and that uses more fuel. Most people cannot do this so feeds can never be correctly prepared.

In India, where 75% of the population live in rural areas, wood, crop residues and animal dung provide 80-90% of fuel needs. In Himachal Pradesh, a relatively better-off state, women typically spend 40 hours a month making 15 trips of about 2km to carry these fuels. These then have to be chopped, dried, stacked and stored. It takes 200g of wood to boil 1 litre of water. A baby needs at least six to eight feeds a day, yet lighting the fire or stove more than twice a day costs more money and time than any poor person has.

Most of you reading this are used to flicking a switch for light, but around 300 million people have no access to electricity. Whereas you can breastfeed easily in the dark, you need light to make up an artificial feed. Torches and batteries are expensive and candles or kerosene lamps dangerous, especially when the whole family shares sleeping quarters, as many do. When you are tired and sleepy you are more likely to stumble. Moonlight can help but you cannot restrict night feeds to around the full moon.[11]

Money: A tin of infant formula is often the most expensive food item a family has ever purchased. Mothers and sometimes older children go hungry in order to buy it. In the first six months of life, a baby needs 20kg of powdered infant formula; that is 44 tins containing 450g each. In Kenya this costs around Ksh3,700 (US$54) a month. Monthly per capita income is KSh2300 (US$34) so you do not need a maths degree to work out that artificial feeding is financially impossible for an average family. In Haiti infant formula costs US$56 a month, about the same as a factory worker's wage. In Bangladesh artificial feeding can cost more than the monthly earnings of a garment worker.*

Even in prosperous areas, artificial feeding can be a financial strain. The booming Indian economy depends on low wages, even for the educated. Artificially feeding an infant costs 43% of the minimum wage of a skilled urban worker. Sometimes mothers and carers who cannot find the immediate cash to buy the next tin, 'stretch' the milk by over-diluting it, causing malnutrition and infection. The feeding bottles and teats cost money too and need replacing when they become scratched and worn. Cheaper plastic bottles have replaced glass, but they are harder to keep sterile and together with the teats contain environmental contaminants. WHO and other international agencies recommend cup feeding rather than bottle-feeding in areas where sanitation and clean water are a problem. Despite this, few governments regulate the sale of bottles and teats.[12]

Education and Literacy: Even in rich societies both mothers and health workers make errors in making up artificial feeds. You certainly need to be able to read the instructions on the label. Continued resistance to female education means that female illiteracy is higher than male, yet it is usually women who do the artificial feeding. Of the 774 million people who cannot read, 64% are women. In sixteen countries the majority of women are illiterate.[13]

Even where female literacy has risen, many babies are artificially-fed by servants who may not be fluent in their employer's language or dare not admit they have problems understanding label instructions. Companies still distribute infant formula and other products labelled in languages foreign to most local people.

There is another aspect to literacy which to my shame only struck me when my own eyesight worsened with age. It is common for

* Garment worker's wage: 1,400–3,200 takas (US$20-US$47) a month. Artificial feeding costs 1,662 takas (US$24) a month.

grandmothers to care for orphans and the babies of mothers working away from home. Sight worsens with age. Many labels are too small to be read by those with sight difficulties. In poor countries even the literate may be unable to afford eye tests or spectacles.

Healthcare: Artificial feeding requires medical services to be nearby. In much of the world, access to medical care is scarce and services overstretched. The economic performance of modern India, much praised by international financiers, has not touched the lives of most of its citizens. There is huge inequality in healthcare. Though Indian doctors are among the best in the world, over 75% of them are city-based – yet 75% of Indians live in rural villages. This means that 620 million Indians lack adequate healthcare.

You need transport to take your child to a health centre: 89% of rural Indians must travel about eight kilometres for medical care and 11% travel even further. And you have to pay. One of the cornerstones of 'structural adjustment', the 20th-century economic dogma of the financial cardinals in Washington DC, insisted that governments make people pay directly for their health services. Unsurprisingly, healthcare take-up fell. In Benin, West Africa just 27% of heads of households can afford healthcare.

The impetus for the UN Millennium Development Goals (Appendix 5) has been hindered by inequality in access to healthcare. You cannot stop women and babies dying if they are too poor to afford health services. In 54 of the 68 poorest countries where 97% of mother and child deaths occur there are glaring disparities between rich and poor. When it comes to maternal and newborn care, over half of the poorest groups have no coverage, whereas most (but not all) of the wealthiest have access to care.

Even if parents get to a clinic or hospital, their children die because the queues are too long and there are simply not enough health workers to treat everyone. In Uganda there is one nurse per 5,000 people and one doctor per 24,700.[14]

An episode of diarrhoea may need only simple, cheap oral rehydration (which can be made up at home), but if your child has a respiratory infection the doctor may prescribe antibiotics which are expensive. Women usually work in informal employment where time off means no pay, so mothers resort to buying cheaper drugs over the counter. These may be unsuitable, out of date or even fake.

Poverty: Nearly half of all human beings live on less than US$2 a day. The wealth of the three richest men is equal to the combined wealth of the 48 poorest countries. In Bangladesh, Ethiopia, Burma and Tanzania the cost of an adequate diet exceeds the incomes of poor families. Such families can never get out of poverty without outside help; their malnourished children cannot develop properly and the whole family is frequently ill. The cruel myth that anyone with spirit can pull themselves up by their bootstraps still prevails. If you have no bootstraps to pull up there is nothing you can do, however strong your determination. If any one of these families attempted artificial feeding, their baby gets ill.[15]

death

The most preventable cause of failure to breastfeed is the death of a mother. If you live in Europe, Australia or North America, it is unlikely that you have lost a sister or close friend in childbirth. A hundred years ago this was common but nowadays, if you have suffered such a loss, there was probably a government inquiry, a court case and maybe even press coverage. It is rare, and when it does happen, health workers as well as the woman's loved ones get very upset. If you live in Sierra Leone or Afghanistan it is highly likely that you have lost a relative or friend this way. Your lifetime risk of dying due to pregnancy or childbirth is one in six. The risk for north-western European women is one in 30,000.[16]

Every year over half a million women (99% of them from the poor world) die from causes related to pregnancy and childbirth. That is 1,370 deaths every day; the equivalent of a jumbo jet crashing every four hours. Unlike plane crashes, these deaths seldom make headlines in our news media.

There is official recognition. Back in 1987 the Safe Motherhood Initiative (SMI) was launched with the support of WHO and it was reported hopefully that "the world began to wake up to a forgotten tragedy."[17] Now, however, though several health agencies and many individuals are doing good work, the world is still dozing. Few world leaders refer to this topic in public speeches.

Another alarm clock has been set. One target of the fifth UN Millennium Development Goal (UNMDG) to improve maternal health, is to reduce maternal mortality by three-quarters by 2015. This can be done by tackling the preventable causes of maternal death. This objective can also help to achieve the fourth Millennium Goal of reducing child mortality. A motherless child is far more likely to die before two years of age than one with a mother.

Why do so many women die? Here are the main reasons:

- Because they are too young: girls aged fifteen to nineteen are twice as likely to die in childbirth than women in their twenties and it is the leading cause of teenage female death in poor countries. In Angola, 70% of women have their first child in their teens.
- Because they are malnourished: 450 million adult women are stunted because they did not get adequate food as children, and 40% of women, a fifth of the world's population, have iron-deficiency anaemia. Being stunted and being anaemic increases your risk of labour complications and accounts for 20% of maternal mortality.
- Because there are no midwives: one in four women gives birth alone or with the help of an unskilled relative or neighbour. In Afghanistan, 86% of women have no skilled birth attendant. In the UK, one midwife per woman in labour is considered insufficient and a shortage of midwives has been partly alleviated by recruitment from abroad, including from countries such as Malawi. In Malawi half the women have no skilled help at birth, but even for the other half there is only one midwife available for ten women in labour.

  Traditional birth attendants (TBAs) can be skilled, but some may be using unsafe practices such as using unsterilised blades to cut the umbilical cord. Others have great knowledge and judgement and know when medical help is needed. Though currently out of favour with the lead health agencies, these women are often the only help available. It seems pragmatic to work with them, rather than try to erase their existence and make them go 'underground'. When they receive supportive extra training and basic equipment, they can provide excellent care, and in some countries, for example Guatemala, they can have a key role in reducing both infant and maternal mortality.
- Because they cannot get skilled medical help in an emergency: obstetricians are not flocking to work in the ill-equipped conditions of rural maternity facilities, even if they exist.
- Because they did not want to be pregnant: 137 million women who want to space or limit their pregnancies use no contraception, usually because they have no access to family planning services; 68,000 women a year die from unsafe abortions. Preventing unplanned pregnancies would save a quarter of maternal deaths.[18]

All these and other related causes are linked to one over-arching reason, expressed by Dr Tariq Meguid, a rare obstetrician working in Malawi: "In the end there is little doubt that women die in Africa because they are poor – really, really poor – and voiceless. They say absolutely nothing. They are women and that is why they die like that. It is a huge, huge scandal. The world knows it and could do more."[19]

His words apply to any part of the world where governments have higher priorities than maternal health. Many governments do not even bother to investigate the causes of these deaths which represent the greatest contrast in health outcomes between poor and rich countries.[20]

In 2008 the reduction in maternal deaths was not on target. Some regions such as eastern Asia made big improvements but in others little changed. Sub-Saharan Africa got worse.[21]

the damaging rituals of birth

The scandal of death through childbirth is not an argument for routine medicalised, interventionist birth, though it is often used as an excuse. The links between hospital deliveries, over-medicalised birthing practices and the 20th-century decline of breastfeeding are strong. Prolonged and traumatic birth has a negative effect. By the mid 20th century in the USA it had become standard for women to give birth in hospital, on their backs, restrained, drugged, deprived of food and drink and without a supportive, caring companion. Actively birthing their babies was impossible and interventions such as forceps became common. Instead of the sense of joy, pride and triumph that women who give birth in respectful, supportive and calm atmospheres feel, women endured an experience they wanted to forget. Indeed the main drug then used, scopolamine, was not an effective painkiller but an amnesiac. Nowadays many psychologists have found evidence that post traumatic stress disorder can be a cause of long-term emotional and physical problems, even when we do not recall the actual trauma. If a horrible experience is blocked out of our memory, then we cannot deal with it or go through a healing process.[22] Millions of women were unable to talk through, understand or even be aware of why they felt bad because the act of giving birth had been suppressed from their consciousness by the drug. Following this model, routine medical interventions and inhumane treatment of labouring women spread around the world.[23]

Many sacrosanct medical practices which humiliated women did more harm than good. Shaving pubic hair was done in the name of hygiene, much to women's discomfort, until someone actually counted the bacteria and discovered that it increased the risk of infection. Another misused practice was episiotomy: cutting the vagina during labour. A 1991 Swedish national survey revealed more complications and pain for women who had had episiotomies than for those with a spontaneous tear, and their pelvic floor muscles remained weaker. The procedure does not protect against perineal trauma or urinary incontinence. Women are often too ashamed to talk about these problems even though they can ruin their sexual and social relationships. Many women think it is birth itself which is damaging and are unaware that it is an intervention which caused the problem. The only good reason for episiotomy is to save a baby's life; it harms women yet it is still common in much of the world.

The Swedish mothers who suffered episiotomy were less likely to be breastfeeding at three months and the researcher speculated that the extra pain might affect their early breastfeeding experience. It seems likely that if you are told that your vagina is so ill-designed that it must be cut open to perform a normal function, you are less likely to believe that your breasts will work well.[24]

Giving birth on your back distorts the pressure of the baby's head, and this makes tearing more likely. Walking about eases pain and helps labour progress, yet watch any Hollywood film and at the first contraction the labouring woman is pinioned into a wheelchair amidst much panic and tension. This slows down labour. Standing, kneeling on all fours, squatting or being supported in a sitting position all facilitate an easier and safer labour. I have visited both rich and poor countries where the lithotomy* position, the woman lying on her back with her legs in stirrups, is considered normal.

Historically women did not deliver flat on their backs, but when 16th century male practitioners began to use forceps they required women to be in this position in order to use them. There is an anecdote that King Louis XIV of France wanted to witness his mistresses giving birth and stirrups provided a perv's eye view. Whatever the origins, several hundred years later, a position used for abnormal birth was adopted for all births. I have walked through maternity facilities in a country where female modesty and veiling were the norm, and yet a lone, labouring woman with her legs apart, strapped in stirrups, could be viewed by strangers. Such humiliation is traumatic. Though I have seen wonderful examples of kindness and sensitivity, I know too much of brutality and abuse. I have seen

* Lithotomy means the removal of a stone from a man's urinary tract.

abdomens pummelled, stretched-out hands disregarded, and have met women who were shouted at and even slapped during labour.

Caesarean sections: In the later 20th century, in some countries – notably Brazil, China and the USA – a 90% rate was common in some hospitals. This does not improve the health of mothers and babies, but it does make obstetricians richer. A C-Section is an essential procedure to save the lives of some mothers and babies and should be available for those who need it. In poor countries women suffer for lack of C-Section, while in rich countries they may suffer from too many. WHO states that no region should ever have more than 15% C-Section births. Studies from rich countries show that C-Section mothers are less likely to be breastfeeding at two weeks than those who delivered vaginally.[25]

Drugs: The drugs commonly used for pain relief in labour can adversely affect the baby's responses and make him reluctant to breastfeed. Though patience and skill can overcome these negative effects, it is an initial blow to a mother's confidence and a cause of early abandonment of breastfeeding. Too many mothers have said, 'My baby didn't like my milk' or 'He wasn't interested in my breast and preferred the bottle' and have been quite unaware that drugs had made their babies behave abnormally. Meperidine (Pethidine or Demerol), an opiate which has often been used routinely without consulting the mother, depresses a newborn's reflexes and impedes the important early suckling episodes. Epidural drugs can also have similar effects.[26]

Continuous emotional support: The single most effective influence on reducing the chance of a complicated labour is continuous support during childbirth. This has more effect than any other intervention. A review of twelve studies in eight countries (rich and poor) found that continuous support significantly reduced time of labour and the need for medication, including synthetic oxytocin. There was a reduction in the need for forceps, vacuum extraction and C-Sections, and breastfeeding was more successful. The presence of a supportive companion could save large amounts of money, time and lives, yet it is still common around the world for health staff to refuse that person her place with the labouring woman.[27]

It has become fashionable in rich countries for the woman's husband or partner to be the birth companion. This has become so expected that couples are defensive if the husband does not attend. This is a mixed blessing because not all men have the qualities needed to support a woman in labour. Some are so nervous themselves that they radiate tension, whilst others adopt a football-coach approach, shouting 'push, push, push' to a woman who needs calm and quiet more than anything. Women are often anxious about their partner's feelings. Michel Odent claims that the father's presence slows down labour.[28]

Until birth was moved into the hospital, almost all human societies had systems of continuous support during labour. Recently, there has been a resurgence in valuing this support. The Greek word 'doula' was reinvented in the 1970s by an anthropologist. It was derived from the Greek word for slave, but is now used to mean the woman who supports and cares for a woman in labour and afterwards. Increasing numbers of women are undergoing doula training to enhance and develop the skills necessary to support women through this important event, and it is becoming an established profession. Regrettably, they are restricted to the private sector and are therefore usually only available to women with money. As far as I know, no government health authority or insurance company acknowledges the value of the doula, despite potential cost savings.[29]

Women must feel entitled to choose the person they know can support them best. The happiest births are when the health workers and these supporters value each others' skills and work harmoniously and quietly together to support the woman give birth as safely and joyfully as possible. When our birthing culture comes to its senses and follows the evidence of what works best, then many breastfeeding difficulties will melt away. As WHO states: "A woman's experience during labour and delivery affects her motivation towards breastfeeding and the ease with which she initiates it".[30]

an anomaly

There is an anomaly in my statements. Women in poor countries may have difficult births but still breastfeed for a couple of years, whilst there are women in rich countries who have given birth easily and artificially fed their babies. This is because culture is so powerful. In breastfeeding societies no one considered doing anything else. In some industrialised countries in the 1960s, when artificial feeding had become utterly normal, even those who practised natural childbirth accepted it as a benign equivalent of breastfeeding.

We know that delayed initiation of breastfeeding kills babies and impedes the establishment of successful lactation.[31] We do not know how much of the casual supplementation in breastfeeding societies is due to difficult births which disrupted the bonding and skin contact we now value so highly. I do know that in the 1970s and '80s many women who had had straightforward, happy birth experiences then stopped breastfeeding at three months because they truly did not know that anyone could breastfeed for longer.

Making birth better makes sense: for the woman, for breastfeeding and for the baby.[32]

10 population, fertility and sex

"The tribe I was with must have used some method of contraception, possibly an abortifacient, although I never managed to find out how they worked it. Anyway, the women had children more or less once every four years and for the first four years of the child's life its mother was never out of its sight."

Crashaw, the anthropologist, speaking in Savages
a play by Christopher Hampton, Faber & Faber 1974

are dead babies useful?

When I started to write this book, a friend asked how breastfeeding could possibly have anything to do with politics. In answer I described a woman living in a shantytown in a poverty-stricken country. Forbidden to take her baby to work, she leaves him to be artficially fed by an older child while she earns the pittance to feed the whole family. Her baby gets pneumonia and dies. My friend responded, "But isn't it a good thing if those babies die as there are far too many of them anyway?" As residents of England, both she and I live in one of the most densely populated areas of the world. In 21st-century Britain over 100,000 families are in temporary sub-standard housing and over a million children live in overcrowded accommodation.[1] Yet if I had suggested we should leave her daughter to die of pneumonia as a contribution to the UK overcrowding problems she would have understandably broken off our friendship.

I quote this story because my friend's reaction is not unusual. It illustrates a common belief about the causes of poverty. She, like many people, believes that there is a problem of overpopulation in the poorer countries of the world and that infant deaths will help resolve this. Linked with this belief is the assumption that somehow the poor are the cause of their own poverty because they reproduce themselves excessively. Overpopulation is seen as a problem partly because of the intense competition for resources, yet the poor use up far fewer of these than the rich. The average North American consumes 17 times more than a Mexican and 100 times more than an Ethiopian. The 13 million babies born each year in the rich world will have a far greater impact on the Earth's resources than the 120 million born in the poor world. US citizens form 5% of the world's population but consume a quarter of the energy.* By her first birthday, a US child will have generated more CO_2 emissions than a Tanzanian does in a lifetime.[2]

Furthermore, whereas every poor person is struggling simply to stay alive, every rich person is energetically contributing to a system of economic 'growth' which depends on increasing production and consumption. This poisons the environment and will eventually exhaust the finite resources of the earth. The poor damage their environment because they have no choice; the alternative is hunger or untimely death. Those of us who live in richer societies pollute the earth because we are part of an economic pattern which must stimulate desires rather than satisfy needs in order to perpetuate itself. Rather than redistribute resources through fairer trading and fiscal systems, we engage in a political economy designed to stimulate and fulfil greed. We damp down the awareness and resolution of these injustices because the acquisition of non-essential consumer goods has become the primary motive of many people's lives. We, together with the richer citizens of the poorer countries, do this on the backs of the world's poorest people. Instead of acknowledging that it is their labour, their raw materials and their debt repayment which provide us with our daily bread, we convince ourselves that they are dependent, incompetent and too numerous. The very dependency and supposed incompetence of the poor is essential for our prosperity. If no one borrowed money, how could 'our' money 'grow' and the financial system function?** I first wrote those words, 20 years ago, in 1988. As I write now the rich world is shuddering from the 'credit crunch', but poor people have been suffering from a 'credit crunch' for years. International finance agencies made loans knowing that repayment would cause suffering to ordinary citizens and that the rich in power could get away with corruption. Even so-called 'aid' gets misused. It is often tied to the commercial interests of the donor government. It also tends to benefit the elite. As an unknown sage remarked: "overseas aid is paid by poor people in rich countries to rich people in poor countries".[3]

If poor people were not diagnosed as incompetent, to whom would the experts sell their expertise? If the birth rates were not so high, to whom would we peddle our contraceptives? Population

* Though a French person generates five times less CO_2 than a US citizen, Europeans are not entirely innocent. Australians are also avid users of energy.
**By 2008 'our' financial system was not functioning and 'our' money was not growing.

growth may be a problem for poor countries, but only because the population explosions of the past in industrialised countries were linked to the establishment of a system which required the continued extraction of resources from those countries at a deliberately maintained low and unfair price.

Until the 19th century in England, and probably in much of Europe, it was the rich who had very large families. Most ordinary people controlled their fertility through late marriage, breastfeeding, and traditional birth limitation methods. These included non-penetrative sex, withdrawal (coitus interruptus), abstinence, vaginal sponges, herbal potions and induced abortion. The last was morally acceptable to religious authorities if it was carried out before the 'quickening' of the foetus (when a mother first feels her baby move) because people believed that was the moment the soul entered the body.

Because most researchers with influence in high places have been men and most of this knowledge has lain with women, there has been an assumption that until recent times people were passively fertile. Most so-called 'primitive' peoples have planned their reproduction more carefully than, until recently, industrialised society has. A Ugandan friend told me how her grandmother had been sexually active all her life, yet only wanted and had one child: "I wish I knew how she managed this", my friend recounted. Awareness of the contraceptive effect of breastfeeding has been used to plan families in many societies, but western ignorance and, more significantly, western infant feeding practices destroyed both the knowledge and the effect.

Wealthy families are still left out of the argument. As George Monbiot has said, "Seldom has the complaint been heard 'people like us are breeding too fast'."[4] A common North American and European attitude is to criticise a low-income family but accept profligate fertility among the rich. The famous US political family, the Kennedys, were known for their numerous children, yet were never condemned for contributing to overpopulation. In the UK, Prince Philip (husband of Queen Elizabeth II) once blamed increasing population as the cause of environmental degradation in Africa.[5] As the father of four children, twice the amount recommended for population stability, resident of several oversized houses in a nation with severe housing shortages and himself a more avid consumer of natural resources than any nomad, his castigation of poor Africans had a curious irony. The 'population problem' has been seen as something that happens in the Indian countryside or a Nairobi slum. It is cited as the cause of hunger and poverty, yet Europe's population explosion reshaped world economic structures to the permanent disadvantage of the now poor countries and of the environment. The idea that more dead babies will reduce world population is nonsense and in fact has the opposite effect. It has been demonstrated repeatedly that when a couple are confident of their children's chance of survival, they willingly reduce family size.

This happened in Europe during the 20th century when public health measures and better living standards made life less hazardous. It also happened in poor regions. In Kerala, India, despite poverty, women's social equality and improved health and education services had a significant effect on birth limitation.[6] These changes often take place within a region on a class basis, which has contributed to the idea of the poor being the principal culprits in the breeding game. The better off have greater access to medical services, health benefits and information, so if a child gets ill they can be confident they can get help quickly (speed of action is more often the life and death factor than the nature of treatment). Poor children die needlessly because they reach the clinic or hospital too late. Rural people may continue to have children because they know several could die. Chances of survival are crucial in decisions about family size which are usually made for sound economic reasons.

However, no region needs to wait to get rich and well-educated to benefit from contraception availability. One of the poorest and most densely populated countries in the world, Bangladesh, is another impressive example of how public health education and widespread contraceptive provision halved average family size. Uptake was excellent and as a result infant, child and maternal death fell. Now even illiterate parents know that fewer, well-spaced pregnancies will protect themselves and their children.[7]

What is more shocking is that I have to justify in demographic terms that babies should not die unnecessarily, implying that if it were good for the world as a whole we should accept it. My friend had never lost a child, but those I know who have, whatever society they come from, never lose the pain, however much joy other children give them. She would have been filled with compassion if my baby had died, but she calmly countenanced the death of 'their' babies. It is this ability to detach ourselves from other people's tragedies that is so dangerous. It is this 'switching off' which allowed the Nazis to deal as they did with another group they defined as a 'problem'.

We are properly horrified when we hear of the deliberate slaughter of children, but when the only cause of a baby's death is that his mother cannot have him near her to feed and protect, this is a kind of murder – a murder through indifference.

breastfeeding and fertility

Some people see the rapid expansion of population as the most serious of the world's problems, while others believe that the attempt to control that expansion is genocide. High populations are seen both as the triggers of beneficial change and as the cause of increased poverty and environmental degradation. Religious and political ideas about population control arouse furious debate and national and international policies can be reversed overnight, often with no consultation with those most affected by such changes. Why does a population explosion happen? There are many and complex reasons and expert demographers will continue to debate them, but I want to examine here two aspects which particularly affect women.

It has been taken for granted that in pre-industrial Europe both birth and death rates were high and that the benefits of industrialisation, such as medical knowledge and greater food supply, led to the survival of more babies thus precipitating the population explosion. Certainly for England this is a false picture. Though overall deaths fell, infant mortality rose during the 19th century in England. The age of first marriage and childbearing began earlier and pregnancies became more closely spaced, probably because unrestricted breastfeeding gradually declined.

Another important factor was that during the 19th and 20th centuries in the industrialising countries there was a fall in the age of menarche, the first menstrual period. In the middle of the 19th century, girls started their periods at about 16 years; the average age fell to about 13 years in the 20th century in most industrialised countries and younger in the USA. This trend has been repeated wherever societies industrialise and urbanise. Theories about the causes include climatic changes, the influence of artificial light and psychosexual stimulation. Earlier menarche is linked to earlier increased height and body weight. The child growth expert JM Tanner states that the causes are probably multiple, but that 'better' nutrition is a factor, perhaps in particular more protein and calories in early infancy. This idea of 'better' nutrition is a controversial claim in relation to women, for early menarche increases the likelihood of health problems such as breast and uterine cancer; it also increases the chances of conception way beyond most women's desired number of children.[8] I do not know whether the development of sexual drive is linked to the onset of menstruation, but I do know that modern teenage girls have problems coping with their own sexual feelings and with conflicting social pressures to appear sexy and be heterosexually active, and yet avoid promiscuity and pregnancy.

Tanner's claim that nutrition in early infancy plays a part in age of menarche indicates that perhaps stopping breastfeeding, giving extra artificial feeds or introducing supplementary foods early might play a crucial part in a girl baby's development and be a disadvantage for her long-term reproductive life. It is now accepted that early infant feeding influences our lifetime's health and that, for example, gaining too much weight in the first years of life may predispose a child to diabetes and other chronic diseases in later life.[9] Ecologist Sandra Steingraber links early artificial feeding with the falling age of puberty.[10] There are anecdotal reports of soya milks for infants being associated with earlier puberty, though interestingly some research has focussed on possible adverse effects on male fertility.[11] It is known that having been breastfed improves kidney transplant acceptance in later life.[12] Obviously if infant feeding can influence long-term biochemistry so profoundly, it seems likely that a woman's hormonal path through life will be affected.[13]

Certainly earlier menarche seems to go hand in hand with industrialisation and 'progress'. It will be interesting to see whether the daughters of today's women who fully breastfeed and delay the introduction of other fluids and foods, will conform to the trend. Because of earlier menarche, the likelihood of teenage pregnancy increased throughout the 19th and 20th centuries and this probably contributed to the rising 'illegitimacy' rates in England. The devastating effects on the lives of millions of teenage girls persecuted for their fertility have not been fully explored. To this day 'underage' mothers suffer discrimination as a result of this effect of 'better' nutrition. Whether surviving children in the 19th and 20th centuries were abandoned to orphanages and 'baby farms' or absorbed into the family, this would have contributed to population increase, for these children would themselves have reached reproductive age while their mothers were still fertile.

Age of childbearing and child spacing are two crucial factors in demographic patterns. It has been calculated that the population stabilising effect of the controversial Chinese one-child policy could be equally achieved by a policy of universal postponement of marriage (meaning first pregnancy) until over the age of twenty-five and two children per family as long as they were born four years apart.[14] The pattern of well-spaced births and late marriage existed in England before the Industrial Revolution and probably in other parts of Europe too. Both late menarche and breastfeeding contributed significantly to child spacing in pre-industrial Europe and still does in the developing world. It is likely that breastfeeding still prevents more births worldwide than all other forms of contraception put together.[15]

Demography is too complex an issue to explore thoroughly in this book, but what is clear is that the industrialised countries' export of artificial feeding and promotion of artificial baby foods, together with the damaging advice from health workers, have had a serious effect on birth spacing. This is a key factor in both demographic trends and in the well-being of individual women, who are at greater risk of birth complications and death if pregnancies are too close.[16] Babies should be born more than three years apart to increase their own chances of health and survival; it is estimated that three million deaths of under five year olds (35% of total) could be prevented if this were achieved.[17] In the 21st century 200 million women who want to limit their childbearing have no access to contraception or family planning services.[18] They live in regions such as India or Sub-Saharan Africa where death in childbirth is common and where child death rates are highest. Unsafe induced abortions kill many women. Breastfeeding is currently their only safe method of child spacing. When this is disrupted through the availability and promotion of baby foods, bottles and dummies, the contraceptive effect ceases.

Excluding China (which practises coercive birth control) breastfeeding provides 34 million couple years of protection in developing countries which compares well with 27 million couple years of protection from family planning programmes. In some African countries birth might increase by 50% if breastfeeding stopped. As I explained in Chapter 9 some international experts considered this to be a feasible strategy.[19] This method of fertility control had been recognised since ancient times, but its importance was forgotten and ignored during the last two centuries because the changes in social organisation and in breastfeeding practices damaged its effectiveness. A 17th-century working Englishwoman married late and had well-spaced pregnancies. She used breastfeeding both to supplement her living and to space and limit her own childbearing. As unrestricted breastfeeding was the normal practice in those days, she would have been unlikely to ovulate. Rich upper class women were discouraged from feeding their own babies in order to reproduce more. Slaves in the Caribbean had their breastfeeding time limited so that they could breed more slaves for their owners. Yet by the 20th century in Europe the use of lactation as a means of child spacing was not considered by doctors or advocates of birth control. The concept survived in folklore, but usually as a warning that 'it didn't work'.

My own mother (born in 1912) recounted that as a child she was shocked to see an Irish relative suckling her two-year-old and said, "I suspect she was doing it to try and avoid getting pregnant but you know that's an old wives' tale." As scheduled and limited feeding times and earlier introduction of other milks and foods became commoner, more women found that breastfeeding 'let them down'. Unaware of the mechanisms that controlled ovulation and of the damage to breastfeeding practices, they believed their grandmothers to be ignorant and mistaken.

kicking the baby out of bed

By the 20th century breastfeeding in much of western Europe and North America was quite different behaviourally from the areas of the world where it had not been disrupted. As the 'men of sense' took over the management from women, new ideas came into vogue. William Cadogan and others thought the "noxious humours of the nurse" was bad for the baby cosily tucked into her bed.[20] By this he meant the odours of her sweaty armpits and her farts. In those days they believed that unpleasant smells actually caused disease. So night feeds were forbidden. Then came the limiting of feeds to an ideal of no more than five a day and eventually a restriction of actual time at the breast (though not by Cadogan). Only someone who did not spend 24 hours a day with a baby could have thought of restricting feeding time. These ideas had arisen from the dread of overfeeding, but they actually caused the problem of underfeeding, as the baby was prevented from stimulating the amount of breastmilk she actually needed. Consequently there was a greater requirement for supplements which in turn decreased the baby's control of the breastmilk supply.

The discouragement of sleeping with the baby at night, which had been the norm since the dawn of human life, spread throughout the 19th century. In England, the early 20th century health visitors handed out banana boxes to serve as cradles in order to stamp out the habit of mothers and babies sleeping together. This was to prevent overlaying, supposedly a common cause of infant death, though this is debatable. This separation increased the risk of infant hypothermia and reduced the important contraceptive protection of night suckling which is crucial to maintain anovulation. A mother sleeping with her baby might not even be awakened, but that occasional mouthing is an important contraceptive. With these reductions in suckling time and the increasing promotion and use of other infant foods, mothers were truly breastfeeding less and less. Even a dummy or boiled water given by spoon can reduce the stimulation needed to maintain infertility.

Most babies sleep with their mothers, because most human households own neither separate rooms nor a bed for each person. However bed sharing has become controversial again in countries where sudden infant death syndrome (SIDS, also known as cot or crib death) is a leading cause of infant mortality. Some national health policies (eg UK and USA) try to ban bedsharing. Not all rich countries share these policies and there is no correlation between societies who customarily bed share and SIDS. Japan loves bedsharing and there are lower SIDS than the west. Meanwhile evidence shows that putting your baby in a separate room increases her risk of SIDS,[21] but there are no national policies to ban separate bedrooms. I can see the UK Department of Health's reasoning. Sharing a bed with your baby is a risk if you smoke (either parent), if you take drugs or are drunk, and if you do not breastfeed. Perhaps the UK authorities judge that so many British parents fall into one of these categories that it is easier to have an overall ban.

SIDS rates fell dramatically in the UK – 1,700 a year between 1986 to 192 in 1998 – after successful campaigns urged parents to put babies to sleep on their backs. Ironically no society ever put babies on their tummies to sleep until doctors recommended it. Because babies have died in adult beds, which are not designed to accommodate babies, there is justified concern, but it is interesting that no one suggested banning sleeping in a cot when 'cot deaths' increased. There is also confusion over diagnosis: SIDS is unexplained death whereas suffocation is an accidental death.

Professor Helen Ball has done ground-breaking research filming mothers' and babies' sleeping behaviours. Breastfeeding mothers, sleeping by their babies in three-sided cribs with the open side joined to the adult bed, respond quite differently from mothers whose babies are in four-sided cribs. It is remarkable how when her baby stirs in his sleep, a mother will turn and pat, stroke and settle him back to sleep without even waking up. When the child stirs in the four-sided cot, the mother does not notice.[22] In the west the culture is to try and ignore a baby, even when she is crying pitifully. In much of China the tradition was to stay alert to the baby's needs. In some regions, little anklets with tiny bells were put on the baby so that the slightest stir would tinkle the bells and wake the mother or carer. The Chinese have lower rates of SIDS than the British even when they do not live in China. Chinese residents in the UK have lower rates than the general population as do other families of Asian origin.

Professor Jim McKenna of Notre Dame University has found that most parents do end up bedsharing with their children at some time and that most of us recall the pleasure of snuggling in with our parents. If it is banned, people still do it because they need to sleep and it is the instinctive way to comfort a baby; they just feel guilty about it but do it in secret. Breastfeeding works better with bed sharing and breastfeeding is protective against SIDS. Not breastfeeding can double a baby's risk of dying from SIDS.[23]

the mechanisms of lactational fertility control

Most women who are breastfeeding do not menstruate and for thousands of years many have known that there is a connection between the resumption of menstruation and fertility. The frequency of the baby's suckling influences the brain's output of the hormones which control a woman's fertility. As long as the baby is suckling at least six times a day, amounting to 65 minutes in total, and including some night feeding, a woman is unlikely to release a ripe egg from her ovary (ovulate). Most women do not ovulate until after they have resumed menstruation. However, about 10% might do so prior to their first period. This is more likely to happen the longer the lactation lasts, so that women who breastfeed for several years are the ones who are most likely to have a pre-menstrual ovulation.

So in the early months, as long as mothers and their babies are together and they can suckle whenever they want, infertility is maintained. The factor which dramatically decreases suckling and therefore increases the possibility of pregnancy is the introduction of other fluids or foods to the baby. This means that juices, water, artificial milk, gruels, dummies or even the baby sucking her thumb or a blanket could alter suckling behaviour and hence the contraceptive effect of breastfeeding. Also breastmilk expression, whether by hand or pump, does not have the same effect. This fact shows how a baby's suckling has a unique power that cannot be imitated. If suckling is frequent then duration of suckling is less important, but the western habit of 'feed' times with clock watching and giving boiled water in between 'feeds' certainly disturbs this biological mechanism. The number of unwanted pregnancies (and miscarriages) will have increased all over the world where medical advice and commercial misinformation have interfered with normal breastfeeding.

This breastfeeding infertility is thought to be due to the suppression of the release of a hormone called gonadotrophin releasing hormone (GnRH), necessary for the secretion of luteinising hormone (LH) which is needed for the maturation of the egg (ovum). This activity happens in the hypothalmus, that part of the brain above the pituitary gland which controls thirst, hunger and sexual function and is also believed to be linked with emotional activity and sleep patterns. The precise mechanism is not fully understood but one theory, derived from animal studies, is that suckling might increase the opiate activity in the hypothalmus and that this suppresses the GnRH release. Interestingly, heroin use suppresses gonadotrophin and causes an increase in prolactin levels just as in lactation. There has been a recent interest in natural opiate activity; breastfeeding does make some women feel great and perhaps this is one reason why. When blood serum levels of prolactin (the milk-making hormone) were measured, investigators noticed a rise that correlated with infertility, which led to the belief that this hormone was itself the inhibitor of ovulation. Now it is believed merely to accompany the process. Prolactin is also stimulated by frequent suckling, so that the levels measured in a woman's blood serum can indicate her likelihood of being fertile. Of course women vary and one woman may be infertile at a certain level of serum prolactin while another is not. Because of this, it is difficult to lay down a norm which could indicate to individual women when they are infertile. There are always the exceptional mothers and babies. Alan McNeilly, who researched this subject, described one woman who had a very fast let-down reflex and a very efficient baby. He took all the breastmilk he needed in two minutes and did not demand more than around twelve minutes' suckling time during the 24 hours. Consequently this woman did not get the frequency of breast stimulation needed to prevent ovulation.[24]

What the practical research has shown is that women with babies less than six months old who fully breastfeed, do not start supplements (but may have given the odd sip or spoon of something) and have not restarted menstruation, have less risk of conception.[25]

Breastfeeding women who are sexually active and use no

contraception at all generally have a baby every two or three years. When I looked at my family tree, I noticed my great grandmother had such spacing between her eight children, except when one baby died soon after birth, when she delivered another a year later.

A lot has been learned about this subject through observations in different communities. The !Kung* women of the Kalahari desert have a semi-nomadic lifestyle and when observed had a completed family size of four to five children, with an average birth interval of just over four years. The !Kung women started menstruating late (at about 15 1/2 years) and reproducing even later (19 1/2). The effect on fertility of breastfeeding was noticed because if a !Kung baby died, the mother soon became pregnant again. Contraception is not used, nor are their any sex taboos during lactation. A baby really does suckle on demand, about four times an hour and all through the night while her mother is sleeping, and this continues for three or four years. The baby stays close to her mother's body and helps herself at will. A woman who feeds like this is not burdened by breastfeeding, indeed it is almost unconscious behaviour. In fact, although she might feed forty-eight times in the 24 hours, in contrast to Scottish or US women's six to eight times, the total feeding time is the same.[26]

As soon as breastfeeding behaviour is controlled, its contraceptive effect is lessened. The Hutterites, a religious community in North America who use no contraception, breastfeed to a schedule for one year and supplement early. Their average family size is just over ten children with about two years between each baby. Then there are examples from 20th-century industrialised society where the custom became either, not to breastfeed at all, or to breastfeed to a schedule, usually (because of the schedule) with supplemental artificial foods. Mrs Margaret McNaught, one of Britain's 'champion mothers', had 22 single children in 28 years, which is a mean interval of 1.3 years between each birth.[27] Mrs McNaught did not breastfeed and was given stilboestrol as a lactation suppressant at each birth. If she had breastfed each child for just three months the McNaught family might have been five fewer, and this little family population explosion would have been reduced by almost a quarter. I do not wish to show any disrespect to the McNaught family, but their example shows how significant lactation suppression can be on one woman's fertility. The health workers who persuaded women around the world to reduce their duration of breastfeeding, and the companies which managed to

---

* !Kung is the language spoken by a group of the San people of Southern Africa, the '!' before 'Kung' represents a click sound.

get women to stop even earlier, have influenced population growth. Yet the presentation of this situation as a problem caused by irresponsible individuals has prompted the unthinking genocidal sentiments of many people like my friend.

What appeals to me about this fascinating strategy of anovulation during lactation is that it destroys the arguments made by some religious and cultural groups that nature designed sexual activity only for procreation.

the nutritional angle

For many years researchers have been investigating the inhabitants of Keneba, a village in the Gambia in West Africa. One of their projects was to supplement lactating women's diet (with high energy biscuits) to see if this would increase their breastmilk supply. The women do hard agricultural work on a much lower energy diet than western women eat and are either pregnant or lactating for most of their lives. The food supplement did not appear to make any significant difference to their breastmilk output as measured by the baby's intake, and the researchers had to conclude that food intake did not influence breastmilk supply. But the food supplement did have an effect: the mothers' prolactin levels went down and some of them ovulated. The scientists were faced with the dilemma that if they recommended more food for lactating women they might be harming their health by creating the risk of a too-early pregnancy. The Keneba women observed strict sexual abstinence during lactation so they were not actually at risk, but the scientists were seeking general data for all women, particularly in poor countries. They wanted to show conclusively that you only had to feed women more and they could produce more breastmilk. Other researchers had claimed this was possible, but they had used flawed study methods.

Some of the Keneba scientists deduced that nutritional status itself influenced prolactin levels, but others thought that the supplement had in fact increased the rate at which breastmilk was made. Consequently the babies had needed to breastfeed less thus decreasing the stimulation so as to make the final quantity of milk the same as before. The babies were 'in the driving seat' and they were deciding how much milk they needed.* This view is borne out by the fact that when comparisons are made between well-nourished English

* This research was done in the days when everyone believed babies should grow faster than they really should. Long before the 21st-century WHO standards. The aim then was to get all babies to grow like artificially fed US babies.

mothers and less-nourished Keneba women, their milk output is the same. The African women suckled more frequently and therefore had greater breast stimulation which maintained infertile status. This makes biological sense because in the food-abundant western environment, a woman whose body is capable of producing lots of breastmilk with minimal stimulation from her baby, can sustain another pregnancy with less risk of death to herself and her child than the mother in the precarious environment of seasonal food shortages.

However this does not mean that fertility is not suppressed in well-nourished women. A study of Scottish women showed strong correlations between night feedings, frequency of feedings and the delayed introduction of supplements and ovulation. Whereas mothers who did not breastfeed at all ovulated, on average, 11 weeks after delivery, the breastfeeders ovulated 40 weeks later. In Chile, a group of 422 middle-class women were informed and helped to use breastfeeding as a family planning method during the first six months after childbirth. The result was a 99.5% efficacy rate which is similar to other modern contraceptive methods and better than some. And the bonus was that breastfeeding was much easier and the babies healthier.[28]

why do we dislike babies?

I have met breastfeeding women, all well-nourished, who have used lactation successfully as a means of birth spacing. Some stopped breastfeeding because they wanted to conceive. Whether a woman wants to use breastfeeding to space her pregancies is her own business; what is more relevant is that women who actually want to feed their babies frequently and exclusively are still viewed as odd in industrialised society. Health workers, relatives and society as a whole pressure mothers to 'get back to normal'. That means not having a baby close to their body or in their bed and most definitely not giving a child free access to a breast. People will accept any means of shutting up a child's crying except a mother offering her breast. Despite more acceptance than a few decades ago, negative feelings are still strong, especially with regard to older babies. The fact that responding to a child's needs by giving her the breast was normal for 99.9% of humans' existence, and ensured our survival as a species, makes current standards of 'normality' questionable.

Why do people in modern industrialised societies feel disturbed by seeing a suckling mother and baby? Perhaps they are experiencing powerful unconscious feelings from their own infancy. Many adults

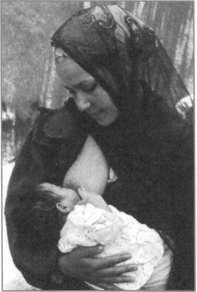

14 Egyptian woman breastfeeding
her baby in the street.
(Photo I Lippman, courtesy of
UNICEF)

around today would not have experienced the kind of cuddly, responsive babyhood that is now known to influence the development of the emotional sector of our brains.[29] Most breastfeeding cultures unthinkingly provided close physical contact and immediate comfort to meet a baby's needs. In societies where leaving babies to cry and physically separating them from their mothers is culturally acceptable, parents can be extremely tense and nervous. Consequently many of us as babies have experienced sadness too early in life, well before we could understand or cope with it. Babies tend to be viewed as insensate beings or even loathed, especially where rigidity in childcare has been well established for several generations. It seems possible that the presence of a baby stirs up feelings of a sad period in our own lives and we can project that onto the baby. Some people feel angry or upset when they think a baby is dominating the attention of an adult, perhaps because it unconsciously reminds them of their own inability to get their needs met as a baby. The 'loud noise at one end and no sense of responsibility at the other' definition of a baby negates the needs and vulnerability of a new child.

In societies where babies are nurtured, not left to cry, and are breastfed whenever they ask, not only are those babies more content and alert, but adults do not view babies with the alarm and revulsion that so many people show in my own society. Also, where babies are cherished, children often appear better socially integrated than in some western societies. One rarely meets the whining 'brat' who so often justifies the exclusion of children from adult company. The extremes of bitchiness and horror shown by some adults when a baby is the centre of attention is more than cultural habit; it has a deeper emotional cause. Attention shown to a new car is tolerated far more.

Here is an account from travellers in Nepal. "We stopped one night in a tea house in the Himalayas. The mother was cooking, but stopped to breastfeed the baby and the father took over at the stove. After the meal, when everything was cleared and put away, the parents began what was obviously a nightly ritual. The baby was lovingly massaged with oil and it was evident that both the parents and the baby thoroughly enjoyed the procedure. The baby was gurgling, the parents were smiling and sharing the task, one doing between the toes while the other concentrated on another area. Eventually the baby fell into a profound and peaceful sleep and the whole family retired contentedly to bed."[30]

It would be nice if western babies gave such pleasure to their stressed and baffled parents. Compare this with a typical British scene where the family are watching television and groan when, via an electric baby monitor, they hear the baby wake up in its expensively equipped nursery upstairs. There might be a bit of bickering as to who should have to go and get him back to sleep. If a few minutes of jiggling does not work, or a dummy or bottle poked in his mouth, then the parents may resort to a pharmacological product. Some will leave their babies to cry until they stop.

Babies who do not sleep 'through the night' alone in a cot, as soon as possible after birth, are seen as a 'problem'. Certainly, I know myself, it can be, but as much because the baby is not conforming to a false ideal as because of a mother's tiredness. Most mothers will endure much discomfort for their babies, the pain is when they are derided for doing so; they should be admired and rewarded. Jim McKenna has found through historical research that sleeping 'through the night', even for adults, is a particularly modern concept linked with industrialisation. We have organised our own lives to fit in with machines, much against our own biorhythms (the short night and siesta schedule is better for our bodies) and we expect our newborns to conform with our own industrialised oppression. Jim McKenna recommends using baby monitors the other way round, so that the baby sleeping in another room will hear the comforting sounds of the household.[31] Because we have lost the art and joy of babycare, parenthood can often be a devastatingly painful experience and a lot of this ineptness may come from our own lack of mothering. Many parents who are physically violent with their infants are found to have suffered the same damage themselves as babies. Most of us did not experience this extreme, but rather a misguided neglect because a few influential baby care gurus dictated childcare practices.

One of the best known was Frederick Truby King, a New Zealand doctor whose ideas gained acceptance during the 20th century. He was both 'pro' breastfeeding and a stickler for rigid routines. Like his predecessor William Cadogan, he propagated a mixture of sensible and ridiculous theories. To his credit he was effective in reducing the infant mortality rate in New Zealand and establishing infant welfare as a topic of importance. Truby King was obsessed, as were many of his colleagues, with 'resting the stomach': "A clean-swept stomach effectively scotches microbes which might otherwise cause fermentation, indigestion, diarrhoea, etc." Like his 18th-century predecessor, he regretted the fact that women were the child carers: "Were the secretion of milk and the feeding of the baby the functions of men and not women, no man – inside or outside the medical profession – would nurse his baby more often than five times in the 24 hours, if he knew that the baby would do as well or better with only five feedings. Why should it be otherwise with women?"[32]

Perhaps it was because many mothers were not as emotionally switched-off as Truby King and his peers to be able to ignore the cries of a child in need of food or physical contact. Whether they like it or not, women are biologically programmed to respond to an infant. I have already described 'the hormone of love' oxytocin in Chapter 3, but the milk-making hormone prolactin may have a role. It is secreted for a period after birth, even if the woman does not breastfeed, and is strongly associated with mothering behaviour in all mammals and some birds.[33] However, because of Truby King's great influence, generations of

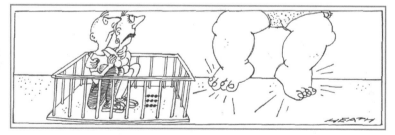

15 Our terror of babies. (Cartoon Michael Heath)

women bravely attempted to deny their own and their child's feelings, and even today many mothers who 'give in' to their babies still meet disapproval in everyday life in the western world. That Truby King still has a following (see page 85) almost a century after he advocated his ideas shows there may be some deep need for some people to control and crush the communication skills of new humans.[34]

These misguided and cruel ideas were able to gain a foothold because of widespread literacy, control of women by medical authorities and the breakdown of traditional support systems. The focus on the mother alone to provide all nurture is an unjust burden. A rural Thai woman remarked incredulously to anthropologist Penny van Esterick, "How can a woman give birth and raise a child without her mother's assistance?" In her society the whole family cared for the baby who was cherished, gave a lot of joy and was never left to cry.[35]

On the positive side of this cyclical/cultural effect of babycare is the response of a mother who told me that she had discovered her own infantile sadness through psychotherapy, but that loving and responding to her own baby's needs through breastfeeding and close physical contact helped heal her own pain. This endorses the fact that babies are born able to take an equal part in their first relationships. If they are not distorted by outside influences the relationship between a baby and her carers can help the adults to grow as well as the child.

sex and breastfeeding

Some societies advocate sexual abstinence during lactation. This taboo was common in Europe from ancient times and was a reason for a husband to hire a wet nurse, who herself was often expected to be celibate. This prohibition is unknown in gatherer-hunter societies, but appears among agriculturalists. Such a taboo indicates that, though aware of lactational contraception, people also knew it became less effective as the baby got older. Long before modern research methods, some human societies had noticed that birth spacing was good for mother and child health.

These sexual taboos might be more common amongst groups who have traditions of early food supplementation which would have undermined the protection. Sometimes the taboo is backed up with a myth: some societies believe that after intercourse the semen travels through the woman's body, gets into the milk and makes it poisonous to the baby. When Dr David Morley first worked in Nigeria, women told him they had stopped breastfeeding because they were pregnant and he believed them. Then he kept records of dates and discovered the women gave birth about 14 months after they had announced their pregnancies. They stopped breastfeeding their babies when they felt ready to conceive another. It was common knowledge that stopping all breastfeeding was precarious for the baby. European colonialists, accustomed to breastfeeding for less than one year, would see sickly looking two-year-olds on the breast and state dogmatically that breastmilk had no nutritional value after a year and that 'prolonged' breastfeeding 'caused' malnutrition. In fact the community recognised that a weak or ill child would probably only survive if his mother continued to suckle him.[36]

Stopping breastfeeding abruptly is a problem in societies with beliefs about semen-poisoned milk or when a woman knows she is pregnant. Many believe that the breastmilk 'belongs' to the new foetus and therefore will harm the suckling toddler. Women may rub chillies or bitter herbs around their nipples to deter the child's suckling or send her away to her grandmother. The process of the journey from the breast to adult eating habits can be made gentle or painful according to cultural approaches. The women who do abruptly deny the breast believe that it is in their children's best interest. It can lead to malnutrition and emotional trauma.

In societies with sex taboos during lactation, husbands may persuade their wives to feed artificially so that sex can be resumed soon after the birth. Under colonial influence and with 'development' there has been a breakdown of traditional customs and authority. As monogamy is encouraged, women may feel pressured to engage in early sexual relations with their husbands in order to deter them from having sex with other women.

Sexual abstinence exists in both monogamous and polygamous societies, and though 20th-century ideas (based on the theories of Sigmund Freud) emphasised the ill-effects of sexual repression, there is scant evidence that periods of celibacy or non-coital sex do much harm. Being sexually repressed is not the same as being celibate. Also, the idea of polygamy being more exploitative of women than monogamy is inaccurate. In many polygamous societies, adultery or promiscuity are as frowned upon as in those that profess to be monogamous. In some African societies, if a man has two wives but both are lactating, he has to be celibate. I was told of one man whose two wives had their babies within nine days of each other five times in succession so that he had a couple of years abstinence between each bout of lovemaking and was the subject of some good-humoured teasing in his village. He survived this ordeal without becoming neurotic.

A friend in Mozambique told me that he must abstain from sex with anyone until his baby was three months old, and then he could have sex with another woman, but not his wife, until his baby was seven months old. His reason for total restraint in the first phase of fatherhood was because he believed that after sexual intercourse the body gives off heat that could damage the baby. There is a wide range of beliefs from different societies. Women in Mozambique laughed at my attempts to generalise about people, and the phrase 'it depends on the person' quashed my attempt to herd individuals into a cultural box. When I asked midwives what lactating women felt about enforced celibacy they said that they accepted it unquestioningly. Who knows how frustrated the women felt? Sexuality is so culturally dominated that often the individual feels what she or he is conditioned to feel and this domination leads people to give 'acceptable' answers to intrusive questions. It is hard enough for those drawn into the western cult of the priority of personal fulfilment to discover their own true desires.

the western taboo

Breastfeeding in industrialised society is closely bound up with perceptions of sexuality. The very reason it is frowned upon in public is that breasts are perceived as objects of sexual attention. The extremity of this attitude was brought home to me when a male friend, responding to my statement that I could not see any good reason for women not being able to leave their breasts showing, stated that men did not walk about with their penises hanging out. He unthinkingly equated breasts with genitals. Breasts are sexually stimulating, but so are legs, lips and the nape of the neck, to name a few focuses of visual eroticism. In societies where there is no shame about breastfeeding, the ordinary man is not driven into a frenzy by the sight of a female breast, but he may be embarrassed or aroused by a woman wearing shorts, as Victorian Englishmen supposedly were by female ankles. Until recently women have been able to breastfeed their babies in the most sexually repressive societies; women who dared not even show their faces could expose their breasts to feed a baby. In Victorian England, famous for its prudery, a respectable woman could feed openly in church,[37] yet in contemporary industrialised society where women's bodies and particularly breasts are used to sell newspapers, cars and peanuts, public breastfeeding still provokes disapproval from both men and women. The fact that

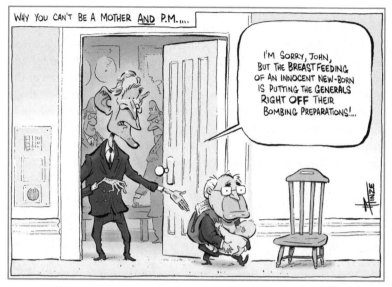

16 Why you can't be a mother and PM. (Cartoon David Pope)
© Hinze/Scratch! Media (www.scratch.com.au)

the USA and some other countries have had to bring in laws to 'allow' women to breastfeed in public places illustrates the severity of the problem. I believe that not only is it a woman's right to respond to her baby's urgent need whenever and wherever it is necessary, but that public breastfeeding is essential to provide a model of normality. It is ludicrous that anxious new mothers pore over books and websites in order to try and breastfeed 'in the correct way'! Where breastfeeding is a normal everyday event women have fewer problems than in societies where it is concealed.

Perhaps the negative reactions come from something more complex than the mere discomfort of unsatisfied sexual arousal.

When I discussed this issue with a successful woman journalist, she expressed concern about the embarrassment of middle-aged men when I suggested that a woman could breastfeed in the boardroom. These same middle-aged men survive the discomfort of erotic advertising hoardings, 'soft porn' pictures on wall calendars and the voluptuousness of classical painting. If they nip through the club areas in their lunch hours they have to resist explicit invitations to voyeuristic activities and be propositioned by prostitutes. In spite of this harassment, which they tolerate so patiently, they survive to run vast enterprises and organise the leading structures of our society. However, if one colleague were to breastfeed during a business meeting the embarrassment would be too overwhelming. The poor dears must be protected from such discomfort.

The feeding of a baby does provoke something far stronger than sexuality. It is a demonstration of power that is exclusively female and perhaps it is unacceptable for a woman who has claimed some of the supposedly male power to show she can have both. A male television producer recounted that a successful and assertive colleague breastfed her baby 'aggressively' during work meetings. He perceived this most tender of human activities as a threat because he disliked the woman. It was as though he could compete with her when she played the political career games, but that by revealing other strengths which he knew he could never match she was attacking him.

The fact that such abhorrence is absent in some societies but not in others may have another foundation. Few of us in industrialised society can remember suckling from our own mothers. Many women have denied themselves the experience of reproduction because they know it handicaps their economic and career advancement. Others have children but do not breastfeed for the same reason, or because it went wrong in the hopelessly unsupportive medical and social systems. When we see a suckling pair it does not summon up associations of tenderness and pleasure, but of rejection, failure and pain both in our relationships with our own mothers and with our babies if we have them. Men who are jealous of their partners' breastfeeding may have had damaged feeding relationships with their own mothers, and seeing the same scene in public may be inexplicably painful.

Women who have not breastfed their own children, especially if they had wanted to, may feel terrible seeing a breastfeeding pair. My sister taught me this when she admitted how angry she felt whenever she saw a breastfeeding couple. She had soon stopped breastfeeding her first baby because, as she realised when it all went well with her second, she had never been helped to position and attach him properly. Until she understood her own experience better she had unconsciously projected her anger at failure, and betrayal by those who should have helped her, on to other, luckier women.

Women report that it is often other women who ask them to stop breastfeeding or leave a café or other public place. In the UK in the late 1990s, Betty Boothroyd, the first woman Speaker of the House of Commons, banned women MPs from breastfeeding in the Committee Rooms on the grounds that food was forbidden there. I wonder whether she forbade diabetics from carrying sugar or anyone the ubiquitous small bottle of water?

libido and breastfeeding: loss of interest in sex

There are endless debates about the state of female libido during lactation, originally sparked off by Masters and Johnson's research in the 1960s claiming that breastfeeding women were more libidinous than bottle-feeders.[38] Much research is contradictory. One male doctor told me that women are desperately randy because of their 'unique hormonal state', but another informed me that breastfeeding induced 'menopausal' signs. Why not say that the menopause induces 'lactational' signs? Some research has linked breastfeeding with post-natal depression citing loss of libido as a symptom.[39] These attitudes reflect a basic assumption in western society, which is that it is culturally desirable for a woman to be libidinous, as long as the libido is directed towards her husband. Researchers have recorded that breastfeeding mothers do not resume 'normal' sexual relations as quickly as artificially feeding mothers. This is assumed to be a negative fact.

In the UK the attitudes of male partners and other family members is a key reason for young women to stop breastfeeding.[40] Some men feel they 'own' the woman's body and her closeness with her baby is more than they can bear. In a way, the modern woman is as oppressed as the 1900s woman who felt she must 'submit' to her husband (see Chapter 14). The modern wife or partner must do more than submit, she must be positively lustful and orgasmic – and no pretence either. The following response to a letter in the problem page of a magazine illustrates this attitude. This letter is quite old, but I still find exactly the same approach in contemporary magazines. Indeed there is an even greater obsession with urging women to 'get your body back for your man!'.

"'Lost interest in sex'

Q: Since I had my last child three months ago I have lost interest in sex. I only make love with my husband when I have to, although when we do, I enjoy it. The trouble is I find myself using every excuse I can to get out of it. So far my husband has been very understanding and hasn't put a strain on our marriage, but I'm terrified that sooner or later he will.

A: A three-month-old baby has a lot to do with not feeling very sexy – not least because babies are very exhausting and constant fatigue is not the best recipe for sexual desire. But also, if you are breastfeeding it's quite likely that your loss of interest is caused by hormonal changes connected with the suckling. As you stop breastfeeding, your interest should return. You only need become anxious if by that stage your sex urge still hasn't returned.

Very occasionally the hormones connected with breastfeeding remain at a specially high level and need to be lowered to their usual level by drug treatment. Even if you haven't breastfed at all, these hormone levels may become too high and require the same treatment. So give yourself a bit more time before panicking, discuss it with your husband, and show your appreciation of him in other ways."[41]

the rampant male and the variability of desire

What is remarkable about the above response is the focus on the supposed needs of the husband rather than of the baby and the woman. The baby is seen as the cause of the problem and breastfeeding is an incidental obstacle to the main purpose of the woman's life which, the agony aunt assumes, is to maintain a sexual relationship with the baby's father. The letter indicates that the husband appreciates the situation more than the agony aunt, presumably because he actually loves his child and his wife. The response shows no awareness that breastfeeding could continue for two or three years. There is an obsession with the maintenance of libido: "You need only become anxious . . ." The woman is exhorted to worry if her feelings do not conform to a culturally approved norm. What about all the thousands of people whose libidos are low (and who defines this?) for the greater part of their lives? Should they become anxious? The implication is that the stability of the marriage rests on the adaptation of the woman's sexual drive to the perceived needs of the man, otherwise he might seek alternative sexual fulfilment and then the relationship is threatened because coital sex above all is the bond that keeps them together. There is no allusion to the woman's sexual needs or her need for attention. There is no suggestion that if simple physical frustration is the problem, the man can masturbate.

I am reminded of the film The Stepford Wives.[42] The topic of compliant and Barbie-doll perfect wives still intrigues the public. The underlying idea is that this is what many men really want. In the film the women are changed into robots so as to conform to the male ideal. In real life, women are not only under pressure to make themselves appear sexually stimulating through clothes, cosmetics, body care and plastic surgery, but must also adjust themselves biochemically through artificial hormones if they do not match up to the required standards of behaviour. Sometimes the pro-breastfeeding lobby have cited the libido-enhancing value of breastfeeding as a sort of sales gimmick to convince the modern couple that it is literally a 'sexy' thing to do, while those who are doubtful about breastfeeding suspect it of interfering with the 'normality' of women's lives. This 'normal' woman must be a responsive partner in a heterosexual relationship where absence of courtship-style passion is viewed as a threat to its stability.

The main goal of the advice in most baby care books, which are invariably directed at women, and from many health workers, is 'how to keep your man happy while you care for the baby', the assumption being that she is supremely responsible for the welfare of both child and adult. If forcing yourself to be libidinous is necessary then you must do it. At all costs (including depriving the baby of breastfeeding) the baby's father must continue to feel cherished and sexually served. The responsibility for both the man and the baby is assumed to lie with the woman. This is profoundly insulting to all those mature men who love their babies and, as women do, are prepared to make profound adjustments to their lives in their children's interest. It also demonstrates the urgent need for changes in the education of boys and men. What if that letter had been written by a man?

"'Lost interest in Sex'

Q: Since I was made inside left for Wolverham Rangers three months ago I have lost interest in sex. I only make love with my wife when I have to, although when we do, I enjoy it. The trouble is I find myself using every excuse I can to get out of it. So far my wife has been very understanding and hasn't put strain on our marriage, but I'm terrified that sooner or later she will.

A: A new football team has a lot to do with not feeling very sexy – not least because football is very exhausting and constant fatigue is not the best recipe for sexual desire. But also, if you are training it's quite likely that your loss of interest is caused by hormonal changes connected with the physical movements. As you stop playing football, your interest should return. You only need become anxious if by that stage your sex urge still hasn't returned.

Very occasionally the hormones connected with playing football remain at a specially high level and need to be lowered to their usual level by drug treatment. Even if you haven't played football at all, these hormone levels may become too high and require the same treatment. So give yourself a bit more time before panicking, discuss it with your wife, and meanwhile show your appreciation of her in other ways."

The original letter writer needed help to see that her husband was showing he loved her and their baby by being understanding. It is taken for granted that a woman should be patient with a husband who is not very sexy when life-changes lower his libido. In fact some breastfeeding women do feel increased sexual desire, but is anyone suggesting hormone treatment to keep their husbands in trim? I can think of many unhappy women confused by the conflicts between their attempts to conform to the social expectations of motherhood and of being a wife. There is the unlibidinous breastfeeder who feels guilty because she prefers suckling her baby to having sex with her partner, and then there is the woman who stops breastfeeding 'for her marriage's sake' and feels guilty about her baby. Sexuality is so culturally conditioned that it is hard to find out what people really feel, but biologically a reduction in libido makes sense and if breastfeeding and low libido cause post-natal depression why are not all women in traditional societies in a permanent state of gloom? In spite of such hard lives many seem less miserable than women in industrialised society. The rates of severe post-natal depression are the same small percentage in all societies. Much of the depression suffered by new mothers in industrialised society arises because they lose social and economic recognition as individuals and are shut up in their homes. In societies where reproduction is admired and women are not excluded from society through childbearing, women are proud and happy to be mothers.

A dominant ideology in many societies is the cult of the permanently rampant male who has to thrust his penis into a vagina otherwise he will experience unendurable suffering. This may sound exaggerated, but one British politician (a woman) publically recommended that businessmen take their wives on foreign trips with them to protect them from the risk of HIV-infected prostitutes.[43] Her idea was that men could not possibly control their desperate biological urges and that a 'clean' wife could spread her legs at the right moment to intercept the lures of a prostitute, and thus protect the poor husband from disease. Why men cannot be persuaded that, if they are desperate, masturbation can relieve their tension and cause no risk of infection is, of course, because sexuality has as much to do with expressing power and dominance as with the relief of appetite.

The fact is that individual sexual drive varies greatly, that penetrative intercourse is not the only means of sexual satisfaction and that celibacy never killed anyone. While at war with Ethiopia (1961–91), the Eritrean People's Liberation Front had a mixed army that remained celibate. These were young, healthy people who had to share tents and whose common ideals made them feel emotionally close. After four years they decided to permit marriage because they did feel the need for sexual and affectionate relationships, but in common with many people throughout history, celibacy had been maintained without health or sanity collapsing, as many individuals know is possible from their own experience.[44]

In modern western society, commercial and cultural images provide a barrage of stimuli to maintain flagging libido in the consumer society. The primacy of sexuality in the marital relationship is endorsed by advertising and the content of magazines, books, films and the internet. Women desperately try to compete with the images of pornography, sales of erotica soar, and men demand that their wives and mistresses wear certain clothes or conform to particular commercial images of sexuality. Breasts must be firm and youthful, stomachs flat and movements frisky.

Sex can be both fun and a profound experience, but for millions of women their sexuality is a trade-off for an illusion of economic, emotional or physical security. Many women must use their bodies to survive in a world where the woman without a man is marginalised, both economically and socially. Breastfeeding and a physically close mother-child relationship conflict with the current values of the ideal, heterosexual relationship. I know of a woman who had no desire for sexual intercourse for a year after childbirth, but who felt guilty and went for advice to her doctor, a man, who prescribed tranquillisers and said, "You'll just have to force yourself." She did, so presumably the doctor can credit himself with 'saving the marriage'.

I happen to believe that a baby's needs are more important than an adult man's. I am also appalled that a woman should have coitus when she feels no desire for it, yet we are still so hooked on the tradition of marriage being a sort of containment of sexuality that these solutions are still endorsed, at the expense of mother-child relationships and by the smothering of women's feelings.

11 from the stone age to steam engines: a gallop through history

"I have ploughed, and planted, and gathered into barns and no man could head me... and ain't I a woman?"
Sojourner Truth (1796–1883) born into slavery, abolitionist and women's rights activist

prehistoric woman

The children's encyclopaedias of my youth were impressively illustrated with the prehistoric family scene. A woman would be sitting demurely at the entrance to a cave, surrounded by a gang of little children, while a large and muscular man, a club in one hand and a large dead animal in the other, would be striding towards them. Somehow I absorbed the idea that our male ancestors dragged 'their' women about by their hair and that the staple food was woolly mammoth.

These distorted images endorse a persistent set of lies. The message is that women in the past were made vulnerable by their burdensome fertility and were dependent on men to feed and protect them. The accompanying myth is that the techniques of fertility control are a 20th-century scientific invention and that all 'primitive' women were more oppressed than their lucky descendants. Fertility is seen as a female 'problem'; whether discouraged or enforced by the vagaries of political, demographic and cultural decisions, it must be kept in its 'traditional' place, preferably out of sight from the prestigious and power-loaded male world. In the same way, breastfeeding is seen as a woman's topic. Though women are often told whether or not they should do it, it is unacknowledged as women's power and viewed as a female handicap and a pretext for discrimination. The idea that women have, in all societies and at all times, been dependent on men for food and survival, because they have been handicapped by the production and nurture of children, is simply not true.

Many of the deductions about our ancestors' way of life come from observations of groups known as hunters and gatherers[1]. I call them gatherer-hunters because that reflects the priority of activity.

It is an oversimplification to assume too many similarities, but groups such as the Australian Aborigines, the inhabitants of the

Amazonian rainforest and the !Kung of the Kalahari desert are believed to have lived, until very recently, as humans have done for the greater part of our existence[2]. It is one of the tragedies of our era that, just as the knowledge of the value of these systems is filtering through to industrialised society, these groups are being destroyed by the process called development[3]. Whereas agricultural society is about 10,000 to 12,000 years old and industrial society a mere 200 to 300 years, gathering and hunting has endured for about a hundred thousand years[4]. The few surviving gatherer-hunter groups occupy marginal lands that have not yet excited the attention of developers. Such groups are under threat from the forces of 'development', a bitter irony, when we have so much to learn from them[5]. Their various economic systems and cultures have certain characteristics in common.

woman the breadwinner

Whether there is equality of the sexes as among the !Kung, or male-domination as among some Australian Aboriginal groups, women in gatherer-hunter societies usually provide the bulk of the food and are indeed the 'breadwinners'. In most societies men do hunt, but this is a precarious method of acquiring food. Hunting for larger game requires a big investment in risk, skill and time, not only in the hunt itself, but in the manufacture of the necessary weapons. Women gather berries, fruits, leaves and shoots, dig roots and tubers, catch insects and small animals and overall provide the bulk of the food for the whole group. They also, of course, suckle their children, usually for three or four years, and overall contribute much more in daily nutrition than the hunting men.

There are several reasons why many women do not hunt, but it is not because they lack the ability or strength. There are of course exceptions and women's hunting skill was vividly illustrated for me in Mozambique where I saw fisherwomen wading through the sea, using tridents to spear fish. Young boys are trained to use smaller weapons, so size is not the issue. It seems that more often women are deterred from 'big game' hunting because something exclusive has to be reserved for the men, to make them feel special. The anthropologist Margaret Mead claimed that men have to do something that women are not allowed to do, supposedly because men lack the power to give birth and produce milk.[6]

Whether women hunt or not, they keep the group alive and well nourished. They use a set of skills and knowledge passed through the generations, using qualities such as dexterity and observation, to find food. There are gatherer-hunter women living today and some of them may be more 'liberated' than many women in industrialised societies. Anthropologist Karen Endicott argues that such women have higher status, greater freedom of movement, more involvement in decision-making and less domestic violence than in agrarian and urban societies.[7]

Many so-called primitive people are not worn down with overwork as so many peasants and urban workers are. A gathering and hunting community will search out the food they need for the present and then relax and play. Wild food is well adapted to the environment and is less vulnerable to drought or pests than agricultural crops. Gatherer-hunters do not need to acquire surpluses, because they have the skills to find food whenever they need it. If they are nomadic there is a disadvantage in carrying too many stores. They might be incapacitated by an accident, such as a snakebite or other hazard of nature, but as long as they can move freely in their accustomed environment their food is all around them and cannot be stolen by other people.

As we saw in Chapter 10, a gatherer-hunter woman would start menstruating and childbearing later, and stop earlier, than women in other societies; her children would rarely be less than three or four years apart. Her way of suckling inhibits ovulation and, even when sexually active, she is unlikely to get pregnant while she breastfeeds for the first few years of her child's life. The lactational infertility may be (no one is sure) reinforced by the marginal nature of her diet. Having been breastfed herself and being slim all her life is likely to be one reason for her later menarche and earlier menopause than most modern women.

the original affluent society

Gatherer-hunters, though usually lean, are rarely malnourished; vitamin or other specific nutrient deficiencies are rare[8]. The customary diet of the desert-living !Kung consisted of eighty-five species of food plant, including thirty roots and bulbs, as well as fifty-four species of animals, and they only needed to work a two-and-a-half-day week to provide an excellent balanced diet.[9] If this is an example of desert dwellers, consider how bountiful was the provision for those living in more fertile regions of the world, the very areas appropriated by colonisers.

The nutritionist AS Truswell found that the !Kung were healthier than people in industrialised countries, with no dental caries, high blood pressure, obesity or heart disease. Anaemia was rare and the majority, including the women, had adequate iron intakes. Iron-deficiency anaemia is a worldwide problem affecting women and young children: women may live in more or less permanent exhaustion and the worst cases lead to heart failure and death. Iron-deficient children have poor growth and development. It is often perceived as an inevitable state for menstruating or pregnant women. Several factors might protect a !Kung woman from iron-deficiency anaemia. Her spontaneous way of breastfeeding would prevent menstruation, a key cause of iron loss. The contraceptive effect would protect her from blood-depleting miscarriages as well as pregnancies. Her varied diet would provide many sources of iron which would be well absorbed because of the plentiful vitamin C and folic acid from fresh fruits, plants and roots. The nomadic way of life would prevent faecally-spread parasites from invading her environment. She would not drink tea, coffee or milk with food, all of which reduce the absorption of dietary iron.

The low-density population of gatherer-hunters, their nomadic habits and absence of domesticated animals meant that the common infections of settled groups were absent or unusual. Tragically, this could result in a lack of resistance to new infections brought by invaders. Truswell observed that diarrhoea (together with pneumonia, the main killer of babies worldwide) was rare amongst the !Kung. Infections such as measles, which thrives in dense populations, did not exist in small nomadic groups until there was direct contact with infected settled people. Semi-nakedness and outdoor existence would ensure maximum vitamin D. The poor bone development and pelvic deformities, which impeded normal childbirth in urban women because of vitamin D deficiency during childhood, did not exist among gatherer-hunter women. Osteoporosis would be rare because the continuous physical exercise of gathering, walking and dancing would have the beneficial effects that obsessive gym-users are now so eager to achieve. Marshall Sahlins, in his book Stone Age Economics, called these societies the 'original affluent society'.[10]

the myth of the traditional woman

Two modern assumptions about traditional female roles were conspicuously absent from many of these groups. Firstly, 'woman's place in the home' did not exist because no one had homes as we know them. A nomad who moves on and constructs a simple shelter at each encampment could not be described as 'domestic' or 'tied to the home'; her work was certainly outside in every sense of the word. Secondly, in many pre-agricultural groups, fertility was not revered as in agricultural societies. There was no pressure on women to produce lots of children, which happened when many hands were needed for the intensive work of agriculture. Gatherer-hunter women rarely had more than five or six pregnancies in a lifetime. I want to draw attention to this lack of emphasis on maternity and fertility because I believe that the interpretation of woman as mother can be harmful if it is perceived as exclusive and excluding. To be a good mother, a woman is supposed to devote herself entirely to her children (and often a dependent and childlike husband) and to do so she must be set apart from 'normal life'. Consequently she is separated from control over her economic survival and social independence.

Though she might have a period of dependency on other women for food after childbirth, during her everyday life a gatherer-hunter woman is self-sufficient and able to support her own children. In most groups, children are well cared for both physically and psychologically, and integrated into everyday life. Children breastfeed and stay close to their mothers for two or three years. After this phase they rapidly become independent, learning the skills necessary for survival and participation in society, at a rate which puts our own ponderous educational methods to shame.

an example of equality: the hadza

One surviving group, the Hadza of Tanzania, live on marginal land and lead the sort of existence that many of our ancestors might have done. A Hadza woman gathers food for herself, eating most of it on the spot, her children quickly learning to do the same. She takes any extra to share with the group. The men do the same, only with meat, and there is no priority of eating or beholdenness in this sharing.

A Hadza woman builds her own grass hut which her husband might share with her, but she owes him no service. She fetches water for herself and her children, she makes skin clothes for herself and her daughters only. The men are not especially saintly and are sometimes violent, but if this happens the women form a band and attack the man. If a husband hits his wife, she will leave him. There is no social pressure to make her stay. Marriages are founded on mutual attraction, affection and companionship, as there is no economic or social reason to maintain the union. It is also normal for older women to marry younger men. It is common for marriages to last a lifetime. The anthropologists James and Lisa Woodburn found that many Hadza couples were still together after twenty-five years. It seems that the Hadza do not consider children to be an essential part of marriage, for men stay with a wife who does not bear them.[11]

I find their lifestyle of interest because this independence, command of skills, and ability to resist male coercion through female solidarity, is what many women would like to achieve. Here are 'primitive' women who have all this and are not exhausted with the effort. They are not better off because the men are especially gentle and kind. The Hadza woman resists potential male oppression through strong female relationships. Because she is not in competition with men nor exploited by them, she is free to care for her babies in the way she chooses. Failure to breastfeed is quite unknown in Hadza society and the very concept astonished them. After the early months, breastfeeding is gradually supplemented by nutritious foods such as bone marrow, soft fat and ground baobab berries. Until her baby develops teeth, a mother pre-chews meat for him. This may protect against disease because the salivary glands are linked to the immune system. Hadza children are healthier than those in surrounding agricultural societies. Derrick Jelliffe and his colleagues found few of the problems of most children in tropical countries. There was no severe malnutrition, anaemia or other nutritional deficiencies, and no ascaris, the roundworms which are so common in poor societies and add to the risk of malnutrition.[12]

Childcare is a straightforward matter in this society and does not conflict with a woman earning her living. Indeed it is integrated into the educational and economic system. Suckling a baby is easy when you can do it while you work or can pause whenever it suits you because you are the one in control of your own work, welfare and survival. This work pattern is more efficient than where a supervisor is needed to ensure that work gets done. Power is control over resources and the Hadza woman has control over her own food supply and her baby's.

the arrogance of the powerful

There is no government in the world that fully respects nomads or other 'Stone Age' people. At best they are ignored; more usually there are clumsy attempts to persuade them into a 'settled way of life'. These attempts are especially energetic if their land happens to contain diamonds or some other valued mineral. Governments claim a desire to provide clinics and schools, but disease and malnutrition increase and the passing on of survival skills collapses. Settlement usually results in alcoholism, drug abuse, a disintegration of culture, and suicide. Authorities may condone or instigate harassment, persecution and even genocide. An unquestioning sense of superiority or patronage accompanies most decision-making by those in authority, although indigenous people can offer modern societies many lessons in the management of resources in complex forest, mountain, and dryland ecosystems.

The destruction of breastfeeding threatens our ecosystem as much as over-fishing, over-grazing or forest destruction. Besides the unacceptable toll of preventable illness and death of children, there are damaging spin-off effects – such as too frequent and closely spaced pregnancies – which those who urged breastmilk substitutes and supplements never considered. We can learn so much from these groups who have breastfed so easily for so long.

agriculture

Agriculture and the domestication of animals changed the relationship of humans with their environment and with one another. Dominant men began to control animals, land, other men and, most especially, women. Perhaps the chance dropping of wild grain seeds that re-grew regularly, or awareness of the habitat of a tasty and easily-caught animal, motivated people to return to the same spot again and again. If it is possible to get food without moving on, why bother to wander? The evidence that agriculture developed after the last ice age suggests that climatic changes may have reduced the food availability from gathering and hunting. Those who had found ways of conserving their food supply may have had more chances of survival. However, it is worth noting that as recently as 1500 (when Columbus had already reached the Americas), a third of all humans were still gatherer-hunters.[13] They did not die out because their systems were unsustainable but because of genocide by invaders who wanted their land for agriculture, cattle-rearing and mining.

Cultivation requires periods of more intensive and sustained work than gathering. There is planting, weeding, pest removal, harvesting and processing to be done. Storage requires a lot of work in the construction and maintenance of silos which are never completely resistant to vermin, fungi or decay. Pastoralism and stock-rearing require constant supervision of the animals. The anthropologists Farb and Armelagos saw increased food through agriculture and animal domestication as a cause of population rise. They claimed that 'better' nutrition in the form of increased availability of energy from large quantities of grain or root crops meant lower infection rates, less death and hence more people.[14] Populations did rise but probably for other reasons, one being a change in breastfeeding patterns due to the intensive pressures of agricultural work. Gatherer-hunters usually had better-quality diets and a less pathogenic environment, and enjoyed better health than agriculturalists. Seasonal hunger and malnutrition and occasional famines are still the experience of many subsistence agriculturalists.

Farb and Armelagos argued that the main advantage of agriculture was that the denser population of a sedentary village allowed for greater protection against enemies and more cultural interaction. Perhaps – but running away and hiding from enemies, unhampered by possessions, might be a better strategy. As for cultural interaction, many pre-agricultural peoples had complex and fascinating rituals, ceremonies, dance, music and art. The beauty of pre-historic rock paintings shows that artistic activity and skill is not a unique benefit of agriculture. The idea that some lesser human had to do all the work while the talented individuals sat around inventing culture is questionable. Many elite non-working groups (usually male) spent time quarrelling, gambling, and devising rituals and rules to maintain their social status. Slaves often produced the art as well as the food. A minority of the elite wrote or produced works of art, but they had the power to define what was art and so their work was exalted. What agriculture seems to have spawned is the oppression of certain castes and groups who were coerced to do more than others. Women in most agricultural societies came under pressure to work harder and to bear more children than was good for their own bodies and for their children's health and survival.

the disadvantages of settlement

The dependency on particular crops and food stores would have made communities more vulnerable to theft, pests and weather, and guarding the stored food or the animals became a full-time job. Men may have devoted themselves more to the task which some see as the very essence of masculinity, warfare.[15] Women might have needed to conserve men's strength for fighting and therefore increased their own share of ordinary work – although men are seen as strong because of their larger size and musculature, women have more stamina. If more men devoted themselves to warfare, then more aggression and easily-provoked conflict between neighbouring communities would have developed. War breeds war. More male deaths meant social pressure on women to bear more sons (and intriguingly more males are born in war time). The pattern of exalting and supporting motherhood, after losses in war, persisted into the 20th century and still exists.

With settlement came more infection from faecal contamination and close contact with animal and parasite disease vectors, and probably more infant death. Closely spaced childbearing led to greater death rates of babies, toddlers and their mothers. Agriculturalist women were under pressure to produce more babies because children were an important source of labour as well as support in old age.

Women may have taken the first step to oppression via the domestication of plants and animals. Both practices are less energy efficient than gathering and hunting, a fact recognised by groups like the nomadic Hadza. They see that the dubious value of attempted food security is far outweighed by the exhausting work input required. You cannot merely plant the foods you gather; only a minority of plant and animal species respond to that control. Many a nutritious 'weed' only grows under certain conditions that humans cannot manipulate. For example, some seeds only develop after passing through the digestive system of a wild animal.

In seasonal climates, planting, weeding and harvesting must take place quickly when the weather is right. As the principal foragers of food it was mostly women who stayed around one area to perform these tasks. In horticultural-hunting societies which represent an intermediate phase of the change to agriculture, women usually grow the staple foods and men continue to hunt. If the crops need frequent attention, someone has to stay near them. Thus domestication of crops, animals and women might have been established simultaneously. Perhaps sustained periods of food abundance and therefore increased energy intake and weight gain did make women more fertile, though it would not have improved the quality of nutrition.[16] Populations have increased with the development of agriculture and pastoralism, but this may have occurred as a result of a deliberate aim to produce more children for labour. The availability of animal milk and supplies of starchy staple foods may have led to their use as substitutes for breastfeeding, particularly during the periods of intensive work. These foods interfere with the frequent suckling that maintains anovulation because they replace breastmilk rather than supplement it.

working mothers

When a woman has to work to produce food and at the same time care for her child, the balance between food provision for the whole group and for her baby is not always easy. The social priorities may change according to the circumstances. What is clear when we look at agricultural or horticultural societies is that women have key economic roles and breastfeed. The Usino in Papua New Guinea could not comprehend the idea of breastfeeding failure, but the women did not live in a romantic cloud of idealised motherhood. While working on their sweet potato plots the women sometimes grumbled about the baby wanting to suckle. As soon as they felt their babies could survive a few hours without breastmilk they might leave them with relatives. However everyone believed that a baby must never cry and breasts were as much used to comfort as to feed. Women in these societies are providers for the whole family and the compromises worked out to suit the baby, the mother's work and the group economy are as complex as any child-minding arrangements made by the western mother who works outside the home; yet breastfeeding lasts for two or three years.[17]

Women in these societies did not sacrifice their children for the good of the group because children *were* the good of the group; women's role as main food providers was organised to fit in with breastfeeding. The rhythms of work interwove with the rhythms of a baby's needs. There is more prolactin in a woman's bloodstream at night, indicating that over the millennia babies have taken more milk from their mothers at night than during the day. To this day most African and Asian, and many Latin American women sleep with babies who suckle sporadically without even waking their mothers, just as our ancestors must have done.

In many modern societies breastfeeding and economic production are still regarded as incompatible. Now that the evidence for the health advantages of breastfeeding is so strong, pump manufacturers are leaping in with marketing techniques to convince the world that bottle-feeding a baby with expressed breastmilk is an exact equivalent to breastfeeding. The sensitive care of our babies is the most valuable investment in the future of all society, but our obsession with the financial markers of prosperity, and our ignorance of the real value of the breastfeeding relationship, over-rides a truly social attitude to childcare, which would involve compromises with other forms of productivity. Scandinavia is the only region where political leaders have accepted the link between meeting the real needs of babies and general prosperity. The world could note that breastfeeding has contributed to the Scandinavian high standard of living. Modern Norway[18] and so-called 'primitive' societies have something in common: the welfare of children is not sacrificed for the good of the group because children are the good of the group.

slavery

The work pressures of agriculture stimulated the strong to coerce the weak, for before the need for such intense work, who would have bothered to force others to slave? Slavery is as much about the psychological control of the master over the slave as of the physical domination, cruelty and exploitation which we associate with the word. Many waged workers have suffered and still suffer the last three and yet are not viewed as slaves. There is slavery in the modern USA and Europe where employers ruthlessly exploit immigrant or illegal workers. In today's world 27 million men, women and children are enslaved ranging from prostitutes in London to indentured workers in Burma. There are also slaves in some West African countries who have such strong personal bonds with their masters that they work abroad and send their wages to them. Presumably the benefits of security from the relationship outweigh the benefits of breaking the bond. Perhaps the idea of 'freedom' within the wage market system of a racist world is too frightening.[19]

Women have been slaves to men in much the same way. Despite the illusion of equality, and despite improvements since 1990, the majority of women are economically dependent on men. The unpaid housewife might joke about being a slave, but it is true.[20] She works for the welfare of her husband and his household for no monetary reward and her status in the world is usually lower than his, often in her own eyes. She is dependent on his whim or that of his family. The fact that some men (and their families) behave decently does not negate the unequal power structure. The fact that many men abandon their wives, when the emotional or sexual bonds have altered, makes many women's situations less secure than traditional bond slaves such as those who belong to the Tuareg in Niger, who may feel obligated to their slaves for life. I am not defending slavery, but I see complacency about women's rights. While there has been a little progress in pay equality in many countries, there are still too many abuses of women which directly relate to their lack of rights. For example, in several countries a widow is not entitled to her late husband's land or property and she has no legal rights when his family evict her. In many countries fathers have more custody rights over children than mothers.[21]

Ideologies developed to sustain coercion. Most slavery was justified by ideas about superior and inferior groups using physical characteristics such as sex and skin colour. Of course most slave ideologies sprang from the imaginations of the dominant group, but often the exploited group internalised the ideology and accepted their lot because they knew no other way. In ancient Greece and Rome as many as 80% of the people were slaves and did all the work, not only the manual but also the bureaucratic, clerical and artistic labour. To the Greek philosophers such as Plato and Aristotle, this was 'natural'. A slave was the property of his or her master as were all the women in his family, and it was argued that both slaves and women were born 'naturally' inferior. Western 'civilisation' has been based on the ideas of ancient Greece, where the concept of 'democracy' (government by the people) assumed that slaves and women should be without political power.[22]

Slavery had a profound effect on childcare. Firstly, powerful women, who usually derived their power through being the wives or daughters of powerful men, could coerce other women to suckle their children for them. Secondly, the organisation of labour took priority over the welfare of a slave's baby.

the caribbean example

I want to illustrate the manipulation of infant and mother relationships to suit the slave owner, rather than the couple, with an account of early 19th-century practices in the Caribbean, because the starkness of the example is reflected in the modern world. Social planners today claim to have the interests of babies at heart, but the organisation of 'wealth creation' takes priority and damages the lives of women and children.

Slave trading had existed for centuries, but as European naval capacity expanded so did the slave trade, in response to the demand for labour in the newly-established colonies. This phase in history produced some of the worst excesses of callousness about human life.

At one stage, particularly in the route between Africa and Brazil, it was cheaper to bring in new slaves rather than provide even the most basic conditions for survival, so child-rearing was considered unnecessary. In 1817 an observer in Jamaica, a Dr Williamson, noted that the rearing of children was not encouraged on some plantations: "on account of the loss of labour incurred by the mother's confinement and the time afterwards required in raising the infant".

Dr Williamson, with the professional detachment of a pig farmer, thought it more efficient to breed slaves on the plantations, rather than continually replace them with newly-transported ones, because "a more vigorous set of labourers than the Africans generally become was brought forward in the course of time". To this end marriage should be promoted and inducements offered to encourage women to have babies. Women were excused certain tasks and given more free time for each child they managed to rear past infancy. The babies were to be breastfed by their mothers, but to be kept in nurseries during working hours. Mothers were allowed two one-hour periods for breastfeeding and if the baby needed food at other times the older women nursery workers gave panada (a mixture of bread, flour and sugar). Women were forbidden to suckle for longer than sixteen months and were separated from their children at this stage. Slave owners wanted the women to start breeding again and they believed that continued breastfeeding might prevent conception.

Stopping breastfeeding so soon was contrary to the women's culture. Dr Collins, who in 1811 laid down his Practical Rules for the Management and Medical Treatment of Negro Slaves in the Sugar Colonies, stated:

> "Negroes are universally fond of suckling their children for a long time. If you permit them, they will extend it to the third year . . . Their motives for this are habit, an idea of its necessity, the desire of being spared at their labour or perhaps the avoiding of another pregnancy; but from whichever of these motives they do it, your business is to counteract their designs, and to oblige them to wean their children as soon as they have attained their fourteenth or sixteenth month . . . If you neglect to do this, you not only lose some of the mother's labour, but you prevent their breeding so soon."

On one Jamaican estate the women slaves performed two-thirds of the agricultural work and did more basic labour than men. Women were reputed to be stronger and "a better investment" than men, living on average four or five years longer. Half the childless women and one-third of the mothers died in their twenties or thirties.[23] This is a horrifying figure, but has to be compared with the expectation of life at birth of 37.6 years in England in 1811. This does not mean that all English women died at 37. In fact if they reached that age they had a reasonable chance of living another 20 years. Expectation of life at birth is calculated by making an average of everyone's age at death, including babies and children who are more vulnerable. Improved expectation of life figures are as much a reflection of the decline in infant and child mortality as of the fact that more people live longer.[24] The point is that modern medical skills, awareness of the ill-effects of poor hygiene and nutrition, and the knowledge that germs can cause disease, did not exist then as they do now. The wife of the plantation owner was as likely to die in childbirth or lose her baby as the slave woman and her child. What is shameful is that with current knowledge of the effects of overwork, lack of health and safety standards, inadequate diet and poor medical care we accept a global system that keeps many workers in bad conditions to maintain economic prosperity . . . for whom?

the continuing coercion

The assumption that fertility control should be manipulated by authorities without respect for the wishes and dignity of individuals still exists. We see this in societies where political and religious ideologies, demographic concerns and class prejudice influence the supply or withdrawal of contraceptive provision and support for mothering. Black women (who as a group are poorer than white women) in the USA and Europe have been coerced into early sterilisation, unsafe contraception and abortion and discouraged from 'breeding'. On the other hand, in some countries where access to contraception and safe abortion had been established policies were reversed on demographic and racial grounds.

In 1967, Romanian President Nicolae Ceausescu, as a means to increase the population, banned all contraception and abortion. Women endured compulsory pregnancy tests and were questioned if the results were negative.[25] By the 1980s over 100,000 babies were in institutions because their mothers could not cope. A woman is the best judge of whether she can cope with a baby. Unwanted childbearing leads to desperate acts of unsafe illegal abortion or abandonment.

In the 1980s the Singapore government gave preferential school admission to the children of mothers with university degrees, while offering less-educated women S$10,000 grants to be sterilised after the birth of their second child. Graduate couples were offered free holidays in romantic places in an attempt to induce them to breed, the authorities apparently believing that graduate status is an hereditary characteristic.[26] In 2005, the French government increased its already generous financial benefits to encourage 'professional' women to have a third child because the existing benefits only "appeal to those on lower incomes".[27] France has one of the highest birthrates in Europe, but as the frank Australian journalist John Ballantyne writes, "this owes much to poorer families of Middle Eastern and African origin who generally have more children than white French couples."[28]

Many 19th- and 20th-century health protagonists were concerned with the tendency of the poor to breed too much. Presumably as they were no longer useful as slaves they should conveniently die out. The irony is that an effective method of birth control, breastfeeding, was deliberately denied to Caribbean slave women to make them bear more children, yet now the fertility of black women is viewed with alarm by powerful white dominant groups.

The modern international economic system – which is principally controlled by giant transnational companies, and the governments who protect their interests – uses methods similar to the early slave traders. It is cheaper and more efficient to replace labour than to reproduce it sequentially by fulfilling the rights of women workers to maternity leave and support for breastfeeding and childcare. Unlike the earlier slave traders they do not have to ship human beings across the globe, but can move their production sites to the sources of cheap labour. When workers ask for fairer wages and decent working conditions, they become 'uneconomic'. A powerful company, with the benefits of the microchip revolution and modern communications, can abandon a mobilising and rights-conscious workforce and move production sites to a more 'pliable' community. This is usually in a poorer country where people may be too scared or too desperate to reject the lowest pay levels. It is commonly women who are utilised in this insecure trade pattern. Core workers are more likely to be men with some job security, but women are hired and fired according to company convenience. In this precarious climate of employment, achieving basic health and safety standards in the workplace is hard enough; to ask for maternity leave and breastfeeding breaks is to ask for the moon. These basic rights, established by the International Labour Organisation (ILO) as long ago as 1919, are still flouted worldwide despite the adoption of the ILO Convention and Recommendation in 2000, consolidating them for all women whether formally or casually employed.[29]

A woman in the Jamaican sugar plantations, or in the cotton fields of the USA, who slaved and bore more slaves for her masters, contributed to the economic prosperity of 19th-century Britain and the USA by producing the cotton, sugar and other crops upon which much of that wealth was founded. Among her descendants today are many of the black women of Britain and the USA who have suffered discrimination in the allocation of education and jobs and are still among the lowest paid. As poor women, their fertility is frowned upon. Black women have suffered more coercion into sterilisation or the use of riskier forms of contraception.[30] In the USA the black infant mortality rate is higher than that of whites, a discrepancy which has stayed the same throughout the 20th-century decrease in infant deaths.[31] US black women are three times more likely to die than white women from causes related to pregnancy and childbirth, and this disparity has widened in the 21st century. US black women breastfeed less than any other ethnic group in the USA, which is likely to be one factor in the raised infant death rate.[32] When the agents of public health lament the fact that poor black women breastfeed too little and conceive too much, they forget that that is exactly what rich white men urged their forebears to do.

before the industrial revolution

The ordinary woman in pre-industrial society did not lead a carefree life, but her lot was not as bad as is sometimes assumed. There was variation between communities and of course suffering and oppression existed, but women had not yet been shoved into the cul-de-sac of the economically invisible 'home'.

There is enough evidence from the world of pre-industrial England to refute some common illusions of school history. The picture of the little woman stirring a pot while her big strong man provided the means of their survival is one such myth. When people refer to the woman's place in the home they forget that before the Industrial Revolution everyone's place was in the home. The household was the work production unit and every enterprise was inextricably bound up with the family. This did not mean that all workers were family members. In England many people went into some kind of service in another household. Wives and children were as vital a part of the whole production system as the tools and manufacturing processes, and as the latter were usually carried out in or near the living quarters, there was no strong demarcation between 'home' and 'work' tasks. The wife who supervised or carried out the food preparation was both 'mother' and cafeteria manager. She was no more and no less economically dependent on her husband than he on her. It was as vital for a man to marry a wife in order to be a full member of society as it was for a woman to marry a husband. Unmarried men who stayed in service all their lives never achieved full economic participation and status and were pitied as much as unmarried women. Women as well as men had worked, learned a set of skills and perhaps saved a little from their wages before they married. Because childhood ended early and marriage was late, most men and women had at least ten years' working life before they established their own economic unit of a new household. The most unfortunate women were often from impoverished families of rank; they were prevented from doing manual labour, yet their inadequate, patchy education did not equip them to earn a living, and they were supposed to be innately capable and desirous of attracting a husband to support them.[33] However the majority of women were workers who participated fully in economic life in a way that was taken for granted.

Capitalism was well established in England before the Industrial Revolution. For example, the wool and cloth industry was run by entrepreneurs who owned and controlled the raw materials and eventual sale of the finished products. The work was done in the countryside by cottagers, who were the great mass of ordinary people. Women, men and children spun, carded and wove for the controllers of their industry. This industrial work was as important to their economic survival as work in the fields. The terrible rural poverty of the late 19th century was due partly to the disappearance of this type of employment. The countryside was a place of production for both food and a wide range of industrial goods. Towns were centres for trade and exchange more than manufacture. Though this society was patriarchal in the sense that men had the authority, women were active participants in economic life and the division of labour was not rigid. The historian Peter Laslett quotes an 18th-century observer of rural life who said, "In the long winter evenings, the husband cobbles shoes, mends the family clothes and attends to the children while the wife spins". Girls became apprentices and women ran businesses in their own right, usually if their husband had died, but not always.[34]

babies and work

In pre-industrial times there was no physical and mental divide between the workplace and the home. Childrearing was an integral part of the system. Even when young people left home, they went into service in other households. There they worked, ate and slept, and loved or hated their fellow workers and employers. Because of this intimacy of working relations it would be uneconomic to ill-treat a woman in the neo-natal period so that she or her baby died because both were part of the long-term production process. A household production unit had a common interest in maintaining acceptable levels of welfare.

Marriage was linked with the setting up of a new household economic unit and production was integrally connected with the activities that are now considered to be 'housework'. Breastfeeding babies fitted into this system: it was simply another task that had to be done, like brewing the beer, making the bread, getting in the harvest or shoeing the horses. Until the land enclosures during the 17th and 18th centuries, most harvesting had to be communal because different families farmed strips: one large field was shared between different households and co-operation was intrinsic to survival.

The land enclosures took away the last shreds of self-sufficiency from poor people. They were carried out both to facilitate 'more efficient' farming methods for the landowner and to force people to hire out their labour. This taking away of people's land, or access to land, has been repeated around the world and is still happening. It is a guaranteed way of creating dependency and is paralleled in infant feeding. By taking away women's primordial right to sustain their own children with their own milk, through the destruction of traditional knowledge and the reorganisation of work processes, dependency on a powerful dominant group is created.

who loved the children?

One school of thought argues that children were universally cruelly treated in pre-industrial times, with facts like the practice (not universal) of swaddled children being hung on hooks while people worked cited as evidence. It is impossible to know the whole truth, but I see little difference between hanging babies on hooks and leaving them for hours in cots or plastic chairs. Certainly I feel that those of us who live in an age where it is estimated that one in five children is sexually abused by adults, and as many physically attacked, have little right to judge. In richer societies hundreds of children are taken 'into care' because their families cannot cope; in poorer regions thousands, many orphaned through HIV/AIDS, are abandoned to the horrors of survival on the streets.[35]

Linda Pollock paints a different picture and shows that tenderness to the young was prevalent in the past.[36] Certainly children were valued, not least for the economic contribution of their work. I want to guard against romanticising the exploitation of children, but their integration into the daily functions of an economic community meant that learning a series of jobs was not a separate process that began at the social recognition of adulthood. Skills were absorbed by imitation and participation over many years. One of the bad effects of compulsory education is not just that children are deprived of this integrated skill learning, but that women become more overworked. This happened throughout the late 19th and early 20th centuries when mothers were condemned for keeping their children out of school, yet never given a new source of assistant labour. Still today, in the world's poorest regions, women work hard on the land to pay for their children's schooling, while being deprived of their much-needed help. Both boys and girls miss vital primary learning in food production, domestic skills and childcare and this contributes to the marginalisation of these jobs.

In pre-industrial Europe a child would have grown up seeing her mother both working and rearing babies. Most children would have handled and played with several babies before experiencing the responsibility of their own. A girl would have learned how to breastfeed by seeing it done a thousand and one times, just as she learned how to stack a corn stook. By the time she had a child of her own, she would have been as confident of mothering skills as she would be of hoeing or spinning. Now, in the 21st century, we embark on tasks for which we have an overload of theoretical knowledge and little practical experience. This may not matter in terms of product manufacture because many processes are divided into components. An individual may be trained to make coat collars but not to tailor a coat; to assemble microchips but not to create computers; to perform kidney surgery but be unable to help someone lead a healthier life. When modern parents have a baby they may be holding a new human for the first time. They may never have experienced a truly multi-faceted job with total responsibility for the outcome. Yet they are assumed to be capable, through books and the advice of strangers, of being the sole carers of their child. In pre-industrial societies the opposite situation existed. A mother had learned throughout her life about the practicalities, rhythms, crises and overall management of the production process and also the same of childcare. Not being able to breastfeed a child or know the optimum time for the harvest would be as incredible as someone from our own society being unable to switch on a television or turn on a tap.

co-operation and exploitation: different baby minding customs

In Britain (and probably elsewhere) before the great changes of industrialisation, women were casual about suckling each other's babies. We can compare this with some of the minding experiences of a modern artificially fed child. Her parents may hire a succession of nannies for daily care, use any available babysitter if they go out at night and the hotel baby-minding service when on holiday. Though psychologists and others might be concerned about the effects on the infant's emotional development, the wide availability of these services indicates that many parents do not believe that their baby suffers from a haphazard selection of carers. Before the Industrial Revolution, a baby might have been suckled by a relative or neighbour when a mother needed to leave him, but it was probably someone both mother and baby knew and trusted well.[37]

Modern reaction to wet nursing has sometimes been condemning of the rich family who may have risked the wet nurse's child's welfare in the interest of their own baby's welfare. I see little difference between this and the fact that devoted middle-class parents in Europe and North America use a whole range of consumer goods, from baby clothes to toys and equipment, which are produced in the low-wage economies of Asian, African and Latin American countries. Many of the practical conveniences of our lives, from our clothes to the washing machine, are produced through the insecure and low-paid labour of women in the global economy who may forego breastfeeding their children to do it. Even within the rich countries, the informal, seasonal and low-wage jobs are usually taken by women who may have to neglect their own children in order to survive. In the USA mothers on 'welfare' are compelled to return to work six weeks after birth or they do not get their social security cheques.[38] Babycare books recommending breastfeeding often suggest 'get help with the housework so that you do not get overtired'. The help may be a Filipina woman who is separated from her own children in order to earn low but essential wages for her family.

There is often an unthinking acceptance of injustice. A European woman who breastfed her own children said to me, "When we were in Bangladesh my servant did leave her baby to be bottle-fed while she worked for me, but it was better for her family as she could help them more with the wages she earned." This woman saw no link between her wealth and the Bangladeshi woman's poverty. The servant felt compelled to leave her baby, a terrible risk in that society. Why should a poor baby be deprived of his mother's milk and closeness so that a rich woman could suckle hers in more comfort? In most circumstances, babies could accompany their mothers to work, but the competition for jobs is so intense that few servants would dare request doing something which might cause minor inconvenience to an employer.

In apartheid South Africa white children were cared for by black nannies who were separated from their own children for years. The white parents were doing what they saw as best for their child. The nanny's suffering was disregarded or denied with such mental gymnastics as, 'they don't feel the same as we do, they are used to being separated from their kids.' I suspect that similar denial existed in those parents who hired wet nurses. It would have been physiologically possible for most healthy wet nurses to feed two children, their own and their charge, but by the 19th century this had become uncommon. The benefits of the added stimulus of two babies were recognised by some early 20th-century doctors (particularly in the USA) and the wet nurse was encouraged to continue breastfeeding her own child.[39]

Before the 19th century, the average English wet nurse hired herself out after her own child could be safely taken off the breast. This may have contributed to the earlier age of stopping breastfeeding that became the norm in England. In most other societies women suckled their babies for two or three years or more, yet in England many babies were taken off the breast at around a year. It is important to add that there were wide differences between regions in infant feeding practices. In certain areas of Europe artificial feeding was already well established before the 19th century, yet in east Lincolnshire women suckled their children until they were seven or eight years old.[40]

women of breeding

A significant reason for wet nursing was that a noblewoman's main function was to produce heirs. A falsehood of history is the myth of the poor 'breeding like rabbits'. On the contrary, it was the aristocrats

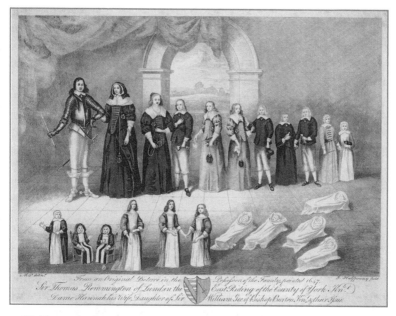

17 The typically oversized aristocratic family of Thomas Remmington
of Lund, Yorkshire, including the deceased infants, 1647.
(Courtesy of Mary Evans Picture Library)

that deserved this comparison. In pre-industrial England eighteen pregnancies were not uncommon amongst the nobility. In the 17th century, the wife of Thomas Remmington of Lund bore 20 children, five of whom died in infancy and are included in the family portrait (see above). During the same era, Ann Hatton, a wealthy heiress, had thirty children: "Five sons and eight daughters, besides 10 who died young and seven infants stillborn." In England, the poorer peasants and artisans married later than the aristocracy. Not only did ordinary women breastfeed their own babies, but they suckled others, both in the day-to-day sharing of childcare and as a waged job. This protected them from the excessive fertility of noble women whose babies were wet nursed from birth. Evidence from 17th-century rural England shows an awareness of the contraceptive effect of lactation. Countrywomen rarely had more than seven children. Records show that their births were better spaced than those of the rich and that their babies were more likely to survive.[41]

Another pretext for wet nursing was the belief that a breastfeeding woman must abstain from sexual relations. This idea persists in some societies to this day. Valerie Fildes, who has researched the history of infant feeding, does not think this was a widespread taboo in England, but Linda Pollock in her book Forgotten Children believes that this was the main reason for wet nursing, and she recounts the belief that semen was supposed to curdle the milk.[42] This concept of semen entering the milk is not so ridiculous; the stimulation of the breasts may lead to sensations in the pelvis and genitals (due in part to oxytocin) so the connection between the two areas of the body and the two white substances is understandable. For several hundred years before the eighteenth century, Roman Catholic doctrine advised wet nursing "to provide for the frailty of the husband by paying the conjugal due".[43] Presumably the conjugal needs of the nobleman (and the state of his immortal soul) were of greater importance than those of the wet nurse's husband or indeed the wet nurse. This conflict between sexual relations and breastfeeding persists. Some western women stop breastfeeding early 'for the marriage's sake', as though a physical bond with the baby prevents a happy sex life.

Wealthy women like Ann Hatton did not have to worry about the harvest, but the vision of an endless cycle of pregnancy, childbirth, and perhaps joyless sex acts, evokes the life of a queen termite whose only purpose is procreation. The ordinary, working woman's life was surely not as bad as the ever-pregnant noblewoman having all her children removed soon after birth.

artificial feeding before the 20th century

Most humans who have walked this earth never drank a drop of non-human milk. Keeping animals and drinking their milk is a very new practice in human history and it probably evolved alongside agriculture. Pastoralists – societies which keep milch animals (such as cows, camels, yaks, sheep or goats) – breastfeed their babies; indeed their knowledge of how important colostrum and early suckling is for the survival of their animals makes them value own-species feeding. However, it must have been those with access to animal milk who first experimented with breastmilk substitutes, probably for a much-loved orphan.

The mummified corpse of such a baby (see picture opposite), judged to be 2,800 years old, was found in the Silk Road region in northern China. Wrapped in beautiful red and blue clothes, with coins on his eyes, this little eight-month-old boy was obviously important enough to merit great care after death. Beside him were placed a horn cup and a feeding bottle made of a ewe's udder.[44] Humans probably tried earlier to imitate breastfeeding and they have been trying ever since. They still have not got it quite right.

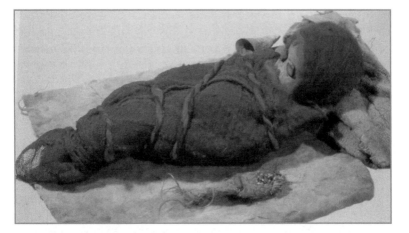

18 Mummified infant from 800 BCE from the Xinjiang Region, China (the Silk Road). Beside the infant is a feeding bottle made of a ewe's udder. (Photo courtesy of the Shanghai Museum)

the fear of syphilis

One reason for the introduction of artificial feeding was that wet nurses were believed to transmit syphilis – and they themselves feared being infected by infants with the disease. Either way, it could spread to other family members.

Syphilis or, 'the great pox' as it was called until the 19th century, appeared in Europe in the late 15th century and became endemic during the 16th. The fear of and reaction to it echoed 20th-century reactions, fear and stigma towards HIV/AIDS. It was horrific. People broke out in disfiguring sores, suffered unbearable pain, and when the infection reached the brain, went mad. Syphilis is transmitted through sexual contact; from mother to baby in the womb, and in childbirth; or through direct contact with sores (chancres) and lesions. It cannot actually be transmitted through breastfeeding if there are no sores on the breast or in the baby's mouth, but no one knew that in those days. Indeed many people do not know this today. It must have been convenient for a family to blame the wet nurse or for a wet nurse to blame a baby for an infection which carried the stigma of sexual transgression. The problem of syphilis is thought to have motivated the various attempts at artificial feeding which included direct suckling of animals, particularly goats, by the baby.[45]

Though a few stalwart individuals, like the beer-swilling baby mentioned earlier, survived artificial feeding, they were exceptional and 'dry nursing', as it was called, was usually fatal. In the mid-18th century, the governors of the London Foundling Hospital assigned children to wet or dry nursing and kept records: 19% of the wet nursed children died compared with 50% of the dry-nursed. This did not deter the continuation of artificial feeding. In 1829, the Dublin Foundling Hospital was closed down because 99.6% of the babies died. They were all 'dry nursed'.[46]

the swinish and filthy habit

There were a few areas where, for no apparent reason, artificial feeding became customary. In southern Germany there was a tradition, which dated as far back as the 15th century, of rearing babies on 'meal pap' (flour and water) mixed with animal milk. There were clear regional differences which were much stronger than any difference between rural and urban life. A 19th-century writer reported that in the district of Oberbayern, "A woman who came from northern Germany and wanted according to the customs of her homeland to nurse her infant herself was openly called swinish and filthy by the local women. Her husband threatened he would no longer eat anything she prepared, if she did not give up this disgusting habit."[47]

Not surprisingly, about half the babies died. As late as 1889 a comparative report in the British Medical Journal on infant mortality showed certain areas of southern Germany with infant mortality rates of over 400 per 1,000, four times the Norwegian rate. The reporter commented that "German nurslings are either particularly delicate or particularly unfortunate in their mode of their bringing up. The difference can hardly be due to climate."[48] Climate probably did play a part in the survival of some infants. In the 20th century in the Punjab, Indian infants artificially fed with animal milks had a mortality rate of 950 per 1,000.[49] Valerie Fildes has argued that artificial feeding only ever became a custom in cold, dry climates where animal milk was plentiful and did not become contaminated as quickly as in hot humid places. She also suggests that because it was the custom, people might have become more adept at preparing the food with some cleanliness.

the neglected babies of nedertorneå

Hygiene and fresh milk were not notable in another part of Europe where artificial feeding had become customary. In Nedertorneå near the Finnish/Swedish border, a Dr Carl Wretholm arrived in 1836 and reported, "I have never seen children so lovelessly treated as those of the Finns. All day they scream in the cradle, skinless due to uncleanliness and vermin. Nobody takes care of them. Instead they are fed with thick and viscous soured milk, given through unclean nipples, which are never washed." Artificial nipples were made of cows' teats and a cows' horns.[50] Valerie Fildes' book Breasts, Bottles and Babies has a photo of a Finnish cradle with a feeding horn in a holder suspended above it, perhaps the original 'propped bottle'.[51] The babies died mostly from diarrhoea. Dr Wretholm employed a midwife to conduct a breastfeeding campaign. By 1851 the infant mortality rate, which had been around 400 per 1,000, had halved because "almost every mother in the town now breastfeeds her children".[52]

No one has found out why these Finnish women did not breastfeed. In other areas with the same pattern of life and labour, women suckled their babies, so it was not because of their work. However, many of the women said that they did not breastfeed because their own mothers never breastfed them. Also they were considered lazy if they stopped their tasks and settled down to breastfeed. These undramatic reasons make perfect sense to me. Most of us do things because they were normal in the household where we grew up. A family friend used to boil spinach in three changes of water and serve up a splodge so revolting in taste and texture it put me off this vegetable for years. When asked why she prepared it this way she replied that that was how her mother had done it. I expect if she had cooked it lightly or even served it raw she would have been called lazy. The overcooking of vegetables is a traditional British custom which carries no nutritional or culinary benefit, but was done because no one thought there was any other way to cook. Then foreign travel broadened the tastes of the middle classes. As with artificial-feeding, those of us who survived such British cooking can say, 'Well it never did me any harm!'

The mothers in Nedertorneå had grown used to horn feeding. Perhaps it had been used years before for an orphan, seemed convenient and caught on. Frequent diarrhoea was probably accepted as a normal part of infancy and because not every baby died the custom continued. However, as soon as someone explained to the women that their babies were less likely to die or get ill if they were breastfed (and presumably helped the women to do it), they changed to the safer method of feeding. How could these communities have accepted such a high infant death rate when the solution seemed so

> *Road crashes are the number one killer of young people between 10 and 24 years of age. Every year 1.2 million die in road accidents which are the seventh biggest killer, ahead of diabetes and malaria. WHO forecasts that by 2020 road deaths will rise by 60% and that between 2000 to 2015 one billion people will be affected by road deaths, injury and bereavement.*
> WHO Commission for Global Road Safety, 2007

obvious? Perhaps, having lost the knowledge of the contraceptive effect of breastfeeding, some parents saw frequent infant death as a way, however painful, of limiting their families. Perhaps, also, in these regions pasturage was so good that there was surplus milk and putting it into babies was less work than producing more butter and cheese. The baby milk industry evolved because there was plenty of spare cows' milk around. Modern health and aid workers still dole out artificial milk to breastfeeding mothers in hospitals, clinics and refugee camps because they do not like to 'waste' free supplies provided by guileful companies and ignorant donors.

These communities may not have assumed a cause and effect between feeding method and death; after all if your baby dies, you do not necessarily perceive that this is part of a regional trend. In the 21st century if parents lose a baby in North America and Europe no one ever tells them, not even the doctor, that their child might have survived if she had been breastfed. As a result many remain ignorant. It seems appalling that the 19th-century Finnish community could bring babies into the world and then treat them so dreadfully, yet there are comparisons within our own times. Good health services save our children, yet thousands of youngsters are damaged or die on the roads, or from the abuse of alcohol, because both the alcoholic drink and car industries are 'good for the economy'. Future historians may ask how our society could have been so callous about the young and be baffled by our contradictory values.

mutilating fashions

Other factors undermined breastfeeding. In Europe until the 15th century, women's clothing was loose and relatively comfortable, but by the 16th century fashionable women wore corsets of leather, bone or even metal which completely flattened their breasts. Grigori Kozintsev's film of Shakespeare's play Hamlet (1964) shows Ophelia painfully laced into such a corset. These corsets could injure internal

> *Around the world, but especially in the rich countries, tens of thousands of women each year have their bodies cut, shaped, stapled, tucked and manipulated to conform to prevailing standards of beauty. A preoccupation with weight and body image has become an intrinsic part of the lives of women and girls. This is particularly so in the USA, but eating disorders are also noticeably increasing in Europe, Japan, and the former Soviet Union. Between 1997 and 2000, breast augmentation surgery increased by 114%.*
> Joni Seager, The Atlas of Women: An economic, social and political survey, Myriad Edition 2003

organs and crack ribs, so they certainly would have damaged developing breasts and nipples. In the 20th century, Dr Cicely Williams noted the same effect in upper-class Chinese women who wore extremely tight and flattening dresses and then found themselves unable to breastfeed. Breasts seem to have gone in and out of favour as a marker of fashionable beauty. Until industrialisation, most ordinary women were relatively unaffected by these trends; being fashionable was confined to an elite who typically had to do extraordinary things to emphasise their eliteness.

Why women should suffer pain, and damage their bodies, to achieve a certain look is a measure of the emphasis of their status as objects. The pursuit of arbitrary standards of beauty has not died out with the abandonment of corsets.

For many young women, cosmetic surgery to enlarge or reduce their breasts has become a rite of passage equivalent to a first party dress. Adolescent girls ask for 'boob jobs' as birthday presents. One mother said "I'm happy for her to have a boob job. It will give her a career."[53] Few cosmetic surgeons routinely discuss their clients' future capacity to breastfeed. In some countries, surgeons advertise without alluding to the pain and risk, charge huge sums and include poor women among their clients. Not only do women jeopardise their ability to breastfeed (though it is possible depending on the type of surgery), but they also may lose the sexual and sensual feelings that they can experience through their breasts. If a nipple has been surgically repositioned, the delicate nerve structures leading to the hypothalamus, and the complex endocrine system involved in arousal, are unlikely to function as before. The tragedy of fashion is that it changes so arbitrarily that a woman can lose the little illusion of power that she has paid for so dearly in both money and pain.

12 other women's babies: wet nursing

"It is not at all in this bargain that you need become attached to my child."
Mr Dombey to Mrs Toodle, the motherly wet nurse he hires to live in and breastfeed his son. Dombey and Son by Charles Dickens, 1847

For thousands of years, wet nursing was a valued profession. There are records from ancient Babylon, Greece and Rome setting out rules, rights and laws about payment, working conditions and practices. Wet nursing was common all over the world well into the 20th century and though it declined dramatically it never completely died out.

Breastfeeding an orphaned baby or shared suckling (usually between relatives) has existed in many societies, but this is different from hiring another woman to breastfeed. The first is an act of support and co-operation, but the second was often carried out to show social status rather than for the good of the baby or mother. In some eras, when a noblewoman breastfed her own child she was seen as exceptional. Blanche of Castile, the mother of King Louis IX of France (1215-1270), was so committed to maternal breastfeeding that when a lady-in-waiting suckled her son when he was crying she made him vomit up the milk.[1] There was variation between individual women, households and regions, but it was certainly accepted for many centuries that important women did not breastfeed their own babies.

Why did upper class women not breastfeed? It was not because of participation in public life, for though a few women had political power, they were the exceptions to the rule. Public suckling was accepted, so modesty was not the reason. It was unlikely to be for physical or emotional reasons, for if overworked and hungry poor women could breastfeed, then noblewomen should have no problems. There are several explanations. A noblewoman had to obey her husband and he would tend to do what family custom ordained. The main reason for controlling breastfeeding was that most people were aware of the contraceptive effect of breastfeeding and the noblewoman had to get breeding again as soon as she could. During the middle ages, wet nursing was common in ruling families and they had the power to pay or oblige another woman to perform this task.

It was a means of earning a living for ordinary women. So there was a supply and a demand which functioned with remarkable cohesion. When it came to the truly powerful such as the royal families, it was a great privilege to suckle a prince or princess. Lactating ladies-in-waiting would compete to suckle a baby prince even only briefly because they could gain status, even a title, from doing so. This shows that posh women could indeed lactate and wanted to.

Class structure is built on the power relationships between people. A noblewoman was expected to delegate all physical work to others to demonstrate her own and her family's high status. Just as today some wealthy people travel by car, even if public transport is quicker, because they cannot be seen on a bus, so some powerful families would stop their women members doing what every ordinary peasant woman had to do. Remember the tale of the princess and the pea? The test of royal blood was proved by the fact that she could feel even a tiny pea through twenty mattresses. I always thought she was very bad-mannered to complain about the bedding, but the story illustrates the belief in and admiration for noble 'delicacy'. As it became usual for the noble baby to be wet nursed, it became more difficult for a mother to defy custom. The exceptional woman who started to breastfeed might have lost confidence because of family disapproval. Eventually the myth that 'high born' women were too delicate and special to suckle would have provided a strong emotional inhibition. How could she believe she could breastfeed if everyone assumed she could not?

So just as in the 20th and 21st centuries some societies have seen artificial feeding as the standard practice, so in the past some saw wet nursing as the norm. And just as with all the fuss about brands and types of artificial milks, there was much discussion about the ideal wet nurse. On the whole wet nursing was like the catering trade, your clients set your status, the chef at the Ritz might be no better a cook than the chef at a Road Stop café, but the wealth and standing of your clients established your rank and reputation.

perfect and celibate, the ideal wet nurse

Views about a wet nurse's attributes stayed more or less the same from ancient times to the 18th century. The required breasts and nipples, hair colouring (redheads were banned), plumpness, personality, sex life and temper, filled pages with pompous statements. People believed that character was passed through the milk so besides being healthy and producing plenty of good milk, a wet nurse must be tranquil, cheerful and virtuous. Sexual intercourse was supposed to contaminate the milk, a belief which survives today in parts of Africa, so the wet nurse was often forbidden to have sex. Some experts then worried she would be frantic with sexual frustration and the resulting hysteria would harm the baby. Whatever she did or did not do might harm the baby through her milk. The great convenience was that families could always blame faults in their children on the wet nurse.

Some cultures were more realistic. Hebrew texts recommended coitus interruptus. Islamic texts had no taboo. The Prophet Mohammed observed that the Byzantines and Persians had sex during the breastfeeding period and their children came to no harm. The contraceptive effect of lactation was well known, but if it did fail, abortion was permitted because the wet nurse's pregnancy might curtail the baby's suckling period and that was the priority.

breastfeeding incest

Islamic texts forbade marriage with the wet nurse's children because breastfeeding made them brothers or sisters. This idea could be backed up by Swedish immunologist Lars Hanson's discoveries.[2] Immunological cells from a mother's milk can circulate throughout her child's life and the 'milk sibling' will have ingested the same cells, so they are slightly 'closer'. This makes the idea of passing on character traits slightly less ridiculous. It may not be our cheerfulness or lustfulness that gets passed on but our immunological profiles.

super wet nurses

Certain regions of Europe were renowned for excellent wet nurses. "Always when the baby cries, we feel our milk returning: acting with energy and speed, we do our duty" sang the famous wet nurses of Casentino near Florence in the 15th century.[3] Confidence, passed on with a bit of technique by other experienced breastfeeding mothers, is still the key to happy breastfeeding. Good wet nurses came from societies where they and their families were proud of their skills. Their good wages probably added to their prestige and respect within their communities. Wet nurses often bonded with their charges; this was well illustrated in Shakespeare's play Romeo and Juliet where Juliet has an easy intimacy with her wet nurse and is formal with her mother.[4]

abandoned babies

Before the Industrial Revolution, abandonment of babies was less common in England, but in Spain, Italy and France, high illegitimacy rates led to the establishment of vast foundling hospitals. A mother placed her baby in a revolving parcel box (called a 'tour') in the door, pushed the box round and rushed off without revealing her identity.[5] Why there were fewer unwanted babies in England is beyond the scope of this book but it has to be said that there were more illegitimate births in Roman Catholic countries than in Protestant ones. During the 16th and 17th centuries, marriage for both sexes occurred quite late in England and illegitimate birth rates were low. Shakespeare's famous teenage lovers, Romeo and Juliet, did not depict English custom but provided audiences with an erotic fantasy about exotic foreigners. In 17th-century England a bride's average age was about 23 years.[6]

During the later 17th and 18th centuries, age of marriage began to get lower and illegitimate births rose. The numbers of abandoned babies increased in England. More foundling hospitals were established, more babies deposited and more wet nurses were needed. The foundling hospitals prevented infanticide or abandonment on rubbish heaps, both common in ancient Rome. Now a mother driven to abandonment could hope that her baby had a chance of survival. Religion influenced feeding practices. In 18th-century Ireland the authorities did not want 'popish' (ie Roman Catholic) wet nurses suckling Protestant babies so babies were artificially fed and died in droves. In 1830, the Dublin Foundling Hospital was closed because 99.6% of the babies died. In 19th-century Austria, Christian wet nurses refused to feed abandoned Jewish babies.

In 18th-century London, philanthropists and doctors, such as Sir Hans Sloane, Thomas Coram, William Cadogan and others, worked, argued and campaigned to improve infant and child survival in a network of foundling hospitals throughout the country. Well organised wet nursing was the key. A 'dry nursed' baby was almost three times more likely to die than a wet nursed baby

who were the wet nurses?

In 18th century England, the new 'lying-in' hospitals, founded through a combination of medical ambition and philanthropy, only allowed

> "One of the most remarkable wet nurses of all time was surely
> Judith Waterford. In 1831 she was written up in both medical and
> lay papers. She celebrated her 81st birthday by demonstrating
> that she could still squeeze from her left breast, milk which was
> 'nice, sweet and not different from that of young and healthy
> mothers.' Judith was married at the age of 22, and for the next 50
> years supplied milk to babies. She fed six children of her own,
> eight nurslings, and many children of her friends and neighbours.
> In her prime she produced two quarts of breastmilk unfailing
> every day, but admitted sorrowfully that after the age of 75 she
> would not have managed to breastfeed effectively more than one
> infant at a time."
> From I Digby and B Mathias, The Joy of the Baby, 1969

respectable poor women with references to give birth there. Later in
the 19th and early 20th centuries these hospitals became feared
centres of cross-infection and death (see Semmelweiss page 195), but
when they first opened, the chance of free food, assistance in
childbirth and rest was attractive. The hospitals also became wet
nursing agencies. Wealthy women would select a wet nurse who
already had a thriving baby, as proof of her quality. However many
people had to find a wet nurse in a hurry, because a mother had died
in childbirth or the first wet nurse proved unsatisfactory. Families
went to these 'lying-in' hospitals where a mother whose baby had died
could hire herself out. Some people are horrified that a bereaved
mother should breastfeed a strange baby but this might have been
helpful. A friend lost her baby at 28 weeks of pregnancy. She started to
lactate and experienced an overwhelming need to hold a baby. She
told me she had asked hospital staff if she could 'borrow' a baby to
cuddle, but they refused and she felt deprived of a means of comfort.
These feelings are common, and bereaved women have suffered
when not allowed to hold either their own baby's body or another
living baby. Some of their sorrow might have been soothed by
breastfeeding and caring for another baby, so that being a wet nurse
in these circumstances could have been a consoling job. But more
than anything it was a decent way of earning money.

Most wet nurses in England had healthy living children. Until the
19th century wet nursed babies were sent 'out to nurse' because it was
believed that country air was better for them. Wet nurses were usually
respectable married country women; they were well paid and

sometimes earned more money than their husbands. They took the babies into their own families, just like modern foster parents today, so the baby was cared for by an experienced and competent mum. The trauma for the child was when she or he returned to her biological family (as with upper class children) or to the foundling hospital which had supervised the placement.

Some wet nurses and their husbands asked to keep a child and sometimes were refused. This may have been to prevent exploitation of the child as a source of labour but, whatever the decision, it was acknowledged that breastfeeding could cement strong ties of affection. Many adults kept in touch with and cared for the welfare of their wet nurses until they died and loved them as though they were their biological mothers, which in a way they were.[7] The bonding effects of suckling can be stronger than giving birth. In 1986 two Irish babies were given to the wrong parents. The mother who breastfed the 'wrong' child was devastated. She felt closer to the suckled child than to her biological baby.[8] The mother who had not breastfed wanted to hand the 'wrong' child back. In 2007, two Czech families found that their 10 month old daughters had been exchanged after birth through a hospital error. One father lamented that his wife had been breastfeeding from birth, implying quite unselfconsciously that this meant a stronger bond.[9] Of all the good reasons to keep mother and babies together continuously after birth, this perhaps is the most emotionally convincing.

fashions in feeding

During the 18th century it became fashionable for upper class mothers to breastfeed their own children.[10] Maternal feeding was advocated to benefit the mother as well as the baby. Dr William Hunter observed that 'milk fever' did not occur if the baby was put to the breast straight away.[11] Early suckling helps expel any fragments of placenta and stems post-natal bleeding; it also prevents engorgement, mastitis and abscesses which could lead to infection, septicaemia and death. Antibiotics have made us forget how dangerous any infection was in the past.

A shift in woman's status had also occurred. Before, aristocratic wives had to obey their husbands and if he said, 'get a wet nurse', she did. Now the doctors addressed women directly reflecting a big social change. Women were making their own decisions about their children. They now realised that breastfeeding could save their own lives and could protect them from another pregnancy. They had caught up with the ordinary countrywoman. But wet nurses were always needed for orphans and for the mothers who still found breastfeeding too difficult or inconvenient.

the decline of wet nursing

Due to the major social changes of the Industrial Revolution, younger, unmarried and less experienced women began to become wet nurses and the status of the profession declined. Such a wet nurse might send her own child to a less caring minder, possibly one of the notorious 'baby farmers' who directly or indirectly (through neglect) caused many infant deaths. As attitudes changed, even married wet nurses were viewed with suspicion.

During the 19th century more wet nurses were expected to live in their employers' houses and were separated from their own babies in case they were tempted to feed them. This showed the misunderstanding of breastfeeding physiology, for two babies would have stimulated more milk. In the USA doctors understood this and encouraged the feeding of both babies. In Britain this ignorance did terrible damage, perhaps contributing to the decline of wet nursing.

Rich people often make scapegoats of the carers of their children. So they could with a wet nurse who had left her own baby to be 'dry nursed' and who had died. They could perceive that a mother who left her own child might not be so good with their child. By focusing on the nurse's inferiority the rich family could avoid confronting the moral dilemma of their complicity in the death of her infant. This unease with the relationship also led to the search for artificial foods: "it's easier to control cows than women," said a 19th-century US doctor.[12]

These attitudes are reflected in many human situations. The quest for technology has often been motivated by the aim of avoiding the provision of decent working conditions and profit sharing. Cows and machines are easier to deal with, because they do not ask for justice. What is important to understand about wet nursing is that before technology and milk surpluses triggered the mass production of artificial milk, this was the only viable option for infant feeding. As with other autonomous skills, wet nursing as a means of economic survival was destroyed by mechanisation and industrialisation. Wet nurses could be self supporting into old age but as demand for their services declined, more women had to resort to the poorest-paid menial tasks or prostitution to the damage of their health and dignity. Over the course of the 19th and 20th centuries a means of employment unique to women began to disappear; both doctors and commerce paid a key role in this redundancy.

Wet nursing culture always varied from country to country. In France where the highest numbers existed, many were exploited, underpaid and subject to abuse. In the European colonies, local woman were often hired to suckle the colonisers' children. In the slave economy of the Southern USA, wet nursing of white babies by black slaves was normal. Hence a slave woman, who normally lived in appalling conditions and could be whipped for a minor infringement of duty, could live in her owner's house and suckle his baby. How astonishing that people who could not bear the thought of intermarriage between people of different races and still believed in the passing of qualities through breastmilk, blithely approved of inter-racial suckling. But then racism has seldom let logic constrain its arguments.

Wet nursing never did die out completely. Some US doctors were quite keen well into the 20th century and they were employed by hospitals. But like a lot of skilled self-employment, wet nursing was never going to make the big share-holder profits of an artificial milk company. The companies had a vested interest in bad-mouthing wet nursing, and they did.

There is a wonderful description in Moira Laverty's account of life in a wealthy Spanish household in 1930s Madrid. Moira, a young Irish nanny, observes that the wet nurse is revered. She gets the best food and must never be upset. To entertain the older children she expresses her milk in an arc across the room. The prim English governess loathes the wet nurse, treats her disdainfully and tells her not to do this. Outraged at being treated with such rudeness, the wet nurse expresses a jet of milk all over the governess's grey silk blouse. Wet nursing had died out in England and Ireland but in southern Europe, there were still echoes of a previous age.[13] It has been claimed that wet nursing ended after the 1949 Communist Revolution[14] in China but I have a different impression. My friend Feng Deming had to choose a wet nurse in a hurry when his wife was ordered to leave their six month old baby and work in another part of China in 1969. He (and the Communist Party officials) considered wet nursing a normal part of life (breastmilk substitutes were hard to get then) and Mr Feng was well-informed about how the wet nurse should be paid, fed and looked after.[15]

21st-century attitudes

Wet nursing remains on the WHO list of replacement feeding options, either for orphans, for babies of mothers with HIV who have chosen not to breastfeed, or for babies whose mothers have developed AIDS when the risk of transmission to the baby is high.[16] In much of the world wet nursing is the safest alternative to maternal feeding; especially in humanitarian emergencies. Screening for HIV infection is advised if it is possible, but if you are fleeing from disaster there may be no choice.

In the rich world commercial wet nursing has made a comeback. In California, USA, staff agencies provide wet nurses alongside butlers and nannies. Perhaps some wealthy celebrities, like the aristocracy of old Europe, find it too burdensome to suckle their own babies. If you live in a culture where paid services are normal you might be under pressure to behave in a certain way or lack the confidence to do things for yourself. There are also women who have had double mastectomies for cancer, or extensive cosmetic breast surgery that prevents them from breastfeeding. This resurgence of wet nursing certainly indicates a new respect for the value of breastfeeding. Nevertheless the sad side of this trend is the account of emotional distance that one modern wet nurse claims to maintain. Asked if she bonded with the babies she suckles, Hollywood wet nurse Tabitha Trotter said: "No, not unless it's my own, when I use breastfeeding as an opportunity to sing to her, talk to her, to marvel at all her tiny features. But when I breastfeed somebody else's child, it's a job. There's no counting eyelashes – I'm watching TV or reading."[17] Mr Dombey would have approved.

13 the industrial revolution in britain: the era of progress?

"No test tube can breed love and affection."
Shirley Williams (b 1930) politician

the history girls

Once more I must refer to the deficiencies of my education, which I share with many of my generation. I was given the following version: The Industrial Revolution happened in the 19th century when George Stevenson invented his steam engine The Rocket. Suddenly, everyone built machines, dropped their pitchforks and rushed to work in factories. So much wealth was created that Britain became prosperous and commanded much respect worldwide. This was all due to the inventive English mind and stable values, endorsed by Queen Victoria's stolid personality and the discipline of the Church of England. The Industrial Revolution was copied by other leading nations as everyone wanted to be like us. We helped by sending red-faced young men to the colonies to teach the natives how to be 'civilised'. This was known as 'the white man's burden'. In the late 20th century, British Prime Minister Margaret Thatcher expressed her desire for a return to Victorian values. I suspect her history education was as appalling as mine.

changes for better or worse

The real facts are less easy to assimilate. Technological change had been happening since the Stone Age. There had been other industrial revolutions, such as the development of wind and water power in the Middle Ages. The 19th-century period of accelerated change was the culmination of many processes reaching a stage of development where they could cross-fertilise. Sailing ships, water pumps, mills and looms had existed for thousands of years and had been improved and refined over centuries of trial and error. This was forgotten, when rapid industrialisation was promoted as the key to development. The internal combustion engine was a major breakthrough, but the development of the motor car utilised hundreds of years of experience of wheel and bodywork construction, from cart and carriage production. Industrialisation was a culmination, not a beginning, and many of its exported 'benefits' have been more than a failure; they have been a disaster. Millions of dollars have been squandered on the import of motor vehicles which were inappropriate for the tracks, climate, skills and economies of poor tropical countries. Similarly, the paraphernalia of artificial feeding has contributed to the damage of babies and national economies. We are only just beginning to realise what the costs of industrialisation are for our own society, but what has happened in some poor countries has been devastating.

controlling the wealth

The original desire of rulers for gold and treasure, as wealth to prop up their dynasties, led to the colonisation of the regions which provided them. As imported raw materials enriched European economies, it became advantageous to influence their production at source, and eventually to seize territorial and political control. Tea, cocoa, sugar, cotton, minerals and numerous other commodities, produced by slaves or indentured labourers, could be acquired in low-priced abundance. As home markets became saturated, exports increased and eventually the producers of the raw materials were purchasing the manufactured goods. Indians who had hitherto developed the finest fabrics were now wearing English cloth made of their exported raw cotton. The management of vast estates made the colonies a well-stocked storehouse for the development of British industry.

The technological breakthroughs were significant, but steam power might have been ignored if there had not been the motive to rush the raw materials to the factories and the finished goods out of them. Ordinary people did not flock to the towns because of the thrill of the night life. As machines were developed to cope with the abundant, new raw materials, there was no advantage for the capitalist owners to continue to distribute wool and flax for spinning, weaving and dyeing in the rural areas where they had been produced. A centre of manufacture in the form of a factory, built near the reception sites of the imported raw materials, was more profitable. Without the economic supplement of the capitalist's outwork, rural poverty increased, and the only way to survive was to go to the towns.

women's shift of power

In the modern world, most country dwellers are worse off than city dwellers. This is sometimes used as an argument to state that rural life was always terrible and that urbanisation is in itself a good thing. What is forgotten is that the very process of urbanisation impoverishes the countryside, because it removes production from the rural areas to the towns. For example, industries such as lace-making and straw-plaiting were thriving women's trades in the 17th and 18th centuries. A woman combined a range of horticultural and domestic tasks with other skilled work. When the eggs had to be collected, the beer brewed or the baby fed she did not have to ask an overseer for permission to stop work. Lace-making by hand requires a small cushion and pins and patient dexterity. Experience increased a woman's speed and ability so that her earning potential would rise over the years, only to decline with her eyesight, by which time she had trained her daughters. With the invention of lace-making machines, demand for her handmade product fell and her lifetime's development of a unique skill became worthless. We know about the Luddites breaking the machines that destroyed their livelihoods*; there must have been many a broken-hearted woman left to an old age of increasing poverty, her very identity as a proud craftswoman dissolved in the tidal wave of 'progress'. People had no choice but to go off to the towns to seek work, and the new organisation of labour did not allow for childbirth and breastfeeding.

who controls the cash?

Because an urban woman could not produce food, she was dependent on her own or her husband's wages to stay alive. A rural woman had access to food. A husband could not hide the eggs or forbid the consumption of potatoes from their shared ground. Excluded from more and more occupations, as the ideology of the 'home' became established during the 19th century, women became increasingly dependent on men, and this altered the power structure of the household. Money paid only to the husband could be hidden or spent before a woman had access to it. Her survival now depended on fate providing her with a partner who earned enough and felt responsible for family welfare. With the rise of factory employment

* The Luddites were mainly weavers who destroyed the new mechanised looms. In 1812 many were executed or transported.

women without children gained more independence, but married women came under pressure to stop work. If they did, and had a mean or drunken husband, they had to resort to demeaning tactics to persuade the wage earner to share his money. In the latter part of the 19th century wages rose, but women, especially mothers, were the last beneficiaries of this economic growth.[1]

increasing mother and child deaths

This change from household to industrialised production was not good for mothers or babies. Rural conditions had not been healthy by modern standards, but urban conditions were horrific. Density of population and overcrowded housing increase cross-infection. When hundreds use one privy or water pipe, as was common in the factories and slums of the expanding cities, diarrhoeal and respiratory diseases thrive.

Maternal mortality was high during the 19th century. Between 1846 and 1876 about one in 200 women died within a month of giving birth.[2] This rate then declined slightly but rose again as the century drew to a close. Childbed (puerperal) fever was a leading cause of death[3]. It spread through bad hygiene, particularly in hospitals where cross-infection was rife. "It would be difficult to imagine any public institution more disgusting", said Dr Charles Bell, describing the Edinburgh Royal Maternity Hospital in 1871. In such hospitals, between 9% and 10% of women left in a coffin. The picture was even grimmer in the Southern USA, and in both nations rich and poor women continued to die from childbirth-related causes right up until the 1930s. The medical historian Roy Porter implicates "careless and cavalier" medical practices in both countries.

Even before Louis Pasteur (1822–95) had demonstrated the germ theory of disease in the mid-19th century, a few thoughtful and observant doctors had noticed a connection between a doctor's personal hygiene and infection. In 18th-century Scotland, Alexander Gordon (1752–99) deduced that childbed fever was caused by "putrid matter" introduced into the uterus by midwife or doctor and recommended washing. The famous US doctor, Oliver Wendell Holmes (1809–94) also believed that birth attendants transmitted infection. The man who can be credited with saving millions of women's lives, Ignaz Semmelweis (1818–65), proved these theories through well-controlled experiments. At the time, however, he was ignored and vilified by his medical colleagues.

Scandinavia and Holland became safer places to give birth long

In the 1840s Ignaz Semmelweis, a Hungarian immigrant doctor, was working in the world's biggest maternity ward in the Vienna General Hospital. He noticed that in Ward One, run by medical students, childbed fever raged and 29% of women died. In Ward Two, run by midwifery pupils, 3% of women died. In an experiment, the two groups exchanged wards and the mortality rates were reversed. Then Semmelweis's friend, Jacob Kolletschka (1803–47) cut his finger during an autopsy, developed symptoms exactly like childbed fever and died. Semmelweis ordered hand-washing with chlorinated water. The Viennese doctors scoffed at his research and ignored its results. They resented this outsider who implied that they killed their patients. Semmelweis returned to Budapest as head of obstetrics in St Rochus Hospital and puerperal fever deaths dropped to less than 1%. In 1865, aged just 47 he had a mental breakdown and died in a lunatic asylum, apparently from an infected cut finger. That year, the renowned Joseph Lister instigated spraying carbolic acid solution in hospitals to kill germs. Lister said, "Without Semmelweis my achievements would be nothing."
reported by Roy Porter and other sources

before the UK and USA. They established high-quality training of midwives and were less likely to use forceps and drugs. Childbirth was safer away from hospitals and doctors, who carried infection. Semmelweis's heartbreaking story confirms my own perception that facts and evidence do little to change the bias of the powerful. As Roy Porter said ". . . gut prejudice and *esprits de corps* prevailed".[4]

Infant mortality had always been worse in the towns than in the countryside. An average figure of 150 deaths per 1,000 live births was typical of the rural parishes of the 16th, 17th and 18th centuries.[5] Compare this with the 235 per 1,000 for Central Bradford between 1891 and 1895. Diarrhoeal deaths rose steadily, doubling as a percentage of infant mortality causes in the last fifteen years of the century. Infant mortality started to fall after 1905, but diarrhoea still accounted for 28% of infant deaths in 1911.[6] An increase in economic activity is usually associated with a decline in deaths, but the reverse was happening. Britain had become a rich and powerful nation, but little of that wealth reached the mass of mothers and babies. As the nation's prosperity increased, the structure of women's lives was disintegrating.

the 'unoccupied' woman

I do not want to argue that everything was rosy until Victorian times, for it certainly was not. Thousands of women and children had suffered poverty, sickness and oppression in the previous centuries. What is important is that during the process of industrialisation, advances were made both in technology and the understanding of public health and medical knowledge that could dramatically improve the quality of people's lives. The construction of sewers and water pipes,[7] the mass production of soap, increased food availability, the discovery of bacteria, pasteurisation and the importance of hygiene, should have made everyone's lives safer, longer and more comfortable, but they did not. Women and babies were left behind in the march of progress. Jane Lewis describes the political framework in her book Women in England:

"As the workplace became separated from the home, so a private, domestic sphere was created for women, divorced from the public world of work, office and citizenship. Moreover, during the early period of industrialisation this separation of spheres between the public and the private was given legal sanction: married women were not permitted to own property or make contracts in their own names. They were thus shut out from the world of business. Furthermore, the 1832 Reform Bill made their exclusion from political citizenship explicit for the first time."

In spite of lip service paid to domestic duties, in 1881 the Census excluded women's household chores from the category of productive work and, for the first time, housewives were classified as unoccupied. Before these changes in policy the economic activity rates for both men and women had been recorded as equal at about 98%; now only 42% of women were officially perceived to be contributing to the economy.[8]

two approaches: dr reid and mrs greenwood

By the end of the 19th century, some doctors wanted to make it illegal for married women to go out to work. In 1901 Dr George Reid, concerned about the discrepancy between the decline in the general death rate and the high infant mortality rate, saw women's employment as the cause of the problem. Dr Reid echoed the sentiments of many doctors when he stated: "Now it is perfectly true that we cannot legislate as to how mothers shall feed their children, but surely we may reasonably expect the State to exercise some control in the case of those mothers who sometimes from necessity, *but more frequently from inclination neglect their home duties and go to work in the factories.*" (my emphasis)[9]

The blaming of mothers for earning their living and neglecting their duties became a well-established principle. The fact that women had earned their living and supported their families since human life began remained unacknowledged. That these women were contributing to the wealth of the nation and to the pockets of company shareholders, including no doubt some of the doctors who exclaimed against them, was ignored then, as it is today. Employers did not take on a particular section of the labour force out of charity. The pottery owners, for example, employed married women because they could make more profit from such a skilled workforce by paying them lower wages than men.[10] Look at the organisation of the 21st century's globalised labour force and uncannily similar patterns emerge.

There were a few people who saw beyond the neglect of duties argument. Mrs Greenwood, a sanitary inspector in Sheffield, published a pamphlet for the Freedom of Labour Defence, which pointed out that: "Such reasons as the love of work and desire for a higher standard of living, or for greater comforts than the husband's wages afford, influence some of the best women of the working class, who are industrious, self-respecting and thrifty, and whose homes are models of cleanliness and order." Mrs Greenwood was aware of the sexual politics of the issue: "Moreover, to prevent women from earning after marriage would be to place them entirely in the power of their husbands, be they good, bad or indifferent, and would practically repeal for many of them the Married Women's Property Act." (This 1870 Act had given women control over any property they had brought to the marriage, and their earnings.) Mrs Greenwood foresaw another aspect of discrimination: "Employers would hesitate to teach girls trades they might not continue in when proficient, and women themselves would not enter industries which would be practically closed to them after marriage."[11]

But Dr Reid was less analytical, and clearly thought mothers were stupid: "If by some means the simple fact could be brought home to mothers that milk, and preferably human milk, is the only permissible diet for infants . . ."[12] He assumed that ignorance made mothers abandon breastfeeding, but women knew that breastfeeding was better and did it when circumstances made it possible. During the Lancashire cotton famine in England (1861–65), women breastfed their babies and the infant mortality rate dropped.[13] The organisation of production was not challenged by doctors. A few were aware of the effects of factory work on mothering and had called for crèches and breastfeeding breaks, but they never developed these ideas into effective political action.

contrasting conditions

Where mothers were not under the intense pressures of urban poverty, breastfeeding could flourish. In Lark Rise to Candleford, an autobiographical account of rural life in the 1880s, the author, Flora Thompson, records how all babies were breastfed: "When the hamlet babies arrived they found . . . the best of all nourishment nature's own . . . No [cows'] milk was taken and yet their milk supply was abundant." This statement shows how old is the myth that drinking cows' milk is necessary for mothers to breastfeed. It is utter nonsense, yet persists in the 21st century.

An artificially fed baby brought on a visit to the hamlet of Lark Rise had its bottle held up as a curiosity. Babies were breastfed casually and publicly, including in church: ". . . or to see Clerk Tom's young wife suckling her baby. She wore a fur tippet in winter and her breast hung like a white heather bell between the soft blackness until it was covered up with a white handkerchief, 'for modesty'." This 'modesty' was not shame; it was taken for granted that breastfeeding in church was normal.[14]

Whereas religious duty and baby nurture could be combined, factory production made such human compromises difficult. When women went back to work almost immediately after birth, some women did bring their babies or the carer brought the baby to be breastfed. There is one account of a weaving mill which had a 'breast hole', a vertical sliding shutter in the wall. The carer held the baby up and the mother held her breast to the hole from the inside.[15] Factories were not like churches; they were noisy, dirty, dangerous places. Mothers who might have taken their child with them to the fields, or to a small, non-mechanised workshop, would be loath to bring their babies into these 'satanic mills'. They were not fit for the workers, let alone their infants. Dr Reid, who felt so strongly about women going to work, suggested an extension of the compulsory (and unpaid) maternity leave from one month to three months. He wanted mothers only allowed back to work if they could show "that satisfactory provision had been made for the care of their infants". The burden was on the mothers and not the employers or local authorities, yet it was the health of the nation, not individual suffering, which was his primary interest. Dr Reid admitted that his concern about infant mortality was not wholly a humanitarian question: "in the face of the decline in the birth rate of the country during recent years it may assume, if it has not already assumed a serious economic aspect."[16]

the motive: breeding the soldiers and male workers

The survival of 'the race' became that era's obsession. Concern about rising infant deaths was motivated by the twin goals of populating the colonies with white people and providing an army. At the time of the Boer War (1899–1902), it was found that 60% of recruits were too small and unfit for military service.[17] The horrified authorities attributed the phenomenon of the shrinking Englishman to a deterioration in long-term nutrition. They were right.[18]

Women had to breed more surviving children and hence healthier workers, colonisers and soldiers, but they were not paid for this contribution to the economy and were impeded from access to it themselves. They were blamed if they needed to work and when they did the very environment contributed to their own ill-health which affected their children.

To this day, telling mothers what to do is seen as a vital part of the maintenance of infant health, but organising society and economic production to make parenthood easy and joyful is still unusual. Where paid maternity leave and related rights have improved greatly in recent decades, women with young children still suffer more discrimination at work than any other group.[19] In 1919 the newly formed International Labour Organisation (ILO)[20] adopted a Convention entitling mothers to six weeks maternity leave, paid for from public finds or insurance, free attendance by doctor or certified midwife and two half-hour breastfeeding breaks a day without loss of pay. These issues were re-addressed several times during the 20th century culminating in a new Maternity Protection Convention in 2000 which reiterates these rights for all women, including those who work in the informal economy. This Convention is more honoured in the breach, for in most deregulated, free-market economies, few women dare demand (or even know about) these rights from employers who can hire and fire at will.

The women who do manage to breastfeed (and here I do not just mean the compromise of expressing breastmilk for someone else to give to the baby) are usually confident, highly motivated and well-educated women, who have control over their work schedules and have financial security. Or they belong to surviving traditional societies where breastfeeding and work have always been woven together. Both these groups are atypical of the great mass of the world's women. Enabling mothers and babies to fulfil this period of vital nurture is not a favour to women; it is a contribution to the whole of society. Yet, almost a hundred years after the recognition of the fact that the organisation of production harmed babies, most workplaces are organised without the needs of mothers and babies in mind.

Many companies have invested profits in works of art, sponsorship of cultural events, political donations, and grants and scholarships to academic institutions. They also have spent vast sums on costly and prestigious buildings; furnishings and entertainment and large, well-publicised gifts to 'charity'. Such acts are often rewarded by generous tax concessions. Yet a well-known woman economist told me that business could not possibly 'afford' to give a little time off for their employees to breastfeed their babies or provide a simple crèche for mothers who wished to feed their babies at work.

the apartheid of mothers

The movement of production from the home to the factory changed the situation of women. The separation of 'work' and 'motherhood' was established and the family unit came to be seen as a group of consumers rather than producers. 'Work' became something that men did outside in the big wide world. If women wanted to participate, their roles as mothers and partners to men were of no concern to the employer. Workers still needed someone to prepare their food, wash their clothes and clean their homes, but it was more profitable if these duties fell upon an unpaid mate. Reproducing the workers was necessary, but if one woman's baby died because her work conditions prevented her breastfeeding, this did not affect the economic unit of the large factory. When the economic unit was a household, poor health and dead babies hindered production; with industrialised production, workers are replaceable. An employer has no economic motive to concern himself with the welfare of the workers.

This situation persists to this day and improvements in welfare have only evolved because of decades of struggle through painstaking and painful organisation and solidarity. The strength for the worker in the new system was in numbers; many men and women resisted, organised, suffered and died to achieve the few basic standards of decency which exist in parts of the world today. Women's role in the development of trade unions has been significant and yet under-recognised. Men have dominated the movement. In the early 20th century, even ardent trade unionists began to internalise and accept the idea that women's role was in the home. Mothers were not dominant in the trade union movement, principally because coping with two jobs left them with no time to participate.

motherhood behind closed doors

Gradually, the idea of motherhood being something that happens behind closed doors, in the private home, became taken for granted and this attitude persisted. The integration of mothers and babies into public life was viewed with ridicule and alarm in many societies. It is worth remembering that this attitude existed towards all women until relatively recently whether they had children or not. In 1918 British women got the vote and could stand as Members of Parliament. Winston Churchill (1874–1965) was horrified at the thought of a woman in the British Parliament, claiming that it would be like having a woman in his bathroom (though why he should be so upset by a woman in his bathroom has always baffled me). The excuses for female exclusion per se are strikingly parallel to those for breastfeeding couples. Women are 'shrill'; babies are noisy; women need special provision (separate toilets and sanitary towels); babies need their nappies changing; women distract people by their looks; babies distract people (gurgling charm); women arouse men and make them feel uncomfortable; babies irritate people and are out of place.

misery and isolation

After the Industrial Revolution the sexual and social division of labour crystallised. No longer could the husband cobble shoes, mend the family clothes and attend to the children while the wife spun (see page 170). In the factories there was no equivalent of the harvest when even the grandest might roll up their sleeves and muck in. Different tasks were allotted to different groups and there was less intermingling of the sexes in the same jobs. The pretexts for this were not just traditional concepts of the division of labour, but an increasing obsession with the control of women's sexuality. Women had worked at heavy jobs for centuries alongside men.[21] They were now barred from heavy, manual, wage-earning labour, only to carry out heavy, physical, unpaid work at home. The zeal with which Victorian reformers worked to 'protect' women from such jobs as mining was more a concern for the effect of sexual opportunity on their souls, than for the effect of heavy work on their health. When industries excluded women, no provision was made for alternative employment and they were angry at being deprived of their livelihoods.[22]

An urban woman about to give birth was often without support. Though this varied from region to region, family and neighbour support structures were hard to maintain when factory hours ruled. Tasks like washing and food preparation had to be done and increasingly a woman had to pay someone to do them. The cities were filthy with factory grime so there was far more cleaning than before industrialisation. Children worked in the factories (and later had to attend school), so they were at the beck and call of the mill owners rather than their immediate family. Female relatives or friends could not leave their own waged labour to help. The old country midwives helped with the washing and household tasks and could always be paid with produce or later favours, but in the towns there was a scale of fees and everything cost money.

pain and humiliation

Maternity: Letters from Working Women, edited by Margaret Llewellyn Davies, depicts the lives of some women at the turn of the 19th and 20th century. As literate members of the Women's Co-operative Guild, they were acutely aware that they were better off than many. The fact that they led lives of unceasing pain and humiliation makes the experience of other women the more horrifying. In most towns and villages there are monuments dedicated to the unknown soldier, and plaques listing the military casualties of war. There are no memorials to the thousands of women who died prematurely through extreme physical hardship. These were the women who produced and serviced the workers who created the wealth and consequent power of Europe and North America. There are no statues commemorating the unknown mother whose baby died because 'progress' made life too hard for them both.

The 'maternity letters' reveal that a life of bad health, overwork, undernutrition and sexual exploitation was the lot of most women. They were unprepared, ignorant, anxious, and self-aware: "Owing to the worry connected with this misfortune [her baby had died], also having to be up so soon after the confinement and for want of rest, I felt my health giving way, and being in a weak condition, I became an easy prey to sexual intercourse, and thus once more became a mother in fourteen months."

During this era missionaries were doing their best to "civilise the savages". In several parts of the world, both prolonged lactation and codes of sexual abstinence protected mother and child from the danger of closely spaced pregnancies. Polygyny* was one way of confining sexuality to a prescribed system which prevented such exploitation of women's bodies, but this was energetically discouraged by Christian missionaries. Meanwhile back in 'civilised' society, Christian marriage allowed a man complete access to his wife's body regardless of her feelings or the effects on her own and her baby's health. Women 'submitted' just to deter their husbands from adultery. Having more than one wife was seen as unchristian, but rape within monogamous marriage was accepted. Female dutiful submission to male conjugal rights was seen as intrinsic to marriage. To this day many legal systems do not yet recognise rape within marriage as a crime.[23]

The women who wrote these letters condemned their own ignorance. All women need practical and emotional support around birth. These isolated urban women suffered the consequences of a changing society where support systems had been destroyed. They missed their mothers or other intimate female support during childbirth. In the 17th century women often went home to their mother's house for several months when they had their first babies, just as some women in Africa and India do today. For these literate women, there was no written information; body functions were taboo in everyday conversation. A townswoman might never have seen an animal giving birth. My own grandmother, a Londoner, was completely ignorant of how babies were born when, in 1912, she was pregnant with her first child.

Women accepted appalling discomforts as normal. The accounts of prolapsed wombs, burst varicose veins, piles, protracted labour and doctors' hands groping for retained placentas without anaesthetic or any pain relief makes the modern reader wince. What is most poignant is how grateful women are for brief periods of health, or if their husband is 'good' – that is, he does not rape them. Miscarriages distressed these women more profoundly than the pain of childbirth. They were acutely aware that 'nerves' and worry were detrimental to their own and their babies' health. If they wanted medical help during

* Polygyny = a man having more than one wife.

childbirth they had to go without food to save the money for the bill. This anxiety would have jeopardised their chances of a straightforward labour and a healthy baby. If they worked outside the home, it was still taken for granted that domestic duties were theirs alone.

the hidden misery of home

Margaret Llewellyn Davies comments:

> "Writers on infant mortality and the decline of the birth rate never tire of justly pointing to the evils which come from the strain of manual labour in factories for expectant mothers. Very little is ever said about the same evils which come from the incessant drudgery of domestic labour."

The Maternity Letters reveal an appalling lack of support: "From the second day [after the confinement] I had to have my other child with me, undress him and see to all his wants, and was often left six hours without a bite of food, the fire out and no light, the time January, and the snow lain on the ground two weeks . . . When I got up after ten days my life was a perfect burden to me. I lost my milk and ultimately my baby." This writer describes her profound depression: "Can we any longer wonder why so many married working women are in the lunatic asylums today? Can we wonder that so many women take drugs, hoping to get rid of the expected child?"

These women found physical hardship more endurable than anxiety, their 'nerves', and the consciousness that their never-ending reproductive state could lead to death. Their fear of being unable to breastfeed probably increased the risk of failure: "Before three weeks I had to go out cleaning and so lost my milk and began with the bottle". However difficult the birth, these women had to get up to wash, cook and clean. Many lived in dread of a husband's sexual advances. Unlike many of the 'savage' societies of the empire, there was no compulsory, socially supported rest period after childbirth.

It is now so well known that stress, overwork and poor nutrition are detrimental to the health of mothers and babies, that we forget that this had not yet been 'scientifically' established. While the medical world railed against the ignorance of mothers, the Maternity letters show women's acute awareness of their needs. Mothers took a shy pride in breastfeeding and knew that artificial feeding was dangerous, so when they failed to breastfeed, yet another sorrow added to their endless misery. "After my second [child], I was very ill with my breasts, but, of course, I put that down to my husband's lack of work." Several women described "a gathered breast" (i.e. mastitis) or an abscess. This revealed that they were not being helped to breastfeed early, frequently and effectively. If their mother or other experienced relative was not there to help, no one could show them how.[24]

The manufacturers of artificial milks have argued that their products kept children alive for all the mothers who could not breastfeed and that there was a 'demand'. These companies were part of the same industrialising society which created the conditions that made women lose confidence in breastfeeding, ensuring that their products would be needed.

an industrial solution for an industrial problem

I have described urbanising Britain but this pattern of change of women's lives and the effect on infant feeding has been, and still is, repeated around the world. The process of industrialised urbanisation appears to cut women off from their support systems and expose them to stresses, both emotional and physiological, which make it difficult to breastfeed. Hard work itself does not impede lactation, as evidence from so many rural societies indicates, nor does living in a city, as thousands of privileged Europeans, North Americans and Australians have proved in the 20th and 21st centuries.

So many changes accompany the process of industrialisation that it is an oversimplification to pinpoint just one as a cause of breastfeeding decline. The common factors that have been repeated around the world seem to be: a loss of support from an intimate family member or neighbour; an imposition of damaging medical rituals onto the private, personal relationship of a woman and her baby, and the widespread availability of products promoted as breastmilk substitutes. The new industrialised production methods, which made life so difficult for mothers and babies, dramatically increased the quantities of infant feeding products on the market. They were widely advertised with extravagant and misleading claims and were extremely profitable for their manufacturers.

the origins of the artificial milks

The 19th century German chemist, Justus von Liebig, was one of the first scientists to apply his talents to the invention of substitutes for breastmilk. Another German, Henri Nestlé, a dealer in mustard, grains and oil lamps, arrived in Vevey in Switzerland in 1843. He invented 'farine lactée' (wheat flour with milk) and claimed to have saved the life of a baby who, having allegedly "rejected his mother's milk and all other food", accepted Henri Nestlé's product. Why this baby was not wet nursed remains a mystery, but the fact he survived a wheat-based product so young indicates a robust constitution.

for infants and invalids

By 1873, Nestlé was selling 500,000 boxes of farine lactée per year in Europe, the USA, Argentina, Mexico and the Dutch East Indies. Despite Henri's concern for babies, the wondrousness of farine lactée did not prompt Nestlé to adjust the marketing of condensed milk for infants when the company merged with the Anglo-Swiss Condensed Milk Company in 1905.

The technique of condensing milk, patented by Gail Borden in the USA in 1865, was introduced to Europe by Charles Page, a former correspondent of the New York Tribune. At the end of the American Civil War he became US consul in Switzerland and together with his brother had formed the Anglo-Swiss Condensed Milk Company. Page's fusion of business interests and political duties was a model for the future of the baby milk business.[25]

The widespread marketing of condensed milk worried British medical authorities. In 1911, an official report was able to collect no fewer than 100 varieties of machine-skimmed, and forty brands of full-cream, condensed milk, and this was not an exhaustive collection. Dr EJH Coutts who produced the report explained the nutritional inadequacies of the product, particularly the skimmed variety. As the techniques for machine skimming improved, more fat was removed from the milk, but all the advertisements claimed these milks to be perfect substitutes for mothers' milk. One product which, under government regulations, had to say 'unsuitable for infants' did so in minute print, while claiming in huge letters: 'FOR INFANTS AND INVALIDS'. Besides the nutritional inadequacies, the manufacturers' claims to 'purity' and 'sterility' were false; one analyst discovered every brand he tested to contain microbes. The report tactfully described each brand by a letter of the alphabet.[26]

Delivering milk to babies grew to be a large-scale task for businessmen, who presented themselves as philanthropists and life-savers. Conveniently, this good work happened to be extremely

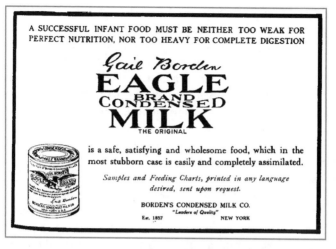

19 Advertisement for Borden's Condensed Milk
in the Journal of the American Medical Association, 1914

profitable. As efficiency in the dairy industry increased and transport communication improved, cows' milk became cheaper and more readily available. In Britain, the introduction of frozen and chilled meat imports lowered home-produced meat and grain prices. Many farmers turned to dairying because, unlike other cheap imported foodstuffs, fresh milk could not be imported from overseas. It had to be sold quickly before it went bad. Another group of people had been philanthropically delivering milk to infants for thousands of years, but they were women, and as many 19th-century scientists knew, they were not to be trusted to do things properly.

the milk depots

The spread of substitute feeding was not engineered entirely by the commercial manufacturers of patent baby foods. In the last decades of the 19th century, infant mortality remained stubbornly high, not just in Europe, but Canada, the USA, Australia and New Zealand. France was particularly concerned about falling birth rates. This became a matter of political and military concern.

The first 'milk depots' were set up in France to provide subsidised fresh cows' milk for the babies of mothers who were judged to be unable to breastfeed. Cows' milk could spread tuberculosis and other infectious diseases, was easily contaminated at any stage in production and delivery, or could be diluted with contaminated water.[27] The milk depots had the declared aim of providing uncontaminated milk for babies and they were also established in Britain, the Netherlands, North America, Australia and New Zealand. Their founder, Dr Budin, sincerely tried to encourage breastfeeding, but, like many of his contemporaries, he dreaded overfeeding and the recommended restrictions must have led to reduced breastmilk for many women. These depots were the forerunners of health clinics all over the world where a cheap or free product has been used to lure mothers to submit to the vigilant eyes of those who know best.

Some have argued that the milk depots saved lives. They certainly must have provided relief for a woman whose breastfeeding was going wrong, to know she could get a supply of cheap milk for her baby. The milk depots spread in regions where the skill to re-establish lactation had been lost, and the change in social relations deterred women from breastfeeding one another's babies. However, there was no evidence that the depots had any effect on the infant mortality rates which only began to fall after 1905. The British Medical Research Committee noted in 1917 that the drop in the infant death rate was the same in widely separated towns, some of which had milk depots and some of which did not. What the milk depots established was the link between artificial milk distribution and the health centres which persists to this day, the world over.[28]

keeping milk safe: the mother's responsibility

The widespread use of factory and household refrigeration has made many people forget what a risky product milk can be. When mothers bought their week's supply of pasteurised or sterilised milk from the milk depots, it still had to be kept fresh. Sterilised milk kept better, but the process destroys more nutrients than pasteurisation. Mothers also used sweetened condensed milk, either whole or skimmed depending on what they could afford. The domestic tin-opener had not yet arrived so the tin had to be opened in the shop and somehow kept uncontaminated in the home. One investigator found that diluted Nestlé's condensed milk, incubated at 37°C (98.6F), contained 11 million bacteria after 24 hours. Dr Coutts's 1911 report found most samples of infant foods contaminated before use. Hygiene was impossible in the average overcrowded, ill-equipped home. Only the rich had water closets and the modern plumbing many of us take for granted today. Working-class people (the majority) in most urban areas used either middens, which were large, leaky, uncovered receptacles, sunk below ground level; or ash privies, which were above ground level and cemented at the bottom. Ash was thrown in at the front and the contents removed from the back. These facilities were often shared by several families. In the Yorkshire city of Hull between 1918 and 1939, 79% of infant deaths due to diarrhoea were in houses with privies or pail closets. Outbreaks of tuberculosis epidemics in 1929 and 1936 were milk-borne, according to the British Medical Association, who issued warnings in the national press. At that time 2,000 deaths a year were due to bovine tuberculosis.[29]

the bliss of rural ignorance

Most mothers intended to breastfeed, but the spreading message to restrict feeding made problems more likely. In spite of continual railing against those unworthy mothers who did not suckle their babies, there was little interest or research into the causes of breastfeeding difficulties. No medical student was trained in the subject, although as a qualified doctor, he (rarely she) miraculously acquired the authority to tell a woman whether she could or could not breastfeed or whether her breastmilk was good enough. Most advice actually contributed to breastfeeding failure and the lucky women were those who escaped the erroneous edicts of the health workers.

Rural women who did not have access to the milk depots had quite different problems.

"We didn't have no bottle for our children. Fed them all ourselves. Every one. All nine. Till they were three years old, some of them. You'd be standing there washing, and they'd hang on to you and want a teat. I didn't know, see. I tried to wean them several times, but then they'd get in again and have another drop. I had no end of trouble weaning my children."

This woman was desperately poor, overworked and often hungry, but she had no breastfeeding problems. She lived close to her mother and relatives and had never learned about 'overfeeding', scrubbing her nipples, or the importance of routines: "I didn't know, see." She lived in a remote area, beyond the ministrations of health visitors, thus remaining obliviously certain that breastfeeding worked: "I had so much milk, I didn't know what to do with it. Drip? It used to run away so, I had no end of milk. But you couldn't afford to bring your baby up any other way."[30]

She was also deprived of the widespread advertising of baby foods. The common advertising style of the day was the personal testimonial:

Saving the Babies.

The Importance of Diet.

Every worker in the cause of saving infant lives has come face to face with the great obstacle of ignorance on the part of so many mothers. This ignorance is one of the tallest barriers which the welfare-worker has to surmount—and perhaps the chief contributing cause of infant mortality.

As in matters of cleanliness and clothing, so does this ignorance wreak great harm upon the infant in the vitally important matter of diet. Welfare-workers know only too well how many infants languish for want of sufficient, correct, and regular nutriment. Particularly is this true in the case of infants whose mothers are prevented from looking to the feeding of their children by occupations other than domestic. With so many women engaged in war work, this difficulty has been vastly aggravated.

For years Corporations of the Midlands, such as Sheffield, Lincoln, and Rotherham, have grappled with the task of conserving infant life. The officials and the welfare-workers have had to face the feeding difficulties in countless cases. Earnest and sincere, these workers have patiently striven to overcome the ignorance of mothers, and have brought knowledge and practical advice to many a hard-worked and worried woman who did not know how to care for her child, scarcely had time to do so even if she knew.

We are proud to say that the diet difficulty has been largely solved in so many of these cases by the use of Glaxo.

Glaxo contains nothing that is foreign to milk. At the source of supply, before any chemical change has taken place, this milk is dried to a powder. The Glaxo process makes the powdered milk germ-free, and prevents the curd subsequently forming a dense clot. Glaxo is packed in closed vessels and is prepared for use by merely adding boiling water. An infant can, by taking Glaxo, obtain a continuous supply of germ-free milk.

Among the many Official Bodies continuously using Glaxo may be mentioned the following :

	lb.
Sheffield Corporation have purchased	137,000
Manchester School for Mothers, over	60,000
Rotherham Corporation, over	85,000
Bradford Health Department, over	50,000
Lincoln Health Department, over	25,000
Birmingham Health Department, over	17,000

Glaxo is specially packed and sold at a special rate to Official Bodies, Crèches, Mothers' Welcomes, and Schools for Mothers.

The address of Glaxo is : Dept. 71, 155, *Great Portland Street, London, W.*

The Proprietors of Glaxo are: Joseph Nathan & Co., Ltd., London, and Wellington, N.Z.

20 Advertisement from Maternity and Child Welfare (Jan 1917) cited in Anna Davin, 'Imperialism and Motherhood', History Workshop no 5, 1978

"Doris until three months old had nothing but the breast: she then weighed only eight pounds and seemed to be wasting away from malnutrition. Then we tried your Frame Food, and she immediately commenced to pick up, until today from a puny mite she has grown to be a fine strong girl with vitality and stamina that is simply wonderful." Mr Polwin, Stanley Stores, PO, Southend on Sea.[31]

In his autobiographical novel Cider With Rosie, Laurie Lee recounts how his mother spent hours writing fictional testimonials to manufacturers (of things she never used) in the hope of earning a few shillings. They often used the letters without paying.[32] Frame Food, like many baby food products, was advertised in the Nursing Times and the company offered free samples. Baby food advertising appeared in the medical journals, as well as newspapers, magazines, cookery books and even children's books. In the Infant's Magazine Annual (1913) Neave's Food is recommended from birth with the endorsement of the Russian Imperial Nursery.[33] As it turned out, Neave's Food could not save the members of the Russian Imperial Nursery from more powerful forces.[34]

Political changes in other places stimulated the marketing tactics of the companies:

"Glaxo, makers of a patent baby food, ask for the attention of welfare workers aware of the terrible obstacle of ignorant mothers (perhaps the chief contributing cause of infant mortality), point out how war work means more babies have to be artificially fed and name some of the many official bodies using Glaxo."

The advertisement opposite was published in Maternity and Child Welfare in 1917, when many doctors were blaming mothers for 'refusing' to breastfeed. The Glaxo advertisement boasted that six city health departments, corporations and a "School for mothers" had used a total 354,000lbs weight (160,909kg) of their dried milk powder.[35] These boasted quantities showed unrestricted sales. Mothers had to pay for the milk in spite of their patriotic war work. British commerce was thriving on the alleged ignorance of mothers, while across the Atlantic industry was creating an even stronger base with the help of doctors.

14 markets are not created by god

*"Markets are not created by God, nature or economic forces,
but by businessmen... There may have been no customer
want at all until business created it – by advertising,
by salesmanship, or by inventing something new.
In every case it is business action that creates the customer."*
Peter Drucker, business and management theoretician,
Management, New York, Harper & Row, 1974

the establishment of the us market: ideal conditions

A market for artificial milk and infant feeding products was created in the late 19th and early 20th centuries. It was conceived through the mutual attraction of manufacturers and doctors. This love affair developed into an enduring and stable marriage which has lasted to this day. Though European industry was playing a significant role, the conditions in the USA were ideal for this relationship to blossom. Several factors contributed to the change from breast to artificial feeding. The USA was industrialising and urbanising rapidly. Any shortfall in workforce numbers could be quickly made up by immigration. Poor Europeans flooded in with little choice but to accept the conditions and wages of the host country, which were not much better than in Europe. The majority of rural women continued to breastfeed, but increasingly urban workers were forced to be separated from their babies, and sought replacement feeds. Though wet nursing was still practised, doctors found they could make money by inventing and promoting substitutes for breastmilk and of course their clients were the wealthier women prepared to pay for them. These women could reject breastfeeding for all the usual reasons and instead of hiring a wet nurse, could pay their doctors for a custom-made feed for their babies, believing that this modern, state-of-the-art concoction was a 'scientific' wonder. The term 'infant formula' was a stroke of marketing genius, it made a recipe based on ordinary old cows' milk seem like something special. At the same time commercial infant milks spread through the market and poorer women, who could not afford doctors' fees, bought them. Family unit labour[1] continued, as in the oyster canning industry where mothers breastfed their infants at work, but increasingly the pressures of industrialised production led to babies being left at home. In 1911, 58% of US babies were still breastfed at twelve months, but the urban rate was lower than the rural.[2]

the fall river study

As would be the pattern throughout the 20th century, mothers who stayed home, as well as factory workers, were also artificially feeding.[3] The 1908 Fall River study of infant mortality in a US textile manufacturing town cited artificial feeding as a significant cause of the excessive deaths from diarrhoea. Other factors associated with this high infant death rate were a high proportion of 'foreign-born' mothers, high female illiteracy and a high birth rate. The stress of rapid change, the absence of supportive female relatives and the attempt to adjust to an alien way of life disturbed the cultural practices which protected mothers and babies. The availability and promotion of commercial foods had a demoralising influence on both individual and social confidence in breastfeeding. If mothers believed that alternative infant foods were good, and no one said they were dangerous, what reason was there not to use them? If absorption into a new society leads to the abandonment of customs of food and dress, it is not surprising if infant feeding practices change as well. If replacement feeds were used, a woman's breastmilk supply would decrease and her need for the substitute foods would become established. This mixed feeding would have made her more likely to become pregnant; more closely-spaced births would have increased the risk of death for women, toddlers and newborns.

'go for the best': hospital childbirth and the decline of midwifery

By the early 20th century in the USA both poor urban workers and the middle classes were breastfeeding less. Doctors were taking over the birth process and hospital deliveries were increasing. Hospital practices sabotaged breastfeeding, as they still do in too many places. It could be argued that this was a small price to pay for an improvement in mother and child health. However, between 1915 and 1930, US maternal mortality did not decline and deaths of babies from birth injuries actually increased. Hospitals advertised widely, urging mothers to 'go for the best', and women believed they were getting just that when they paid the high fees. Even for healthy, low-risk women, the routine use of stirrups, restraining straps, shaving, episiotomies and forceps made the majority of births abusive experiences. The use of the amnesiac 'twilight sleep' drug meant that women embarked on motherhood having suffered a trauma they could not recall and therefore deal with. Babies were separated at birth and given artificial feeds, and any breastfeeding was delayed and restricted. No wonder breastfeeding was declining.

Midwives were eventually outlawed, although they continued to serve poor women who could not afford doctors. The denial of orthodoxy and disappearance of the profession of midwifery in the USA led to the loss of skills which survived in Europe, where midwives increased their status during the same period. Midwives generally understood breastfeeding better than doctors. Most had done it themselves and midwifery usually involved continuous intimate post-natal care where they could learn by observation. Also, a midwife's role was to work with nature, whereas a doctor was trained to seek out its defects and remedy them. The majority of doctors then, as now, were woefully ignorant of the practicalities of breastfeeding. Sadly they managed to convince the maternity nurses of the rightness of their ideas.[4]

health, wealth and status

The major 19th-century discoveries, such as the role of bacteria in infection, had generated a new optimism about the conquest of disease. It was perhaps inevitable that a reverence for all things 'scientific' should be accompanied by some scorn for 'natural' processes. Improved living standards and public health measures, such as safe water provision and sanitation, contributed more to the decline in killer diseases, such as diarrhoea and tuberculosis, than medical knowledge. But this knowledge was increasing, and doctors communicated their faith in their new skills to the public. In the USA, the 'specialist' came into vogue and paediatrics was a speciality gaining in reputation.

The wealth of the rising middle and ruling classes changed the role of woman, from producer to consumer. The joke of the wife spending her husband's hard-earned money survives to this day. What is forgotten is that the cult of excessive expenditure by the rich was, and is, necessary for economic growth when workers' low wages restrict their own purchasing power. Someone had to be buying the products, and the wealthy wife, devoting her life to the selection of household goods, clothes and other status symbols, was an important spoke in the capitalist wheel. Her conspicuous consumption reflected her husband's financial success and helped retain confidence in his market skills. A breastfeeding wife might be as demeaning to a successful industrialist as a wife who reared chickens. Why do it yourself when you can afford to buy an expensive and modern 'scientific' substitute?

the cult of female frailty

To conform to her caste etiquette, the rich, fashionable lady must be a fragile creature:

> "It was as if there were two different species of females. Affluent women were seen as inherently sick, too weak and delicate for anything but the mildest pastimes, while working-class women were believed to be inherently healthy and robust.
> "The reality was very different. Working-class women, who put in long hours of work and who received inadequate rest and nutrition, suffered far more than wealthy women from contagious diseases and complications of childbirth."[5]

While women workers were struggling to keep their children fed and alive, their leisured sisters were convinced by doctors that they were too delicate to do anything, let alone breastfeed babies. Though doctors advocated the superiority of breastmilk, they did not believe that upper-class women were able to breastfeed, and they despised the lower-class wet nurse. In the past, rich women had frequently delegated childcare to a wet nurse. As doctors and companies began to promote and provide artificial milks, this practice began to be abandoned. A bottle would be less of a rival for the child's affections: "the physical defects of the bottle we can understand pretty well, and can to a great extent, guard against them. Its moral qualifications compared with those of the wet nurse, are simply sublime," stated the influential Dr Thomas Morgan Rotch. The great problem with breastmilk was, in the minds of many doctors, that it came out of women's bodies. Dr Rotch's ambiguous attitude was typical of the medical thinking of the time, but it survives in the 21st century:

> "Also the mere fact of the milk being obtained from the human breast does not preclude many dangers which arise from it as a

food, owing to the highly sensitive organisation of the mother allowing the mechanism of the mammary gland to be interfered with. When this mechanism is interfered with good milk may also become a poison to the infant . . . It is evident, therefore, that there is nothing ideal about breastmilk."

Whereas, of course, Dr Rotch considered his own formulas (or 'formulae') ideal.[6]

technology and the new products

During this era, technological innovations were welcomed and 'modern' methods of feeding paralleled the railway, the motor car and plumbing as the way to a comfortable future. Women could be relieved of the burdens of nature through the wonders of science, and many welcomed this liberation. Improved dairy farming led to milk surpluses in the industrialising countries and new methods of preservation were invented. Condensed milk was first developed in 1853 and evaporated milk in 1885. Dr Rotch set up the Walker-Gordon Milk Laboratories in 1891 and by 1907 they formed a chain in twenty cities in the USA and Canada. Cows' milk was modified according to complex rituals, supposedly made up to match the varying 'formula' prescriptions of each doctor, and then delivered directly to the consumer. In reality they were not so accurately made, the laboratories were not always as clean as they claimed to be, and the service was expensive. Nevertheless, for the first time in history a baby could be fed cows' milk without the family having direct access to a cow.

Most innovations arise more out of the desire to profit from waste or surplus products than the quest to meet human need. Whey surpluses from the increasing production of butter and cheese prompted the search for market outlets; thus they became the base for artificial baby milk (as it is today), not because research proved it to be the most suitable substitute for breastmilk, but because it was plentiful and cheap. New materials and production methods also enabled easier manufacture of feeding bottles and teats, which became widely available. In 1897 a bottle was patented that could be suspended over the cot for the baby to feed alone, and another had short legs so that it could stand on a baby's chest. These, together with a wide variety of foods advertised as 'ideal for infants', flooded the market. Artificial feeding had become a money-maker.[7]

$$M = \frac{Qb-bC}{b} \qquad C = \frac{L(b^1F-a^1P)}{ab^1-a^1b} \qquad C = (2F+S+P)\times1\frac{1}{4}Q$$

21 Highly complicated formula used in infant feeding.
(Cited in Jelliffe and Jeliffe, Human Milk in the Modern World)

the 'formula' cult

Doctors were in the market too. The focus on the 'problems' of the rich was more profitable and less distressing than trying to tackle the insurmountable troubles of the poor. The cult of the uniquely frail infant digestion was less of a fraud than the cult of female frailty for, deprived of breastmilk, a baby certainly did need close medical supervision. As knowledge about the constituents of human and cows' milk increased, doctors devised recipes for imitating human milk. They experimented with different proportions of ingredients and different experts led heated arguments about the relative virtues of different theories and methods.

Because rigorous exactitude was a part of scientific respectability, these experts presented their recipes in the form of complex mathematical and chemical formulae. A successful cake is also a complex chemical reaction depending on precise proportions of ingredients, but cake is not called 'formula', whereas artificial milk for infants is, to this day. It is a ridiculous word, reminiscent of the pseudo-science of those doctors, and it is a measure of the triumph of marketing that this promotional jargon is now used as a scientific term.

At first each baby (and of course only the rich could afford this service) would have an individual 'formula' made up to suit its particular digestion. This individual tailoring for each baby was seen as a matter of life and death. Charles Warrington Earle stated at an 1888 meeting of the American Medical Association: "One food nourished a given baby well, but may, if administered persistently, kill the next baby." A variation of 0.1% of an ingredient was considered crucial. The mother had to return every few weeks to have her baby's formula adjusted.[8] However, when this cult of individuality became commercially inconvenient to the doctors, it rapidly went out of fashion.

ethical marketing: a brief tussle and a long happy truce

While doctors were insisting on custom-made preparations, more mothers were buying commercial infant foods over the counter. These products were widely advertised in newspapers, domestic magazines and medical journals and were easier to prepare than the paediatricians' formulae.* Nestlé's Milk Food (the life-saving 'farine lactée') and Horlicks's Malted Milk only needed to be mixed with hot water. Doctors at first objected to commercial infant foods, supposedly on nutritional grounds. The mother who bought ready made milks was less likely to visit the doctor, which meant a loss of income. It also meant a loss of prestige. In 1893 Dr Rotch wrote:

"The proper authority for establishing rules for substitute feeding should emanate from the medical profession, and not from non-medical capitalists. Yet when we study the history of substitute feeding as it is represented all over the world, the part which the family physician plays, in comparison with numberless patent and proprietary foods administered by the nurses, is a humiliating one, and one which should no longer be tolerated."

The manufacturers realised that conflict with such an influential body as the doctors was against their own interests. They began to court the doctors, who actually found it difficult and time-consuming to make up these artificial feeds and saw the advantage of an alliance with the manufacturers. One doctor negotiated with infant food manufacturer, Mead Johnson, to produce a product he favoured, Dextri-Maltose, and it was tested in 1911 at the Babies' Ward of the New York Post-Graduate Hospital. The development of the infant food industry has depended on the repeated testing of unproven products on unsuspecting consumers without their informed consent. If a scientific team wanted to set up today the experiment that has been carried out on babies over the past hundred years, an ethical committee would throw out such a proposal.

Doctors began to recommend certain commercial foods. They did not prescribe them like a drug, but the manufacturers agreed to put no directions on the package and to instruct the mother to consult her doctor before using the product. This was called 'ethical' marketing. However the infant foods were still widely available with no attempt to restrict sales to prescription only. Mead Johnson gave doctors feeding

* Note the Latin plural which attaches an air of learning and science to the product.

calculators and other items which made "it easier for the general practitioner to obtain better cooperation from the mothers".

Mead Johnson advertised publicly while boosting the doctor's position: "When Dextri-Maltose is used as the added carbohydrate of the baby's food, the physician himself controls the feeding problem." For the doctor to flourish, feeding did indeed need to be a problem, for if it were not, why should the mother visit him? In the days before immunisation, antibiotics and rehydration methods, there was little a doctor could do for a sick baby. However, with carefully supervised artificial feeding the doctor could maintain the illusion, to himself as well as the mother, that he was useful. Perhaps a good side-effect of the reverential 'formula' making was that better hygiene was maintained. A doctor's control had to be skilled, the baby must not die, but nor should it be wholly without feeding problems. By 1923 Mead Johnson could boast with all honesty that their "ethical" marketing policy was "responsible in large measure for the advancement of the profession of paediatrics in this country because it brought control to infant feeding under the direction of the medical profession."

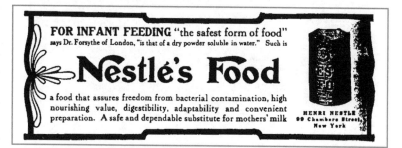

FOR INFANT FEEDING "the safest form of food" says Dr. Forsythe of London, "is that of a dry powder soluble in water." Such is

Nestlé's Food

a food that assures freedom from bacterial contamination, high nourishing value, digestibility, adaptability and convenient preparation. A safe and dependable substitute for mothers' milk

HENRI NESTLE
99 Chambers Street,
New York

22 Advertisement for Nestlé's Food in the
Journal of the American Medical Association, 1912

enlightened self-interest and cooperation

The infant feeding product companies and the doctors now became the best of friends. In 1915 SMA (Synthetic Milk Adapted) was launched at a meeting of the American Pediatric Society. It had been tested on another batch of babies conveniently ready for experiment in the Babies' Dispensary and Hospital, Cleveland. The advertisements in the popular press directed the consumer to a physician; in the medical press they extolled the ease of preparation which "rouses the parents' enthusiasm and adds to the prestige of the physician". The commercial success of this approach convinced more

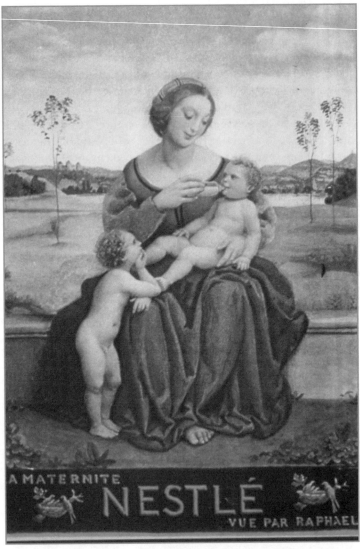

23 La maternité, Nestlé advertisment,1935

companies that this relationship with doctors could be profitable. Nestlé had been advertising to the public for decades, offering free samples and booklets, but in 1924 it launched Lactogen in the US, "only on the prescription or recommendation of a physician. No feeding instructions appear on the trade package." Horlicks launched their milk modifier with the same message. That poor mothers could not afford both the product and a physician's fee did not appear to be a matter of concern.

Many paediatricians advocated breastfeeding and some were uncomfortable with the relationship with commerce. The Philadelphia Pediatric Society believed that advertising through medical channels implied "recommendation by the members of the American Medical Association" and undermined the doctors' attempts to educate the public "to the fact that infants cannot be fed in this indiscriminate manner."

a committee of inquiry

In 1924 the American Medical Association (AMA) set up a committee to investigate infant food advertising. By now the use of commercial foods was so well established that it seemed impossible to recommend their withdrawal. The benefits of breastfeeding and the dangers of 'unsupervised' artificial feeding were reiterated, but the committee applauded the 'disposition on the part of many manufacturers of proprietary foods to cooperate with the medical profession and its medical journals'.[17] The scruples of the Philadelphia paediatricians could not withstand the force of commercial interests. However, the balance of power did not weigh solely in favour of the industry. When Horlicks refused to change its labels and advertising of Malted Milk, 'for infants, from one week to 12 months', they were banned from advertising in the medical journals and Horlicks lost its place in the infant foods market.

By this time the AMA's Committee on Foods controlled the acceptance of advertising copy. Mead Johnson described the economic benefits of cooperation with the medical profession with disarming candour:

> "When mothers in America feed their babies by lay advice, the control of your paediatric cases passes out of your hands, Doctor. Our interest in this important phase of medical economics springs, not from any motives of altruism, philanthropy or paternalism, but rather from a spirit of enlightened self-interest and cooperation because [our] infant diet materials are advertised only to you, never to the public."[9]

When I was researching this topic I looked for original advertisements in the old medical journals and could not find them. Many libraries had discarded and destroyed advertising material in order to lower the book-binding costs. Thus the evidence of this medical commercial liaison was not visually apparent to an historical researcher. This screens out the more questionable activities of the medical profession. If you are confronted with the old advertisements interspersed throughout the medical text, you realise that the medical profession shamefully endorsed products that did more to relieve patients of their money than their suffering. The librarians' part in this censorship is, I believe, innocent, but outrageous. They are like amateur archaeologists who destroy the ancient cooking pots because they believe that only the jewelled swords are important.

the resilience of breastfeeding

This medical/commercial relationship in the US became a model for similar relationships the world over. It has undermined breastfeeding wherever it has been established and continues to do so. Companies will capitulate over direct advertising to the public if they are pressured, but they fight tooth and nail if they are kept apart from their beloved doctors. In the 21st century, the most robust evidence has been published revealing the risks of artificial feeding and the key role of breastfeeding in child survival and long-term adult health. However, just as in the early 20th century, this evidence is ignored if it disturbs the harmony between industry and the established medical hierarchy.

Of course there were maverick doctors who defied the trend. When Dr Cicely Williams was imprisoned in a Japanese internment camp in Malaya (now Malaysia) during the Second World War 20 women gave birth in the camp. All the babies were breastfed, all survived and all were healthy. These mothers suffered malnutrition and extreme physical deprivation; they did not know whether their husbands were alive or dead or being tortured and had no certainty of their own fate or that of their children but they still breastfed. They did have Cicely Williams's support, and with her experience of ordinary African and Asian mothers, she knew that breastfeeding worked. Her faith in the process was the only supplement needed. Women need confidence in their bodies, not products which destroy this.

killing US babies

In the early 20th century, the infant food industry expanded while some concerned doctors researched the risks of artificial feeding. A study in Boston in 1910 found that artificially fed babies were six times more likely to die than those breastfed. Another study in eight US cities, carried out between 1911 and 1916, found the same sixfold mortality risk for babies in low-income families and a fourfold risk in high-income families. These high mortality rates were due to diarrhoea, pneumonia, measles, whooping cough and other communicable diseases.[10] This six-fold difference is the same today wherever children are born into poverty.[11] Most children are. Even as late as 1924, when medical knowledge, public health and living conditions had improved, the same pattern of mortality persisted. A Chicago study of 20,000 infants, all from poor families, all under the supervision of local welfare clinics, revealed that at nine months of age the artificially fed infants were 50 times more likely to die than those who were still breastfeeding. The custom was noted of "trying to make the baby regain its birth weight by ten days old. To do this the child was bottle-fed in addition to breastfeeding. It is difficult to insist on breastfeeding because nurses and physicians are eager to have the infant show the greatest possible gain."[12] It was the medical staff, not the mothers, who resisted the idea that breastfeeding worked.

Later, in the 1970s, Dr Natividad Clavano in the Philippines also found that persuading the medical staff of the importance of exclusive breastfeeding was far harder than convincing the mothers.[13] Babies freely fed in the early weeks usually gain weight rapidly, but delayed breastfeeding, routines and supplementary feeds cause breastfeeding difficulties and reduce milk production.[14] Of course a baby will not stimulate or take in enough breastmilk if she is not allowed to suckle whenever she wants – or if drugs used in childbirth have suppressed her reflexes. As I write, these destructive practices continue today. The medical/commercial relationship needs to keep it that way. In the USA, the American Academy of Pediatrics (AAP) accepts artificial-milk company money and promotion which defies the WHO Code.[15] The 2008 Chinese melamine-laced milk scandal could not have happened if the medical establishment in China had not succumbed to the blandishments of all the big companies. Paediatricians who endorse or supervise artifical feeding should be regularly checking the quality of the milk on the market. This could be organised through their national paediatric associations. It is not just the dairy producers who have been corrupt.[16]

who had the power?

Back in the 1920s, well-informed paediatricians would have known about the research results, yet there was no effective protest against the companies' activities. Throughout this era most articles about infant feeding started with the ritual praise for breastfeeding, like the prayer of grace before a meal, before the author launched enthusiastically into a discussion of the various merits of different artificial foods. As in Europe, there were few attempts to discover the causes of breastfeeding problems or failure, though there was criticism of women who refused to breastfeed. The arbitrary, irrational rules of the maternity wards were rarely questioned and the doctors' authority was absolute.

Most pioneer women in the USA (and of course every Native North American) had not only breastfed but had also provided most of the food and necessities for the household, spending only a few dollars a year in the market economy. The wealthy industrialist's wife depended on her husband economically, was beholden to another man, her doctor, for the skill to keep her child alive and to an industrialised product to replace her banished breastmilk. The enforced uselessness of her existence often led her into a cycle of depression and psychogenic ill-health which, along with damaging management of early breastfeeding, led to an almost inevitable lactation failure.

For the poor women who contributed through their work to the wealth creation of the US, heavy labour in home and factory, poor nutrition and bad living conditions precipitated greater rates of birth complications, stillbirths and smaller, more sickly babies. Many mothers would have needed special encouragement and skill to establish and maintain lactation; this support was just what urbanisation destroyed. The commercial and medical pressures to use artificial milks would have kept breastmilk supplies low. Breastfeeding failure, infrequent feeding and early supplementation would have meant a greater likelihood of closely spaced pregnancies, thus burdening women more and increasing the risk of their own deaths and that of their newborns and existing children.

Commercial baby foods were acknowledged to be dangerous when used without instruction, yet few doctors and no manufacturers attempted to restrict or control their distribution. Ignorance was a mother's crime; as long as she was able to buy a doctor's knowledge she would be absolved, but most mothers could not afford this means of absolution.

expanding the markets

Eventually better living standards, education and medical care in Europe and North America offset the more lethal effects of artificial feeding. After the Second World War immunisation was developed and became available in the industrialised countries, conquering epidemic childhood diseases such as polio and diphtheria. Measles, still a major killer in Africa, became preventable. Antibiotics came into widespread use and a minor respiratory infection could be treated immediately and the risk of pneumonia avoided. Almost all mothers could read feeding instructions and an expanding army of health workers taught them how to prepare bottles with some hygiene. There were still risks in artificial-feeding, but resulting problems could usually be dealt with by the medical services at hand. The economic costs of this vast medical back-up were ignored until the late 20th century. In 1979, in a middle-class US suburb, medical costs for artificially fed babies were fifteen times that for breastfed babies. In 1991, in an English town, the costs of treating just 150 artificially fed babies hospitalised for diarrhoea was estimated to be £225,000 (US$382,500).[17] Hospitalisation for diarrhoea is almost unknown for exclusively breastfed babies.

As industrialised society created a healthier environment, mother and babies could contribute to the prosperity of the baby food manufacturers without having to sacrifice so many infant lives. However, there is an illusory complacency about the effects of artificial-feeding in post-war Europe. At many a conference someone will say confidently, "Most of us here were bottle-fed and we are all

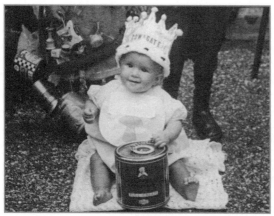

24 First prize for fancy dress at 1945 Victory party (the baby was actually breastfed).
(Photo courtesy of the Brewer Family.)

healthy!" This was often untrue: the long-term effects of not being breastfed are only beginning to be understood. Blood pressure, cholestrol levels, overweight, diabetes and academic performance may all be linked in part to how we were fed as babies.[18]

I have a personal interest in this statement because, according to my mother, I developed gastroenteritis during an epidemic in 1947. Diarrhoea was still a problem of artificially fed infants and there were major outbreaks of gastroenteritis throughout the 1930s and 1940s in Great Britain, Ireland and the USA.[19] The disease was linked with artificial-feeding, though in the USA scientific comparisons were weakened by the universal practice of supplementary feeding. Research comparisons have been obscured by the fact that until recently there were so few exclusively breastfed babies. At the very least parents were instructed to give babies boiled water 'in between feeds'. I survived artificial feeding because my mother had a telephone and could call a doctor quickly, but many parents could not.* When blasé academics point to our universal health, they pass over many petty histories of distressed parents and babies whose fortunate outcome means they are not included in the statistics. It is rarely the medical researchers who are wiping the sore bottoms and washing out the soiled sheets in between anxious attention to the miserable, wailing child. My mother, like most women, had wanted to breastfeed, but a helpful doctor, a family friend, had told her that she had insufficient milk and must put me on the bottle. No one encouraged her and, like her doctor friend, she was quite ignorant of how breastfeeding worked.

If the artificially fed child was more prone to illness, at least medical skills were improving apace and this meant the doctors were becoming increasingly important fixtures in infant life. So there were more jobs, more careers and more sales of drugs, even though public health measures should have decreased the dependency on medicine. Defenders of our society may say that all this was worthwhile, as now the appalling 19th-century contrasts of misery and wealth have been eliminated. But they have not. The extremes of poverty have now moved to remoter places and there are more horrifying contrasts than ever before. The international organisation of labour and capital echoes the social and economic differentials of 19th-century Manchester or New York; so do the urban squalor, the inadequate public hygiene and the commercial morals. The foundations of this system were consolidated during the days of colonial expansion.

* In that era the effective home treatment of oral rehydration had not been developed.

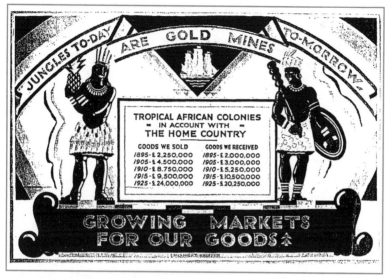

25 Empire Marketing Board Poster (Poster: McKnight Kauffer 1927; courtesy of Public Records Office, London)

The British Empire was founded on commercial interests. Not only were the colonies sources of cheap raw materials and labour, they also formed new markets for the sale of British products. In the late 1920s, the Empire Marketing Board (EMB) boasted that the Empire overseas purchased almost one half of British manufactured goods. The EMB poster in 1927 (above) claimed, 'Jungles today are gold mines tomorrow,' and under a drawing of two traditionally dressed black men was the statement, 'Growing markets for our goods.' In 1910 Britain sold just over £8 million worth of goods to the African colonies and imported £5 million worth. By 1925 these figures were £24 million and £20 million respectively.* Artificial milk was taken along with Christianity, tinned fish and plantation managers to forge the economic links that were the principal goals of colonisation.[20]

the example of the baby milk market in colonial malaysia

Low paid women worked long hours on the profitable rubber estates of British colonial Malaysia. One rubber product was the bottle teat, manufactured in Europe and sold to the rubber tappers to artificially feed their babies.[21]

* 2007 values: £5 billion, £3 billion, £7 billion and £6 billion respectively.

Just as the organisation of factory labour in Britain had disrupted breastfeeding, so did plantation employment. Traditionally in Malaysia, suckling continued for two to four years and babies were carried on their mothers' backs with constant free access to the breast. Plantation labour changed this and to this day women plantation workers work in difficult conditions.[22] In a 1983 study in Penang, estate women said they felt too exhausted to breastfeed after a normal 5.30am to 4.00pm day, tapping 600 to 700 trees. Work burdens increased during the 20th century. Older women reported that intensive methods with more trees to be tapped did not occur in the old days.[23]

The colonial administration set up infant welfare clinics and British nurses energetically converted mothers to the idea of the clock. In a 1925 report on infant feeding there was the regretful statement that "some mothers had not even seen a clock and those who had, could not understand what it had to do with the feeding of an infant".[24] The zealous British nurses soon remedied this deficiency and by 1926 "the majority of mothers understand the clock and feed their children regularly by it and the boat-shaped bottle is accepted in most homes".[24] The devotion to strict routines in nursing practice had sprung from the establishment of the profession by Florence Nightingale during the Crimean War, so that army conventions influenced the running of hospitals and clinics outside the military sphere. This was and is disastrous for mothers and babies because flexibility, spontaneity and a relaxed environment are vital for breastfeeding. Unlike traditional midwives, few of the British nurses who bossed the local Malaysians had themselves experienced breastfeeding and their training had instilled in them an unquestioning acceptance of disastrous 'rules of management'.

Most of the British administrators' wives had also been subject to this medical sabotage, so wherever they took their infants, there was a demand for a supply of artificial milk. The companies were only too glad to use this to stimulate a local market, with the help of the misguided infant welfare nurses. In Malaysia, the Straits Times was carrying advertisements for tinned milk from the mid-1880s onwards, and by 1900 there were four brands available. From 1896 Mellin's Infant Food – "the perfect substitute for Mother's milk" – was advertised weekly and by the start of the First World War Allenbury's, Nestlé's Milk Food, Milkmaid, Infantina and Fussell's were being advertised specifically for infants. Glaxo joined them in 1915 and competitive advertising continued throughout the war. By the 1920s these six brands were still among the eighteen different brands featured in the thirty to forty advertisements per month in the Straits Times. Feeding bottles and teats were also promoted. These were originally aimed at the colonial elite, but local language advertising started towards the end of the l920s.[25]

the nutritional value of the substitutes:
the case of sweetened condensed milk

Even though mothers have been going 'out to work' for thousands of years, the milk companies have claimed mothers were giving their babies inppropriate breastmilk substitutes because they 'had to go out to work' (separation from their babies being an incidental act of God); therefore the marketing of commercial breastmilk substitutes was a useful and good thing to do. Did the companies have the babies' interests at heart? It had long been recognised in Europe and the USA that there were more cases of diarrhoea and more deaths among artificially fed children during the summer. It was well known that tropical climates were riskier for infants. This did not deter the manufacturers, who advertised their products without warnings, whatever the environment. Besides the higher contamination risk of the bottles, teats and milk, some of the milk sold for babies was a nutritional disaster.

Sweetened condensed milk has a high sugar content (about 45% by weight) which reduces the concentration of important nutrients and makes the milk highly unsuitable for infants and young children. Later some sweetened condensed milks were fortified with vitamins A and D, but those used before the Second World War lacked these vitamins. In Malaysia, sweetened condensed milk was highly recommended by doctors and manufacturers and was widely used as a breastmilk substitute, even though in Britain by 1911, doctors published reports to the government recommending that the tins carry labels warning against use as an infant food. The companies had to change their European marketing so they were well aware of the facts.

Of 21 babies with rickets (vitamin D deficiency) seen by Dr Cicely Williams in Singapore, twenty had been fed on sweetened condensed milk. Vitamin A is vital for eye health and babies fed on sweetened condensed milk have gone blind. Vitamin A had been identified and named in 1915, yet in south-east Asia in 1936 Nestlé circulated a diary for doctors with two pages of statements from infant feeding experts. These recommended sweetened condensed milk for infants, with accolades such as, "Sweetened condensed milk is the food par excellence for delicate infants."[26] The British government regulations had made the harmful effects well known so this marketing was cynical and callous in the extreme. This situation prompted Dr Cicely Williams to deliver her speech "Milk and Murder" to the Singapore Rotary Club in 1939, where she said:

> "If you are legal purists you may wish me to change the title of this address to Milk and Manslaughter. But if your lives were embittered as mine is, by seeing day after day this massacre of the innocents by unsuitable feeding, then I believe you would feel as I do that misguided propaganda on infant feeding should be punished as the most miserable form of sedition, and that these deaths should be regarded as murder. Anyone who, ignorantly or lightly, causes a baby to be fed on unsuitable milk, may be guilty of that child's death."[27]

Marketing of Nestlé's sweetened condensed milk as an infant food continued until 1977. After that date, label instructions for infant feeding were supposed to be removed, though tins with these labels continued to be found in developing countries for years afterwards. The problem is not just one of illiterate mothers in developing countries. In 1980 6% of UK mothers were feeding their babies unmodified milk (such as sweetened condensed milk, evaporated or whole fresh cows' milk). In 1982–83, health visitors discovered that some mothers still fed sweetened condensed milk to their babies (as their grannies and mothers had done), believing it to be safe as there was no warning on the label (unlike dried skimmed milk). The Health Visitors' Association (HVA) was advised by the UK Department of Health (DOH) to contact Nestlé who told them that "the incidence of use of condensed milk for infant feeding is so low that there would seem to be as little justification for this move as there would be for a similar statement to appear on 'doorstep milk'".[28] Nestlé has a reputation for giving large sums for nutrition research, especially in the field of infant feeding, yet it refused to spend the small sum needed to protect babies at risk from a product marketed for decades as the "infant food par excellence".

The UK DOH advised health visitors to explain to mothers individually that sweetened condensed milk was unsuitable. Health workers paid by the British National Health Service (NHS) were not only expected to promote new infant feeding products for no extra pay, but also to debrief the customer who followed a dangerous practice instigated by the marketing tactics of a previous generation.

In Malaysia, advertising of all milks continued to increase until the Second World War when breastfeeding rates went up because of the unavailability of artificial milk. The infant mortality rate dropped during this time of 'hardship'. When the British administration resumed control they saw a 'need' for large-scale imports of milk and intensive advertising was resumed.[29] Whenever manufacturers claim to be responding to a 'need', it seems that people have to be reminded through advertising in case they have forgotten what they craved so desperately.

after the second world war

After the Second World War artificial feeding had become quite normal in the USA and to a lesser extent in Europe. In the USA the breastfeeding initiation rate fell by half between 1946 and 1956. By 1967 only 25% of US babies were breastfed on leaving hospital. Damaging hospital practices made breastfeeding a near-impossible procedure and only women with alternative sources of support and knowledge were able to do it. It became common to administer routine lactation suppressant injections immediately after birth.[30]

Doctors trained in this ambience and with little or no knowledge of normal lactation were among the 'experts' who went to help the newly independent countries establish their health services. Until this time, the majority of rural mothers in these regions were continuing to breastfeed; they knew no other way and had fewer problems than European and North American women. Western-style maternity services were unavailable, so they avoided the damage of the medical environment. The standards of living in most of these countries were not rising as they had done in the west. The salesmen arrived with all the tricks of their trade ahead of the sewer construction, the water treatment, the education and the comprehensive medical services which had alleviated some of the risks of their products back home.

Commercial skills were not inhibited by the absence of a modern infrastructure and salesmanship quickly adapted to a new situation. Newly independent countries were attempting to 'develop' and as the colonial administrators withdrew, the business negotiators moved in, though sometimes they were the same people. The potential markets were irresistible to the companies, whose home markets were reaching saturation point. "The high birth rates permit a rapid

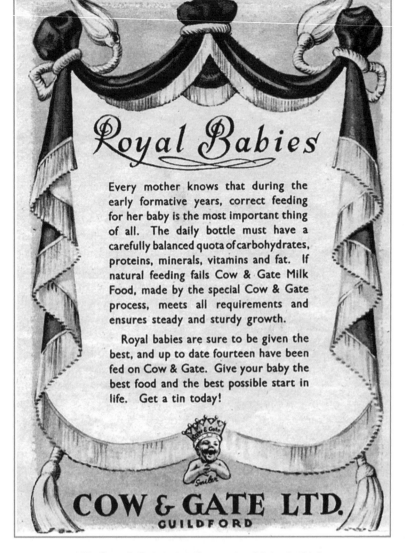

26 Cow & Gate advertisement published widely
in 1940s and 1950s UK

expansion in the domain of infant nutrition," wrote Nestlé in 1970, when planning marketing in Thailand.[31] Growth and expansion were sacred words in commerce and with improving communications and transport, the new shop counter could stretch round the globe.

the great protein fiasco

In 1932, Dr Cicely Williams described and identified kwashiorkor, which means in one Ghanaian language 'the illness the child gets when the next baby is born'. It is the disease of the child displaced from the breast. Unlike the form of malnutrition then called marasmus, when a child is thin and hungry, the child with kwashiorkor is swollen and without appetite. Dr Williams (who spent her later years trying to debunk the protein/kwashiorkor theory) found that cows' milk could have a therapeutic effect on a child with this illness. She speculated that 'some amino acid or protein deficiency cannot be excluded' from the possible causes. To this day no one is certain of a specific cause of kwashiorkor. In spite of this uncertainty, kwashiorkor is still described as a 'protein deficiency' disease in many textbooks. Like most manifestations of malnutrition, kwashiorkor is prevented by adequate food intake and protection from infection. It is a disease of poverty.

Nowadays marasmus and kwashiorkor and the combination of the two are called severe malnutrition. The medical management of severe malnutrition involves the well-supervised re-feeding of the child with a specialised therapeutic food with a carefully made-up balance of nutrients, and milk is usually the basic ingredient. Ironically many of the children who need this treatment have developed severe malnutrition because they were not exclusively breastfed.[32]

Back in the 1930s and 1940s nutritionists developed their focus on protein. Kwashiorkor was common where cows' milk was not a significant part of the diet and appeared to be alleviated or prevented by its consumption. So the concept of milk being a 'protein food' and the answer to malnutrition became well established. Milk is actually a multi-nutrient food, so it was rather arbitrary that 'protein' was seen as the magic ingredient rather than calcium, zinc, various vitamins or indeed the energy in the fats and lactose. However, protein at that time was the nutritionists' favourite nutrient, they knew there was some in milk and when children got better they found a dramatic vindication of their faith in its powers. Anyone dealing with children in the 1930s and 1940s worshipped cows' milk and was sincerely convinced that it was the answer to most nutritional problems – and it happened that there was a lot of it about.

After the Second World War, dried, skimmed milk became "a fortunate by-product of a domestic surplus-disposal problem." It was more satisfactory to dump it in developing countries than to bury it, a solution contemplated by the US Department of Agriculture. Besides planning dried skimmed milk distribution, the authorities formed committees to manufacture 'protein-rich' food supplements from dried skimmed milk, but in the end they failed commercially so were abandoned. During these post-war years, scientists and health planners obsessed about the 'world protein gap' and the 'impending protein crisis'. This led to the allocation of resources to find ways to combat this 'problem'. Then nutritionists thought a bit more, redid their calculations and, oops, they discovered that the problem was not there. Almost overnight the 'protein gap' ceased to exist and became the 'great protein fiasco'.[33]

It is still hard to convince people that it is actually quite difficult to become protein-deficient if you get enough to eat of a range of foods. Most foods contain some protein and you would have to eat a very peculiar diet to meet your energy needs and yet be protein-deficient. Malnourished children are deficient in all nutrients, including energy. The so-called 'high-protein' foods such as meat, fish, milk and eggs are also rich in fats, vitamins and minerals. Some adults spend their entire lives on a vegan diet, consuming no animal products, and they are not protein-deficient. As long as they can afford a wide range of plant foods they can live long healthy lives. Children do need more protein than adults but in conjunction with all the important micro-nutrients which are essential for health.

In some cases high-protein diets may even have negative effects; a high-protein supplement given to pregnant women resulted in an increased rate of premature delivery.[34] Also a high protein diet is not good for a young infant. The main task of making cows' milk into an 'infant formula' is to reduce the proportion of protein and minerals through dilution. Breastmilk is low in protein.[35]

It was during the phase of the imaginary 'protein gap' that the international agencies embarked on distributing tons of dried skimmed milk around the world. The attitude of the nutritional establishment was this:

"Largely through the good offices of UNICEF many thousands of tons of DSM have been distributed to children in countries which are short of dairy cattle. The improvement in health of children receiving this milk has been demonstrated in controlled experiments and vast numbers of children have benefited."[36]

Non-human milk, though a useful product, is not an indispensable food, and after infancy, children can stay healthy on diets without it as long as they have a plentiful range of other foods (including some animal products). In poor countries, many children do not get enough good food and any controlled experiment where deprived children are given extra nutritious meals would show improvement in health. The idea of countries being 'short of dairy cattle' illustrates the ethnocentric bias of nutritional scientists, many of whom have strong links with the food production system of the industrialised world. Avocado pears are a useful food crop in tropical climates, producing a high-energy, vitamin-rich food, yet there are no vested interest groups persuading industrialised cold countries to invest in expensive technology because we are 'short of avocado trees'.

It was cheap dried skimmed milk, though, not the whole dried milk that was favoured for worldwide distribution, because there were non-nutritional advantages: "We aim not only at improving the standard of nutrition but also, as a necessary corollary, at expanding the market for milk."[37] In Nigeria, where Fulani women had always bartered milk for grain, the British residents became interested in organising milk collection when their butter supplies from Europe were cut off during the Seond World War ('Cynthia, I'll be damned if I'll have my omelette cooked in palm oil, we'll just have to teach these natives to churn'). The leftover buttermilk was discarded and in 1954 UNICEF recommended that it should be roller-dried and distributed via the medical service. This milk obsession went hand in hand with scorn for breastmilk. A WHO consultant who visited Nigeria in 1955 referred to mothers' "impoverished milk". Mothers were confronted by health workers, told to reduce the number of breastfeeds and then encouraged to supplement with substitute milks.[38]

In the Caribbean, mothers had been positively discouraged from breastfeeding in the second year (called 'over-nursing') by the Colonial Health Administration:

"Their mothers keep them at it for sixteen to eighteen months, during the last seven or eight months the children draw an abundant supply of a highly unnutritious fluid from the breast . . . No amount of advice will prevent the women from carrying on this deadly habit."

This was written in 1917, but the attitude was still around in 1952 when clinic nurses were advising mothers that seven to nine months was the desirable length of time for breastfeeding. Nurses also instructed mothers not to let their babies fondle their breasts.[39]

Fortunately for British sensitivities, UNICEF dried skimmed milk was soon to put a stop to all this fondling.

By the early 1960s UNICEF was distributing 900,000kg of milk annually. This was going to babies as well as mothers and children all over the world and was used to entice mothers to clinics, just as the infant milk depots had in Europe. In Sarawak in 1954, dried skimmed milk donated by UNICEF and government-supplied evaporated milk was seen by health workers as 'bait' to attract mothers to the clinics. In Singapore, 22,590kg of free powdered milk were given out by clinics in 1959.[40]

Dried skimmed milk is high in protein and calcium, but unless it is artificially fortified it lacks the fat-soluble A and D vitamins. Rickets is not a widespread problem in sunny countries but vitamin A deficiency is. Its occurrence is linked with frequency of diarrhoea, which itself is more likely with the use of dried skimmed milk. During the 1950s and 60s blindness in children due to vitamin A deficiency was widespread. Although vitamins A and D may be added to dried skimmed milk, these can deteriorate in storage. In 1991 the European Community (now the European Union) produced 40% of the world supply of dried skimmed milk and sent out 83,500 tonnes as food aid.[41] Many children who suffer from periods of marginal malnutrition recover and go through a phase of catch-up growth with no long-term ill-effects, but eyesight has no comparable recovery. With all food aid it is notorious that any donated food inevitably replaces home meals. In many areas of the world where dried skimmed milk was distributed, the traditional diet included leaves, oil seeds and fruits high in vitamin A. By zealously promoting this 'protein supplement' there might have been an accompanying reduction of other important dietary components such as vitamin A. In the 21st century UNICEF distributes high dose vitamin A pills to children and these programmes have dramatically reduced deficiency.[42] It is a poignant thought that vitamin A deficiency might have been worsened by the changes in dietary practices, due to the earlier distribution of dried skimmed milk.

Dried skimmed milk was distributed in countries where the use of animal milk after breastfeeding was not customary. As children were suckled for three or four years, they were not deprived of a balance of nutrients but they needed more of the share of family foods. In many societies any non-human milk donation was interpreted as a health message to replace breastfeeding, an idea often endorsed by the resident foreigners' custom of giving artificial milk to their babies. From the 1950s onwards, the 'normal' practice in most industrialised, cows' milk producing countries was for any breastfeeding to last for a token three to six months, followed by either whole or modified cows' milk. Health workers and milk distributors spread this pattern all over the world, to the delight of the artificial milk industry who could then persuade mothers to replace the inferior dried skimmed milk with their expensive products.

UNICEF now energetically promotes breastfeeding, but sadly this is part of undoing its own terrible mistake made in the name of nutrition.[43] It was not the only misguided organisation; all major charities, church missions and other relief agencies did untold damage to breastfeeding and to the economic and health independence of newly independent countries through energetic milk promotion. This practice persists to this day in refugee camps and other focal points of international aid which become sinks for dumping milk. This depresses local food production and purchase, discourages breastfeeding and appropriate local dietary habits, creates a need for imported products and often a black market. It may accelerate the economic and social breakdown which may have precipitated the refugee problem in the first place.

Any country that has imported dried milk on a large scale worsens its economic problems and sees small local dairying decline. Local fresh foods are replaced by the multinationals' products.[44] When the baby food industry protests that they are not wholly responsible for the decline in breastfeeding they are right; the aid agencies as well as medical misinformation prepared the market by helping to create a need. By the 1960s the marketing campaigns of Nestlé, Cow & Gate, Wyeth, Bristol Myers and others were advancing all over a developing world where charity had helped map out the roads.

15 the lure of the global market

"No significant manufacturer introduces a new product without cultivating the consumer demand for it. Or foregoes efforts to influence and sustain demand for an existing product".
JK Galbraith, The Economics of Innocent
Fraud Truth For Our Time, Allen Lane, 2004

selling to the shack as well as the mansion

The companies' boast of 'ethical' practice – "To be used only under the direction of a physician"[1] – disappeared when promotion reached the developing countries. They used every possible method to persuade mothers to use their products, including huge billboards and frequent radio and newspaper adverts. Nestlé created their famous 'milk nurses', saleswomen dressed as nurses, described by Cicely Williams to be "dragging a good lactating breast out of the baby's mouth and pouring in baby milks".[2] A few were trained nurses, but qualifications were irrelevant because they were employed to promote and sell artificial milk. The recruitment of qualified nurses drained emerging health services of badly-needed staff. They were usually paid on commission, earning more than in the health service and, qualified or not, their uniforms carried the prestige of a health worker. An investigation in Nigeria in the early 1970s showed that 87% of mothers used artificial milk because they believed that the hospital staff had advised to do so. In reality they had been advised by saleswomen disguised as nurses on the hospital ward.[3]

The advertising messages undermined confidence in the rival product: "When breastmilk fails, choose Lactogen." Like a bad spell the words put the idea of failure into a mother's mind where it had not existed before. She only had to use one or two bottles of artificial milk and her replete baby would suckle less. The mother, unaware that filling her baby's stomach with other milks would reduce breastmilk stimulation, would then find her own milk decreasing and become dependent on the artificial milk. The radio was a good way to reach the illiterate. In August 1974, in Sierra Leone, 135 30-second advertisements for Nestlé's Lactogen were broadcast over the Sierra Leone Broadcasting Service. In December 1974, there were 45 30-second ads for Cow & Gate baby milks and 66 for Abbott-Ross's

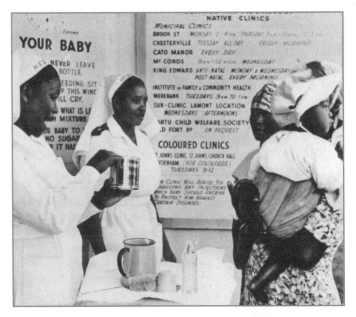

27 Nestlé milk nurses in South Africa in the 1950s
(Photo from Nestlé in Profile)

Similac. On one day, 14 separate advertisements were broadcast
(three Similac, four Cow & Gate, and seven Lactogen). In the local
Creole language Nestlé proclaimed: "Now Lactogen a better food cos
it don get more protein and iron, all the important things dat go make
pikin strong and well. Lactogen Full Protein now get more cream taste
and Nestlé den guarantee um . . . Lactogen and Love." Ironically, more
protein and iron are dangerous for a small infant's body.

Research showed that the advertisments were effective: "Depth
interviews brought out very clearly the mother's positive attitude to
bottlefeeding."[4] Many mothers were convinced that artificial milk was
a medicine, especially as it was endorsed and distributed through
healthcare channels. That it was an imported product, used by the
colonial elite, added to its status.

No single manufacturer had a monopoly on immoral promotion,
but the giant food company Nestlé was the world leader in artificial
milk sales. It had been the proud innovator of the most effective
promotion techniques:

"The advent of television as a universal means of
communicating with the shack as well as the mansion permits
the standardisation to an increasing extent of advertising and

promotion. Nestlé uses the medium extensively wherever it can. Where it still can't, the company relies on newspapers, colour magazines, billboards and other outdoor displays. In less developed countries, the best form of promoting baby food formulas may well be the clinics which the company sponsors, at which nurses and doctors in its employ offer childcare guidance service. In the less developed countries, effective distribution may call for unusual, imaginative techniques."[5]

These claims were not confined to artificial milk promotion. By 1970, mothers in the Ivory Coast were giving Nescafé to their toddlers because a radio advertisement proclaimed: "Nescafe makes men stronger, women more joyful and children more intelligent."[6]

whistle blowers, doctors and the united nations

In much of Africa, doctors were dismayed by the numbers of younger infants suffering from the diarrhoea and malnutrition that came to be called 'bottle-baby disease'. It was increasing in areas where previously the only reason for not breastfeeding had been a mother's death, and in that case a relative breastfed the baby. In a tactful article called Commerciogenic Malnutrition, Dr Derrick Jelliffe pointed out the harm of the promotion of infant feeding products in developing countries. He proposed a dialogue between the baby food industry and the doctors. Dr Catherine Wennen had already described the problem in 1950s Nigeria. While trying to cope with the numbers of babies sick from artificial-feeding, she was surrounded by widespread, aggressive publicity. She heard frequent radio slogans and saw images of healthy babies smiling down from giant billboards. The companies were well aware of the risks for, as Dr Wennen noted, they had initially refrained from promoting to the 'unsophisticated market'. She became aware of the excellent public relations between the companies and top figures in the medical profession, the free artificial milk for doctors and the gifts to hospitals, so she approached the Nestlé manager in Lagos "to point out the sad consequences of their indiscriminate sales promotion". He did not want to talk.[7]

By this time many health workers had written to Nestlé to explain the dangers of artificial feeding in poor societies. The complaints were ignored unless there was adverse publicity. In 1965 in Jamaica, a young nutritionist, Ann Ashworth Hill, had written to Nestlé about the dangerous labels on their sweetened condensed milk tins. Nothing happened. Then Ann's husband, Member of Parliament Winston Hill, asked questions on the issue in the Jamaican Parliament. Immediately Nestlé executives flew into Jamaica, talked with Ann and the labels were changed.[8]

More and more doctors were witnessing the same practices around the world and their concern led, in 1970, to a meeting of the UN Protein Advisory Group ad hoc Working Group (its name a reflection of the protein obsession described in Chapter 14) where paediatricians, the baby food industry and UN agency representatives discussed the problem. The proceedings were never made public, but it is known that the industry refused to accept that the promotion and availability of artificial milk had any impact on the decline of breastfeeding.

This is one of the great feats of double-think in business. While marketers and advertisers attribute rising sales to their strategies and earn huge rewards for their efforts, if the industry is challenged over its harmful effects, it quivers with innocence and protests that people never buy anything they do not need. Some public relations men have even claimed that their advertising had no effect, though why a company should squander investors' money on ineffective promotion is difficult to understand.

Further Protein Advisory Group meetings which, needless to say, no breastfeeding women from poor countries attended, resulted in a sort of marketing declaration for artificial milk: "In any country lacking breastmilk substitutes, it is urgent that infant formulas be developed and introduced." Governments should support investment, promotion and measures which disseminated the use of these products. From the industry's viewpoint the meeting had gone well. By 1979, a World Health Organisation survey had found that fifty brands and 200 varieties of breastmilk substitutes were being distributed across 100 countries. About half the companies had established factories in developing countries and their distribution networks were spaced across a broad economic spectrum.[9]

'the baby killer'

The result of the 1970s Protein Advisory Group's meetings echoed those of the 1924 American Medical Association's meeting with the infant food industry. You cannot expect the representatives of business to accept damage to their sales without a struggle. If a squeamish employee resigns on a moral issue, there is always a new

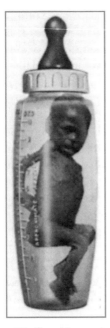

28 Graphic used on the front cover of The Baby Killer by Mike Muller 1974. (Courtesy of War on Want)

delegate to fight for the company's interests. One company (Abbott-Ross) did call for 'restrained promotional practices', but their developing country markets were small so they had less to lose. While these discussions were continuing, the ordinary woman or man in the streets of the industrialised countries knew nothing about the problem. When there were earthquakes, hurricanes or wars, pictures reached most newspapers and TV networks and emergency funds were set up – for example the child victims of the Nigerian Civil War (1967–70) aroused widespread compassion – but this other quiet slaughter was unreported. Then, in 1973, the magazine New Internationalist published an interview with two paediatricians with long experience in Africa, Drs David Morley and Ralph Hendrikse, who described the problem in everyday language. This was followed in 1974 by a publication, by the British charity War on Want, called The Baby Killer. This explained the issue vividly including pictures of the conditions of poor people's daily life as well as the promotion and its results. The cover design conveyed the pain and the problem in the powerful visual message of a malnourished baby inside a feeding bottle. This was how I first learned about the issue. Twenty thousand copies were distributed and it was widely translated.[10]

some business tries to do good

In response to The Baby Killer the British company Cow & Gate sent an investigative team to both Asia and Africa. It offered to withdraw its products from these areas, but government authorities and paediatric experts advised against this, claiming that "better techniques of education and better controls on promotional activities were required". This decision is understandable when you consider the identity of 'government authorities and paediatric experts'. They were the elite, who had a lot to lose from company withdrawal. They were the recipients of gifts of equipment and grants for hospitals and medical schools. Their high standards of living enabled their own children to be more safely bottle-fed with the free milk the companies gave them. The cultural influence of the retreating colonials survived among some elite families, who spurned 'peasant style' breastfeeding. The Jelliffes pointed out that in the ex-colonies artificial-feeding was associated with authority, and breastfeeding with oppression.[11] The paediatric 'experts' were usually western-trained and consequently ignorant about breastfeeding. Some sincerely believed that artificial milk filled a 'breastmilk gap', but its withdrawal together with bottles and teats would have saved many lives.

Some international business thinkers considered the idea of restricting the distribution of breastmilk substitutes. In 1979 the Journal of Contemporary Business published an article proposing the "demarketing of infant formula" in parts of the world where lack of safe water, sanitation and education made it a dangerous product.[12]

the nestlé trial

Within two months of publication, The Baby Killer had been translated into German by a Swiss group (AgDW) with the title Nestlé Tötet Babys meaning Nestlé Kills Babies.[13] Nestlé quickly filed a libel suit against the group. In Switzerland the company was known for product quality and paternalistic fairness. To say it killed babies was akin to accusing the little red hen of laying poisoned eggs. In fact the image had to be carefully nurtured, because Nestlé had already been taken to court as a defendant concerning questionable practices. In 1948, it had been convicted in Swiss courts of false labelling of condensed milk sold to the Red Cross and of a chicory/coffee product, Nescore.[14]

During the preparation of its libel suit, Nestlé offered to settle out of court if AgDW apologised, destroyed the report and paid all costs. AgDW refused and the case proceeded. Nestlé had originally issued proceedings on four counts, namely against:

- the title;
- the accusation of immoral and unethical practices;
- the accusation of responsibility for the death or damage of babies through its sales promotion policy;
- the accusation of dressing its saleswomen as nurses to give a false scientific credibility.

However before the final hearing, Nestlé withdrew the last three. The case had already gone through three hearings. Internationally respected doctors had testified about the effects of commercial promotion on infant lives and had shocked all who heard them.

The judge found the AgDW members guilty of libel in the title because:

> "The adequate causal connection between the sale or any other type of distribution of powdered milk and the death of infants fed with such products is interrupted by the action of third parties, for which the complainant, in terms of criminal law, cannot be held responsible. In this sense, there is no negligent or even intentional killing."

The defendants were fined 300 Swiss francs (US$150) each, but the judge took the opportunity to state that Nestlé's advertising in developing countries went considerably further than in industrialised countries and said:

> "The need ensues for the Nestlé company fundamentally to rethink its advertising practices in developing countries concerning bottle-feeding, for its advertising practice up to now can transform a life-saving product into one that is dangerous and life-destroying. If the complainant in future wants to be spared the accusation of immoral and unethical conduct, he will have to change advertising practices."

If Nestlé had accepted the spirit of the judge's verdict, acknowledged its mistakes and changed its marketing of artificial milk immediately, it would have been a coup for the defenders of big business and a rebuke to those who claim that transnational companies are inevitably immoral. But they could not admit to unethical practices. The managing director stated, "I was able to see that they [the advertising practices] were normal and usual advertising methods, used by manufacturers of such products all over the world," and, "We must affirm that we have full confidence in the ethical basis of our actions."[15]

Yet Nestlé itself had, after 1924, proudly adopted a policy in the USA (where conditions were better than in poor countries in the 1970s) of selling Lactogen "only on the prescription or recommendation of a physician". Artificial milk accounted for a small percentage of the overall sales of Nestlé, at that time the world's second largest food company. It was advised at one stage by an advertising agency to pull out of the breastmilk substitute market because it was damaging its public image.[16] Who knows what motivated which individuals to resist change so stubbornly? There was conflict between the company's diehards and those who were shocked to discover the extent and effects of its promotional practices. The fact, as the executive director had stated, was that it only did what was normal for all companies. Why should it adopt a commercially disadvantageous strategy and stop what everyone else would continue to do anyway?

The Protein Advisory Group meetings had brought the companies together and enabled them to form the International Council for Infant Food Industries (ICIFI), a group of nine companies including Nestlé. As though galvanised by the publicity from the Nestlé trial, the ICIFI proposed a code of ethics and published it just before the end of the first hearing of Nestlé's libel suit. This code was so weak regarding advertising in the developing world that one company, Abbott-Ross, decided not to consolidate its ICIFI membership.

an attempt at shareholder pressure

In 1975 a group of Roman Catholic nuns, the Sisters of the Precious Blood, filed a lawsuit against Bristol Myers, a US company, charging it with 'making misstatements in its proxy statement'; in plain English, lying. When the nuns, as shareholders, challenged the company to provide detailed information about its practices abroad, they were informed that there was no promotion where chronic poverty or ignorance could lead to product misuse. Bristol Myers marketed in Latin America, in countries such as Guatemala where about half the population had no access to safe water. 40% of Enfamil (a Bristol Myers artificial milk) sales were outside the USA. In 1974 advertising and promotion had cost it US$296 million, almost three times as much as it spent on research and development.[17] Other investors could see the contradictions between the evidence found by the Interfaith Centre for Corporate Responsibility (ICCR) (set up to monitor church investments), and the Bristol Myers statements, but the company refused discussion. The nuns and the ICCR collected evidence from 18 different countries which proved the falseness of the statements. Nevertheless, the judge dismissed the case because the nuns had not suffered irreparable harm from the company's statement. This judgment implied that only malnourished babies themselves could sue, and that companies were free to lie if it did not hurt their

> *"Well, as we were about to leave, one of the Sisters said, 'Tell me, if you stop selling to people who are too poor to use the product safely, will you still make a profit?' There was absolute silence. It must have been a full minute. Finally one of the corporate executives picked it up and said, 'That is the crux of the problem.'"*
>
> Exchange at a meeting between the Sisters of Mercy and Abbott-Ross in Chicago. Reported in The Bottle Baby Scandal: Milking the Third World For All It's Worth by Barbara Garson, Mother Jones, December 1977.

shareholders. The sisters gathered support from other shareholders and appealed. They also had the backing of the US Securities and Exchange Commission, the statutory body which governs shareholder transactions. Eventually Bristol Myers decided to settle out of court, to send shareholders a report of the nuns' evidence and to halt direct consumer advertising and the use of 'milk nurses'.[18]

the nestlé boycott

In spite of the publicity and the lawsuits, the companies, including Nestlé, continued their widespread promotion. Then in 1975, Peter Krieg's film Bottle Babies made a profound impact. People who had read descriptions of the problem, admitted that they had never really felt involved until they saw the shot of a woman scooping water from a visibly filthy pool to mix with her baby's powdered milk; or the wasted, malnourished baby screaming as a drip needle was placed through a vein in her head.[19] Hundreds of viewers from study groups and organisations concerned with world poverty felt exasperated by the companies' indifference. From the country where the most energetic marketing methods had evolved came the commitment and the ideas to challenge them. Whenever Bottle Babies was shown, people spontaneously vowed to boycott Nestlé's products. In Minneapolis, USA, a group calling themselves the Infant Formula Action Coalition (INFACT) responded to these avowals by deciding to co-ordinate a boycott and launched it in July 1977. It was one of the few actions they could take, for at that time only Swiss nationals were permitted to own Nestlé shares so US citizens could not use investor influence. In the USA, the mainstream support for the Nestlé boycott came from the churches. Many did missionary work in poor countries and could verify the facts of the marketing abuses. INFACT's demand to Nestlé was that it should halt all promotion of artificial milk. This meant no milk nurses, no free samples and no direct advertising. The boycott spread to Europe, New Zealand and Canada.[20]

a tale of three babies

Ben and Bradley: In 1979 two American babies, Ben and Bradley, were rushed into hospital suffering from alkalosis, a condition where the body's alkali/acid balance goes awry. If untreated it may be fatal. Their condition was caused by their food: two infant formulas (Neo-Mull-Soy and Cho-free) deficient in chloride, made by Syntex. Their parents, Carol and Alan Laskin and Lynn and Larry Pilot, turned to the US Food and Drug Administration (FDA) to see if any other reports linked the disease to use of these products. They discovered that there were no requirements for infant formula manufacture, except that it must be manufactured under sanitary conditions and the label state the ingredients. Syntex made some attempt to recall the formula from its retail outlets, but months later there were still tins on sale. The Laskins and the Pilots contacted the press and the politicians and, as a result of the ensuing publicity, received 60,000 queries. Congressional hearings were instigated and a parents' pressure group, FORMULA was set up. By 1980, legislation was drafted setting nutrient standards for infant formula, requiring routine testing by manufacturers, as well as immediate notification of any problems which might present a health risk. Is this tale an accolade to the US system, its principles of freedom and the power of the individual?

There are some more details to this story: Carol Laskin was a health care management consultant and Alan Laskin a management consultant with contacts in the media. Lynn and Larry Pilot were both attorneys, she with experience in Congress and he employed by the FDA as a specialist in food and drug law. In spite of Ben and Bradley having a hand-picked team of experts for parents, it was still hard for the Laskins and the Pilots to influence powerful bodies. Thirty years later formula 'mistakes' are still occurring. A Congressional subcommittee asked the Justice Department to prosecute the company for their poor recall of the dangerous formula. By 1984 this had not happened, because the Justice Department argued that criminal prosecution was not necessary to prevent similar incidents in the future. As Maureen Minchin said, "Would you not prosecute a burglar because after a crime he had lost his ability to steal?"[21]

The 1980 Infant Formula Act could be seen as a step forward for the protection of infants, but its power was yet to be established. The manufacturers agreed to the act in principle, but when the FDA drafted stringent recall procedures they disagreed. The FDA has no powers of coercion, and in the drafting of consumer protection laws there is always the hazardous journey between proposal and final draft, where the vested interest groups are waiting at every turn to influence the wording. We are talking about potentially lethal products which have damaged babies, yet manufacturers were trying to evade the responsibility of maintaining safe standards.

The companies complained about the regulation proposals in the first draft of the law. They were supported by the American Medical Association (AMA) who saw no need for regulation because it believed the industry should and could regulate itself. The Syntex company had removed salt (sodium chloride) due, they claimed, to 'consumer pressure' because of a theoretical link between dietary salt and high blood pressure. The chloride content was one-fifth of the amount recommended by the American Academy of Pediatrics (AAP). Here is an example of nutritional 'fashion' influencing the content of a product which is supposed to be based on scientific principles. When you next see a new infant formula with a claim to unique health benefits, think of Ben and Bradley and ask yourself whether a new ingredient or composition is based on fashion or impartial scientific evidence.

I do not know how the AMA explained away the fact that the companies had repeatedly proved themselves incapable of self-regulation. Once again doctors and industry were found in cahoots. The AAP supported industry too, because "regulations might make formula unaffordable and reduce the number of specialised formulae *available to doctors*" (my emphasis).[22] The AAP, an organisation supposedly concerned with child health, considered quality control an extravagance, whilst millions of dollars were, and are, spent by the baby food industry on advertising and promotions such as free lunches, conferences and services to doctors. In the early 1980s, the AAP received a renewable annual grant of US$1 million from the baby food industry.[23]

In 1982 the FDA was still drafting the regulations (and being chivvied by President Reagan's administration to weaken them), when it announced that Wyeth was recalling half a million cans of Nursoy Concentrate and Ready-to-Feed because they lacked vitamin B6 and contained excessive vitamin B1. A week later they recalled half a million cans of SMA, but only after debate with the FDA. Deficiency of B6 can cause irritability, convulsions and even brain damage. When asked by the press why they did not pre-test the formula to ensure content quality, Wyeth replied that it was not required by law to do so.

That same year the FDA published its quality control regulations as a compromise between the original strong control proposals and the companies' interests. FORMULA and other parents' groups filed a lawsuit charging the Reagan administration with violating the Infant Formula Act of 1980 by leaving the specifics of quality control to the manufacturers. Lynn Pilot commented that the supposedly explicit regulations did not even rise to the level of the FDA rules for cold remedies, yet were dealing with an infant's sole source of nutrition. Thousands of babies had received the two chloride-free formulas. Perhaps we can say this was all a sad mistake, that modern medical skill saved the babies' lives and that all ended well. It did not. Lynn Pilot and Carol Laskin investigated the thousands of cases that parents reported to them. Children suffered from slow motor development, speech delay, kidney problems, reduced muscle tension (hypotonia), convulsions and dental problems. Learning difficulties and intellectual impairment were linked with the use of the product. One study showed that the longer the child had received the formula, the lower the score in an intellectual measurement test. Ten years later these children had recovered growth but still had behavioural and language problems. An estimated 20,000 to 50,000 children had received the formula in 1978 and 1979. Such was Syntex's concern for infant health, they applied to the authorities for permission to 'donate', for export, the batches of the formula that had damaged so many babies. Just so that you do not collapse into complete cynicism about the state of US commercial morals, you may be relieved to know that permission was refused.[24]

Debbie: In 1982, a Filipina baby, Debbie, was taken to the public hospital where she had been born six weeks earlier. She had a high fever and had not responded to the antibiotics and antipyretics which a private doctor had prescribed. An upper respiratory infection was diagnosed and she was prescribed four further types of medicine for fever, colds and oral eruptions. Because there were no vacant beds she could not be admitted, so her mother, Cely, took her home.

Debbie had been delivered by Caesarean section and weighed 3kg, an adequate birth weight. Though Cely had planned to breastfeed, Debbie was put in the nursery and artificially-fed, the normal practice in the Philippines where hospital practices had followed the US model. Debbie was discharged a day ahead of her mother and cared for by her grandmother. The health staff told her to feed the baby with infant formula until Cely joined them. Cely's parents lived in four badly-ventilated rooms with no ceiling under the metal roof, which made it extremely hot. Water came from a public tap outside and they shared a toilet and bathroom with three other families. Cely, her toddler daughter and the baby slept in one room, her parents and two sisters in another. Her husband stayed in their own flat in another part of the city, but visited often. Cely attempted breastfeeding, but because her breasts softened quickly during a feed she believed she had insufficient milk, brought about, she decided, by the drugs used during her surgery. She fed Debbie with infant formula and cleaned the bottles and teats with salt and water and boiled them for two minutes.

After her baptism at one month Debbie became ill and after the initial consultations, she got worse. Cely took her to the private hospital where she was admitted and given oxygen and dextrose. Tests showed that she might be suffering from salmonella septicaemia with concurrent meningitis and she was put in intensive care. She died and because her parents did not allow an autopsy the exact cause of death will never be known. Debbie 'lay in state' for a week before she was buried. Cely suffered from engorged breasts during this time. The money that Debbie's god-parents had given at the baptism paid for her funeral expenses.

This account is a shortened version of Debbie's history related in *Seven Infant Deaths* by Lorna P. Makil and Mayling Simpson. They analyse the reasons for Debbie's death and note that the family and hospitals did everything in their power to save her. She may have died from an infection or the side-effect of a drug[25] or both. The crux of the matter is that if she had been exclusively breastfed it is highly unlikely that such a well-sized baby would have contracted a severe infection so early. The hospital's endorsement of early artificial feeding conveyed the idea that it was a safe feeding method. It also prevented Cely's breastmilk being stimulated by Debbie. If a baby is strong enough to suck at a bottle she can breastfeed. Debbie was a good birth weight so it would have been safe to give her nothing at all until Cely came round from the anaesthetic. If she had been 'roomed in' with her mother they would not only have established a good breastmilk supply together, but saved money and staff time on feeding her in the nursery. The hospital was too overcrowded to admit Debbie when she was ill later. It was doubtless dealing with the problems of other babies whom they had started on artificial-feeding. Cely had never been told that giving bottles and formula could reduce her own milk supply. When the hospital discharged Debbie a day before Cely, they indicated that separating a newborn from her mother was an acceptable practice and even advised infant formula.[26]

who dupes whom?

Ben, Bradley and Debbie suffered because their parents had trusted that a commercial product could be as good as breastmilk. Skilful marketing and medical complicity had created that trust. Millions of other parents believed in the images projected by the baby food companies and endorsed by the medical profession. Lynne Pilot breastfed Ben for three and a half months, which is still longer than the US average and at that time was recommended as sufficient by most paediatricians. For years, doctors recommended new products with unquestioning faith in the competence and integrity of industry. They were as duped by the companies as any poor, illiterate woman. How many doctors and paediatricians actually get their free samples laboratory tested and give them thorough 'scientific assessment'? The AAP's 1976 guidelines had recommended 29 millilitres per litre for chloride, yet when tested the Syntex formulas contained nil to two millilitres per litre. It had been that low since 1978, yet as far as I can discover, no pediatrician had reported or publicly discussed the possible risks of such a drastic change in ingredient proportions. In the 1979 edition of Nelson: Textbook of Pediatrics there is a chart of commercial food composition; a footnote states that data are supplied by the companies.[27] It seems that it always takes infant illness or even death to expose faulty products as the 2008 Chinese Sanlu milk scandal has illustrated. Twenty two other brands also contained melamine, yet no company ever made publicised recalls before the Chinese tragedy. (see Appendix 6).[28] If paediatricians are not alert to these problems and their source of facts comes from the fallible manufacturers, where is accurate, relevant information to be found?

In the case of Ben and Bradley it took the concerned, and as it happened, highly trained, parents to confront a company and the official bodies with the links between a product and a serious illness. In the case of Debbie, her parents had neither the skills, nor the access to information, that would have made them realise that a product disseminated through the health system had caused their daughter's death. If paediatricians had been doing their job properly they would have tested the Syntex infant formula and questioned the advisability of low chloride levels, by checking through the available evidence, long before these tragedies occurred. In the hospital where

Debbie was born, responsible paediatricians should not have allowed anything other than breastmilk to be used, except in special circumstances. Doctors, however, are just as vulnerable to marketing tactics as the rest of us; companies merely use different methods to seduce them.

In the USA, most ordinary women who return to employment after childbirth still find it difficult to arrange breastfeeding. The same country that has such weak regulations (and they are among the best in the world) of the artificial milk market has restrictive practices against breastfeeding. The USA has no federal legislation concerning maternity protection, let alone breastfeeding breaks, and despite some high profile companies supporting breastfeeding employees, many women workers are barely allowed food and toilet breaks let alone permitted to breastfeed. In the 20th century women could be arrested for breastfeeding their babies in public, though in the 1990s several states brought in protective legislation. The Syntex managers were never arrested for distributing a product that proved poisonous (several poisons work by depriving the body of an essential nutrient) for many babies.[29]

Cely came from a country which had formerly been a US colony and, just as in British-controlled Malaysia, the Philippines had adopted the appalling infant feeding culture of her former rulers. In 1909, the US had forced a 'free' trade arrangement on the country which gave an advantage to the US, restricted the Philippines' international trading relations and stifled self-sufficient development. This legacy allowed freedom of marketing to the baby milk companies, a policy which conveys little economic benefit, even when milk is produced in the country. Many raw materials were imported and the profits went back to foreign companies. In the early 1980s, over half the Filipino population lived below the absolute poverty level. It cost over a third of the minimum wage to feed a two-month-old on Nestle's Nan infant formula. An artificially fed Filipino baby was forty times more likely to die, yet in 1988 only 22% of one-month-olds were exclusively breastfed.[30]

But Debbie died in 1982, a year after the International Code of Marketing of Breastmilk Substitutes had been adopted by the Philippines. This should have changed things. Let's go back to the 1970s and pick up the story.

a public hearing

> *"Whose responsibility is it to control the advertising,*
> *marketing and promotional activities which may create*
> *a market in spite of public health considerations?"*
> Senator Edward Kennedy's opening speech at the 1978 Senate Hearing

As more people in the industrialised world learned about the needless illness and deaths of infants in poor countries, they joined the groups who had discovered that Nestlé continued to lead the market and engage in aggressive promotion. According to Fortune magazine, Nestlé was probably the most profitable food company in the world in 1977, superseding both Unilever and General Foods. Nestlé could have afforded to pull out of the infant feeding market, but as the boycott grew, rather than reform their marketing methods they invested more resources in public relations (PR). For example, they paid a US $1 million fee to the PR firm Hill & Knowlton, who sent 300,000 glossy booklets to the clergy and religious bodies, explaining that Nestlé was not aggressively marketing the baby milk in the developing countries. This was how many of the churches learned about the issue for the first time. Swiss journalist Jean Claude Buffle has estimated that the boycott cost Nestlé US$2billion in PR expenditure and a loss of turnover which may have amounted to US$1.5billion.[31]

As concern grew, Senator Edward Kennedy, chairman of the US Senate Sub-Committee on Health and Scientific Research, proposed and set up a hearing on the promotion and use of infant formula in developing countries. This brought the issue into the public spotlight. Representatives from industry, the health field and non-governmental organisations (NGOs) gave evidence. Kennedy asked Oswaldo Ballerin, President of Nestlé Brazil, whether his company should market a product in areas without clean water and where people were illiterate. Ballerin evaded the question by reciting the nostrum that all the instructions were on the tin, but Kennedy persisted and Ballerin answered, "But . . . we cannot be responsible for that." Kennedy asked if Nestlé was able to investigate the use of its products in poor areas and Ballerin agreed that it was, but that it had not. Then Ballerin declared, "The US Nestlé Company has advised me that their research indicates that this [the boycott] is actually an indirect attack on the free world's economic system." This statement provoked laughter and Kennedy explained that a boycott was "a recognised tool in a free democratic society".[32] In its own report, Nestlé claimed that Kennedy "was able to overwhelm the inexperienced witness new to the spotlight". Few of the other testifiers were practised witnesses and no one else there had reached such a pinnacle of power and wealth, yet Nestlé's account depicts Ballerin as a poor little chap and regrets that it overlooked Kennedy's "lack of sympathy for big business and his commitment to the economically disadvantaged".[33]

Why should big business, which prides itself on strength, competence and PR skills, be in need of 'sympathy'? As for the commitment to the economically disadvantaged, Nestlé claimed to share this: "I hardly need to emphasise that we are all equally distressed by this sad situation and we are also equally anxious to help in finding a solution," proclaimed Carl Angst, General Manager of Nestlé, in a keynote speech at the 13th International Congress of Nutrition in 1985, referring to poverty in the developing world.[34] The concept of the Nestlé boycott being an anti-capitalist conspiracy was laughable. The boycotters included nuns, clergymen, business people and lawyers, parents and childless people, teachers, health workers and students, all having different individual political and philosophical opinions. It was an issue which drew together many strange bedfellows, and as the boycott spread to other industrialised countries, it attracted support from many shades of political opinion.

good capitalism: the paradoxes of US society

As a European, I was fascinated that so many US citizens, who were neither Marxists nor socialists, had such a strong and active commitment to the Nestlé boycott, and through this I learned something about the paradoxes in US society. Although the USA embodies industrialised capitalism, there is in fact a long-established tradition of resistance to the big corporation when it behaves badly.

A bulwark of the power of the giant corporation in the USA is the 14th Amendment to the US Constitution. The original aim of the 1866 Civil Rights Act had been to give equal rights to black citizens; "citizens of every race and color were to have equal rights to make contracts, to sue, and enjoy full and equal benefit of all laws and proceedings for the security of person and property." This legislation did not change the position of black Americans; they were excluded from basic political participation in society until the 1960s, and are still economically and socially oppressed by white racism. Instead, however, the corporations were able to increase their power by claiming the same rights as individual citizens. In 1886 the Supreme

Court ruled that corporations were "natural persons"[35] and therefore entitled to the protection of the Bill of Rights. Whenever a state government tried to use laws to curb corporate action which hurt people, the federal courts invalidated any legislation by citing the 'due process' clause of the 14th Amendment. This prohibited a state government from depriving any person of life, liberty or property without due process of law. In the eyes of US law, a legal entity such as a corporation is treated as a person, so that any attempt at restriction of company activity was interpreted as taking away the "life, liberty and property" of the anthropomorphised corporation.

Globally, by the turn of 19th and 20th centuries, industrialised capitalism had a soured reputation. The oppression and exploitation of workers by the owners of capital led to revolutions in Europe, but to legislation and regulation in the USA.[37] Both Republicans and Democrats attempted to restrict the more unwholesome activities of big companies. The 1890 Sherman Antitrust Act was designed to prevent monopolies and cartels from price-fixing, maintaining inferior goods and services, and suppressing competitors and innovation. The Sherman Act was used to break the stranglehold of the oil, steel and tobacco monopolies in the early 20th century. Despite the tide of deregulation since the advent of 'Reaganomics', the Sherman Act was used to confront Microsoft in 1998. Despite the government winning the case, it failed to take strong corrective measures which perhaps illustrates how even a fine constitution and good laws can buckle under a political culture. As this book goes to press, the world is learning some harsh lessons about the effects of lax regulation.

Of course the big question throughout the 20th century was whether there was a boundary between the big corporations and government? Did the dog wag the tail or the tail wag the dog? Historical analysts have shown that quite early in the century, powerful corporations used clever methods to influence policy. This was not just through the bankrolling of political candidates, but by the use of PR tactics to shape government decisions. This 'engineering of consent' was an admitted aim of corporations and still is, but now the bland initials PR (significantly these have replaced the words in full) cover activities with the same purpose. It is that very 'PR' that has renamed 'capitalism' as 'the market system' because it sounds nicer.[38]

The idea of government interference contradicts the US concept of liberty, yet such was (and is) the power of the corporations, that their interests and the government's can be the same. Despite of the myth that any US citizen can become President, only those who have the backing of the controllers of capital can get into politics.* Corporations possess capital because the development of the law has provided the fiscal advantages that enable them to accumulate wealth while avoiding punitive taxation. That fiscal advantage was won through corporate PR influence on politicians. This is one of the reasons why so many US corporations were able to grow so large and why the USA came to dominate the world economy.

US citizens take these Goliaths for granted, but they have always loved their Davids, those individuals or small groups of citizens who challenge the practices of the big corporations. There are also those US politicians who resist the pressures of big business and fight to end the exploitation of the ordinary US citizen and consider their well-being. The dynamic between the state and big business, and the actions of the ordinary citizen who challenges what she or he sees is wrong, is fundamental to US life. It was a faith in the possibility of 'good' capitalism that motivated many activists in the infant feeding issue. The very name of one group, the Interfaith Centre for Corporate Responsibility, indicated that many US citizens believed sincerely that the large-scale capitalist enterprise could be induced to act morally. Nevertheless, it was a fusion of corporate and political interests which was to override these moral considerations when the US government came to a decision on the Code that its own committee had proposed.

the involvement of the international health agencies

The aftermath of the Kennedy hearing was a decision to draft an International Code to regulate the marketing of commercial infant feeding products. The US Committee's decision had triggered the process. It required the involvement of the WHO and UNICEF, who convened the WHO/UNICEF Meeting on Infant and Young Child Feeding in October 1979. This was welcomed by everyone involved in the controversy. Of course mothers in poor countries, for whom little had changed, remained unaware of all this activity on their behalf. They continued to take home their free samples and to cope with the diarrhoea, the debt and the funerals.

The baby food companies were put out that some participants at the WHO/UNICEF meeting were from the very groups (the Berne Third World Group, ICCR, INFACT, International Organisation of Consumer Unions, OXFAM and War on Want) who had criticised them. The companies had almost a hundred years of experience in

---

* Or survive in politics? I remain open-minded about this topic and would love to be proved wrong.

dealing with doctors, but were nonplussed by these groups: how could they manipulate people who were not careerists, were uninterested in making money and had nothing to lose in the battle themselves? The outcome of the meeting was the decision to form an international code for the marketing of breastmilk substitutes.. Though accepting the idea in principle, the companies expressed doubts about an international code, as opposed to local codes, because they feared it might lead to a loss of national sovereignty. This patriotic and philosophical problem had never worried them when they produced their own International Council of Infant Food Industries (ICIFI) Code at the time of the Nestlé lawsuit in 1975.[39] Another outcome of the 1979 WHO/UNICEF meeting was the foundation of the International Baby Food Action Network (IBFAN) which enabled the groups struggling to halt the aggressive marketing of baby foods to maintain the links forged during this period of hard work.

At this stage WHO, whose task is to improve world health, and UNICEF, which is concerned with the welfare of children, fell into the role of mediators between the pressure groups and the baby food industry, rather than defenders of infant and young child health. This diversion of skills gives an insight into the vulnerability of these international agencies. They have to be cautious about taking strong stands on sensitive issues because they are beholden to the world's most powerful groups for their survival. This is not a direct relationship, or at least it was not at the time. (In 1987 the successor of ICIFI, the International Assembly of Infant Food Manufacturers, achieved the status of an NGO within WHO, which changed the relationship.) It was significant at that time that the USA paid 25% of WHO's budget and that the other major industrialised countries made up 70% altogether. Delayed payment could be used as an implicit threat to pressure WHO (and other UN organisations) if the organisation attempted any action perceived to be against the interests of these governments. As the US government represented the interests and principles of big business, it was unlikely to support moves that restricted the activities of these companies. Nestlé may have been Swiss, it may have been the market leader in milk and baby foods in the developing world, but it was only doing what the US-based companies wanted to do, namely, dominate the world market. Like any government, the different factions within it, were not all motivated by the same agendas. At the time of the Kennedy hearings, the US government was proud to show its caring face. It was bad luck that the Code vote happened to coincide with a change of government and values.

the USA rejects the code

After a year of revision and consultation between governments, infant feeding experts, the baby food industry and the NGOs, the International Code of Marketing of Breastmilk Substitutes (the Code) was produced. At the World Health Assembly[36] in May 1981 it was overwhelmingly approved by 118 countries. There were three abstentions and one vote against.[41] The US delegate, Dr John Bryant, under new orders from the US State department, had reluctantly voted against the Code.

This was an extraordinary event because the drive to bring in an international code had come from the US Senate Committee's decisions, and US delegates had led much of the drafting process. WHO and UNICEF staff who understood that the legal status of the Code would affect implementation had pressed for the Code to be a WHA Regulation. Under UN protocol, a Regulation is stronger than a Recommendation because it has to be implemented within a set period of time. The US delegation had argued for the Code to be a Recommendation because it would be accepted back home more easily. Though other delegates were troubled by this, they pragmatically accepted this compromise because they knew it was important for the USA to be on board. The Code was on track to be born in this form when, a couple of days before the vote, the newly appointed President Ronald Reagan* ordered the sudden change of direction. He had been lobbied by the US baby food industry.

This sudden shift of policy brought to light the corporate/political fusion of US politics. Other countries with strong industrial interests against the Code, such as milk-producing New Zealand and European countries, had more to lose economically than the US, but their votes were based on moral and health grounds. Political ideology played little part. The UK, under Prime Minister Margaret Thatcher**, was a bastion of free-market economic policies and she was close to President Reagan. Nevertheless, she approved the common sense of regulating marketing which harmed children, and the UK wholly supported the Code's adoption. This is significant because it was Thatcher and Reagan who together promoted a brand of capitalism that put inordinate power into the hands of corporations.[42] It seemed that even the Iron Lady (as Thatcher was called) saw the need for limits to rapacious marketing that harmed babies. The US

* US President 1981–1989.
**PM from 1979–1991.

government's decision shocked and embarrassed many US citizens. There was extensive newspaper coverage and two leading US Agency for International Development (USAID) officials resigned in protest. Public demonstrations were held and 10,000 letters and telegrams were received by the White House and the State Department. Both the House of Representatives and the Senate approved resolutions expressing dismay at the vote.

The pretext for the US vote was that the Code's provisions would "cause serious and constitutional problems for the US itself". This was nonsense. The Code was a recommendation so that each country would be free to use its customary methods of implementing public health measures. Neither WHO nor UNICEF are law-enforcing bodies; they cannot coerce any country to implement the Code. There were no constitutional problems. If there were, why had the USA proposed the Code and supported its delegates throughout the drafting process? The Code does not restrict the sale and availability of breastmilk substitutes. It bans all advertising, but endorses the provision of scientific and factual information for health workers. The US government decision did not represent the will of the US people, who rejected the idea of their own companies, as well as Nestlé, being implicated in infant illness and death. But the Reagan administration, under industry pressure, acted to keep the door open for the companies to push their products wherever they could, regardless of their effects.[43]

History has shown repeatedly that the infant feeding product industry has never controlled itself voluntarily and that the medical profession, in spite of its supposed authority, lacked the solidarity, the will or the skill to deal alone with the marketing practices. It took the energy and dedication of a mixed band of people, brought together through their common sense of responsibility, to say 'this cannot continue', and to do something. The baby food activists were conspicuously moderate in their protests and there is no illegal or violent action on their record. The Code was produced in an open forum, respected and accepted by governments spanning all shades of political colours. There are international rules for sports, and players agree that following them is the only workable way of running tournaments. US government representatives declared the Code to be against the interests of free trade and 'competition', because they realised that an international code of marketing concerning any product might restrict their own companies, who wanted to be free to change the rules as they went along so that they could always 'win'.

16 what is the code?

"That's why I have never done a commercial. Never. Ever. Because if I have any quality on the screen, it's that people will believe that what I say is true. Or at least, they certainly believe that I believe it's true. Now if you do a commercial, it's palpable that you're saying this is the best margarine because somebody has paid you! That's all."
Broadcaster and naturalist David Attenborough interviewed by Esther Teichmann, The Guardian, 4 November 2006

the key points

Reluctantly, I am going to devote a few pages to the International Code of Marketing of Breastmilk Substitutes (the Code).[1] Rules, codes and laws rarely make good reading because the need for a definitive clarity stretches them into boredom. They are often misunderstood because few of us have the patience to read them. Lawyers are well paid because they have the tenacity to plough through documents which make the ordinary mortal collapse into a coma. The Code is not too bad, but it is no adventure story and its very moderation crushes any dramatic possibilities.* It is important because it is the only tool there is for establishing a basis for consistent, international, ethical marketing practice to protect all babies, whether breastfed or artificially fed. It also protects parents, carers and health workers from commercial pressures which undermine the impartiality essential for making decisions about infant and young child feeding. Here is a brief explanation of the Code's main points.

why the code is necessary

Most babies are less likely to get ill or die if they are breastfed, so breastfeeding must be protected. To do this, accurate information about breastfeeding must be disseminated and false information stopped. The promotion of breastmilk substitutes damages breastfeeding. For good and bad reasons, many babies are fed with

---

* The Code is remarkable in that it was the very first international 'consumer' code. Its formation provoked ideas of other international marketing codes for products such as pharmaceuticals. This alarmed big business.

> "The marketing of breastmilk substitutes requires special treatment, which makes usual marketing practices unsuitable for these products."
> Preamble to the International Code of Marketing of Breastmilk Substitutes, 1981

breastmilk substitutes. This is a high-risk process so the carers of these babies must be well-informed about the use of artificial milks and other breastmilk substitutes. The marketing of milks, bottles, teats, dummies, drinks, cereals and solid foods or anything used instead of breastfeeding should not threaten babies' health and survival, nor undermine breastfeeding as the normal mode of infant feeding.

aim, scope and status

a. The Code's aim is: "To contribute to the provision of safe and adequate nutrition for infants, by the protection and promotion of breastfeeding and by the proper use of breastmilk substitutes, when these are necessary, on the basis of adequate information and through appropriate marketing and distribution."

b. The Code regulates the marketing of all breastmilk substitutes (not just infant formula), whether suitable or not, and infant feeding utensils. These include:

- Any product marketed for baby feeding, whether suitable or not, during the first six months.
- Any product marketed for baby feeding after six months which replaces the breastmilk part of the diet.
- Any feeding bottle, teat or dummy.

In practical terms this means: infant formula; special formula; follow-up formula, any other milk or pseudo-milk (eg soy-based) products, infant 'teas', juices and bottled waters; complementary foods before six months, feeding bottles, teats and dummies and any other new products which are marketed for babies.

A country may add any other product to its Code, especially if there is evidence that this product undermines breastfeeding: for

> *"If advertising simply provided information, it would be hard to object. But a lot of advertising makes us feel we need something that we previously didn't need. The advertiser may have only wanted us to buy his brand rather than another. But the overall effect is to make people want more."*
> Economist Professor Richard Layard, Happiness, Penguin, Allen Lane 2005

example Brazil includes nipple shields in its Code because their promotion and use can do harm to breastfeeding.

Countries may also extend the age to which the Code applies and add extra provisions. For instance, in Malaysia they ban infant feeding product companies from involvement in baby shows involving children up to three years old. A country can add a provision to prevent any marketing activity which undermines breastfeeding and responsible artificial feeding.

c. The Code was designed to function internationally and:
- Applies to companies and governments;
- Is a minimum baseline: governments and companies may strengthen it to make it more effective;
- All companies should implement it even where governments have no regulatory measures;
- To have any real 'teeth', it should be implemented through government regulation or law.

d. The Code is a World Health Assembly (WHA) Resolution which is a collective international decision to tackle a global health problem. Since 1981, twelve other WHA Resolutions on infant and young child feeding have been adopted. These have clarified misinterpretations of the Code and addressed new threats to infant and young child health. All of them restate the importance of making the Code work. For example, the 2002 Global Strategy for Infant and Young Child Feeding was adopted as a WHA Resolution.

The Code's purpose is transparent; like international football rules, it aims to make the game fair for everyone – except that infant feeding is not a game, but a matter of life and death. The drafters of the Code had the vision that if you removed marketing pressure from the arena of infant feeding, everyone involved, including the companies, would find it easier to behave ethically. Fewer babies would get ill or die and the world would be a healthier place.

Here are some explanations of the twelve main provisions:

1. No advertising of breastmilk substitutes, feeding bottles or teats.
If advertising did not work, designers and copywriters would not get paid. Why waste money on ineffective sales tactics? Advertisers claim they provide information, but most artificial milk advertisements are uninformative. For example, the additives used in infant formulas are not proven to be safe for babies under 12 weeks old, yet no advertisement has ever told us this.[2] The Code bans all advertising and promotion to the general public. Any company information directed to health workers must be restricted to scientific and factual information and not be promotional.

Parents and carers who artificially feed do not 'need' advertisements, which persuade the use of one brand. These cloud the information and make decision-making difficult. Most parents and health workers find it difficult to get the truth about product quality and safety. Until recently even health workers were unaware of the dangers of the intrinsic contamination of powdered infant formula. No advertisement informed them of this risk. Artificial feeding requires impartial information and guidance from well-trained scientists and health workers.[3] Many health workers are influenced by advertisements and the persuasive arguments (and gifts) of marketing personnel which maintain the normality of artificial feeding and censor the risks.[4] If the companies behaved ethically they would publicise the risks, give warnings and disseminate safer feed preparation instructions.[5]

2. No free samples or free or low cost supplies.
Health workers who give free samples of breastmilk substitutes reinforce mothers' doubts by demonstrating their own lack of confidence in breastfeeding. Artificial milk satiates a baby's appetite, so he cannot stimulate the quantity of breastmilk he needs. His mother's body gets the message that her baby does not require much breastmilk and reduces production. If given during the early 'calibration period' just after birth, this may set breastmilk production at a low amount for the rest of her lactation. Most women who end up artificially-feeding stick to the brand given in hospital, which is why companies are so keen on this form of promotion. How can a woman make an informed choice to breastfeed if the process is damaged at the start? The free sample has been implicated in the deaths of thousands of poor babies when its use reduced their mothers'

SUMMARY OF THE CODE'S MAIN PROVISIONS

1. No advertising or promotion of any breastmilk substitutes (any product marketed or represented to replace breastmilk), feeding bottles or teats.

2. No free samples or free or low cost supplies.

3. No promotion of products in or through healthcare facilities.

4. No contact between marketing personnel and mothers (including health workers paid by a company to advise or teach).

5. No gifts or personal samples to health workers or their families.

6. Labels should be in an appropriate language and have no words or pictures idealising artificial feeding.

7. Only scientific and factual information to be given to health workers.

8. Governments should ensure that objective and consistent information is provided on infant and young child feeding.

9. All information on artificial feeding, including labels, should explain the benefits of breastfeeding and warn of the costs and hazards associated with artificial feeding.

10. Unsuitable products should not be promoted for babies.

11. All products should be of a high quality and take account of the climatic and storage conditions of the country where they are to be used.

12. Manufacturers and distributors should comply with the Code (and all subsequent WHA Resolutions on infant feeding) independently of any government action to implement it.

Source: WHO European Series No 87, 2000, p150

breastmilk and made the purchase of artificial milk necessary. Too poor to buy sufficient amounts, mothers 'stretched' the milk by over-dilution so that their babies gradually starved, succumbing to inevitable infections. If a mother is not helped to re-stimulate her own supply (and a sick, weak baby may be unable to suckle effectively), she is in a desperate situation. She cannot afford the replacement product and she may be unable to re-establish her own milk in time.

Once a doctor from a poor, tropical country said, "But I must have free samples. I have to have something to give a poor mother to take away."[6] He saw the consulting room as the boundary of his responsibilities and believed he must hand over a token gift to maintain the doctor/patient relationship. In his country he might as well have handed a mother a lump of bad meat for her baby. Handing out a free sample is taking a stand against breastfeeding.

Infant formula samples are placed in 'discharge bags' full of promotional products. These are presented as attractive gifts when in fact they are snares to entrap women at their most vulnerable. Why do even the most intelligent and well-informed women accept these 'gifts' and tend to believe what promotions convey? Well, there is evidence that the glorious 'hormone of love', oxytocin, makes people extra trusting, so it is possible that women are more vulnerable at this time.[7] Companies pay hospitals for the privilege (and profit) of distributing discharge bags. When a woman goes home without support for breastfeeding, she will inevitably go through a period of doubt and that is when she turns to the free sample.

In the 1980s and 90s some companies purposefully directed their free samples in a special discharge bag directed 'for the breastfeeding mother'. Through market research they had discovered that mothers who had wanted to breastfeed but given up through lack of support continued to use infant formula for longer than the mothers who had planned to artificially feed. They made more money out of 'the breastfeeding mother' than the 'formula feeding mothers', so they pushed free samples towards the former.[8]

A major source of free samples has been the free or low-cost supplies to maternity hospitals. These exploit an ambiguity in the Code which permitted charitable donations to institutions. The drafters of the Code intended free supplies to be for orphanages, but companies claimed that maternity facilities were institutions.[9] Supplies are such an effective marketing tool that companies pay thousands of dollars to induce hospitals to accept them. When free milk is readily available, health workers tend to hand it out.

The Code does not prohibit the donation of milk in special circumstances. What it does stipulate is that if a baby needs artificial feeding, then whoever provides the milk must ensure a continuous supply for as long as the baby needs it: that is, for a year or more. I have never yet met a health professional who handed out a free sample and then took responsibility for ensuring a supply of free milk for a year or more for that individual baby.

A 1986 WHA Resolution clarified this Code ambiguity and banned all free supplies, stating that any breastmilk substitutes needed should be purchased through "normal procurement channels".[10] A 1994 WHA Resolution made this edict clearer by banning all free and low-cost supplies in any part of the healthcare system. Interestingly, this was the first WHA Resolution which included full Code implementation that the USA endorsed.[11] There had been a change of government and President Bill Clinton's* administration seemed less hostile to the principles of the Code, though nothing was done to implement it in the USA. Free supplies persist in many countries, with three-quarters of the major companies flouting this rule.[12] Health workers' collusion in this practice cannot be denied, but ignorance and intimidation exonerate some.

3. No promotion of products in or through healthcare facilities.
Since the advent of the milk depots clinics and hospitals have been associated with the provision, supply and even sales of milks, bottles and teats. This undermines breastfeeding. Many health workers are so used to their hospitals and clinics being plastered with company posters, calendars, notepads, pens, diaries and electronic gizmos that they do not perceive their function. Each time a health worker scribbles a note or writes a prescription on a paper with a company logo they endorse that company's product. Many claim that the notepad does not link them with the company, but how many doctors would write prescriptions bearing the name or logo of an alcohol or tobacco company, a casino or lap dancing club?

Though direct corruption can exist, many health workers are unwitting participants in this game and receive little personal benefit through acting as salespeople for the companies. As Dr Natividad Clavano (1932–2007), the Paediatric Chief at Baguio General Hospital in the Philippines, said, "We allowed the companies to touch the lives of our babies, not because we did not care, but because we did not realise the consequences of granting such a privilege."[13] When Dr Clavano decided to do something about breastfeeding, her most difficult task was persuading the hospital staff that you could run a maternity ward without company endorsement. Health worker practices have proved hard to change, because the commercial links have become such an intrinsic part of their lives.

The record from the USA in the early 20th century shows how vital it was for companies to establish themselves within the healthcare system. This is still the case and it is an area where companies struggle fiercely to resist Code implementation. They know medical endorsement is vital for sales.

* US president 1993–2001.

4. No contact between company marketing personnel and mothers.
After the publicity from Nestlé's infamous 1970s lawsuit, companies phased out the notorious 'milk nurses', only to replace them with such devices as telephone 'carelines', direct mailing with free DVDs and other babycare advice materials, email marketing and internet websites. In China in 2005, Nestlé positioned doctors in 'Nutrition Corners' in supermarkets to promote products to pregnant and breastfeeding women.[14] Using qualified health workers inspires trust. In many countries, health workers and hospitals sell the names and addresses of clients to promotional agencies to facilitate direct mailing to new mothers.

Careline telephone numbers are widely publicised in parents' magazines, the internet and on the products. Mothers usually seek outside help when they are most worried and there appears to be scant regulation of the content of company advice. Monitoring shows that company advisers have given misinformation about safe feed preparation. In 2007, long after the UK Food Standards Agency had issued new advice on making up each feed with boiled water that had not cooled to less than 70°C and using it just before a feed, a Cow & Gate* Careline adviser told a caller, "Prepare bottles of sterile water in advance. That stays fresh without refrigeration for 24 hours. Take from the bottle and mix. That formula is good for an hour."[15] Such laxity echoes the practices of the milk nurses of the 1950s and 60s who promoted artificial milk regardless of the safety of babies.

5. No gifts or personal samples to health workers or their families.
It is hard to go against the workplace norm. If one health worker tries to take a stand by refusing to use notepads or diaries, she or he might be viewed as petty or sanctimonious. Resisting company pressure when your superiors do not implies criticism of their principles, and in the hierarchy of health systems this makes working life difficult. The Code makes it easier for everyone because it provides a clear, realistic base for practice; everyone can refer to it and know where they stand.

The issue of receiving small gifts is often viewed as a trivial matter. Where low wages barely cover basic needs, an object's value may not be so small. Any gift makes us feel cherished and loved by the giver. A health worker can feel obligated, even affectionate, towards the salesperson who has given an attractive or much-needed pen, notepad and diary, and of course this is why it is done. There is no such thing as a free biro; a profit-making company is just that and it is

---

* Cow & Gate is now owned by Danone.

"In 2001 and 2002 I worked in a hospital in Gabon, West Africa. There was no hot water, soap, disinfectant, toilet or hand towel paper, syringes, bed linen or food or even the most basic medical equipment. Throughout, Nestlé offered free conferences and study days. It supplied posters, textbooks, prescription pads and pens all displaying its logo. All staff were invited to a monthly ward-based pharmaceutical presentation that included promotion of Nestlé Nan and Pre-Nan artificial milks. The midwives and nurses were poorly paid and often did two jobs to support their families. One day the ward manager came in wearing a gorgeous necklace. It was a gold chain with a central, solid gold motif of a mother bird and her young on a nest: the famous Nestlé logo. It was a gift from the Nestlé salesman."

Sue Saunders, Lactation Consultant (IBCLC).

very inefficient and unbusiness-like if it spends money on PR tactics that do not improve sales. An analysis of the effect of sponsorship on doctors showed that 61% of physicians believe that promotions do not influence their own practice, but only 16% believed this about other physicians. Small gifts have as potent effect as large. "The sheer ubiquity of trinkets . . . is evidence of effectiveness; why else would profit-minded companies continue to provide them? Thus policies against gifts should not be limited to large gifts." The recipient's bias towards the gift-giver is unconscious and unintentional. The authors found that all gifts subliminally influenced and undermined the quality of clinical decision-making. They state that a policy of prohibition is the only answer.[16]

Of course the big gifts go to the big people. Between 1983 and 1991, the AAP received contributions from infant formula companies which amounted to US$8.3 million, in addition to the income from journal advertisements and design costs of hospital paediatric clinics.[17]

Individuals may be offered irresistible deals. Nestlé offered a highly-respected professor an exceptionally large sum of money for the privilege of translating his book and distributing it in China. All they asked in return was that Nestlé's name was on the book cover. The book is a best-seller about the use of medication during breastfeeding and provides useful information for health workers. The professor resisted the offer, but he is unusual.[18]

This problem has been addressed by WHA Resolutions in 1996 and 2005 which urge member States to ensure that financial support for

> *"I would not suggest that a woman sees a fluffy duckling and thinks 'right, I'll give up breastfeeding'. But if she is having trouble feeding her baby, the packaging appears to offer reassurance. 'Closer than ever to breastmilk' might be just close enough."*
> George Monbiot, 'Not what it says on the tin', The Guardian 19th June 2007.

professionals working in infant and young child health did not create conflicts of interest.[19] This is a particular problem within the health professions because the practice has become so entrenched that few see it as bribery or corruption. These Resolutions were aimed at governments like that of Canada which pressured hospitals to accept payment for free supplies to make up public budget deficits. The fact that companies pay substantial sums to 'donate' free supplies indicates their high value as a marketing strategy.

This does not let individuals off the hook, but it is clear that governments should not allow systems of career advancement to depend on company sponsorship. We trust David Attenborough's words (see start of this chapter) because he has never taken money from a company. In contrast, there is a shadow over the work of many researchers. Dr Ranjit Chandra's Nestlé-funded work was published in the BMJ during the 1990s, widely cited and underpinned the launch of a new Nestlé product. In the 21st century it was discovered that his research was fraudulent and it brought his University, his profession and the BMJ into disrepute.[20]

6. Labels should be in an appropriate language and have no words or pictures idealising artificial feeding.

The Code has detailed instructions about labels, the principal ones being that they must provide all necessary information about the product and should not discourage breastfeeding. For example, they should state the possibility of the intrinsic pathogenic contamination of powdered infant formula and the new instructions for safer feed preparation.[21]

It seems obvious that you should be able to read instructions in your own language, but astonishingly, companies have fought to evade this rule. In Malawi, Nestlé did not provide local language labels for seven years. From 1993 campaigners and the Malawi government repeatedly requested fulfilment of this Code requirement. Nestlé claimed 'cost restraints' prevented it from action – Nestlé, one of the

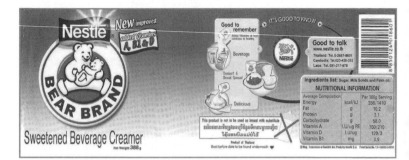

29 Bear Brand Coffee Creamer

THE BREASTFEEDING BEAR

In impoverished Laos, health workers discovered that babies were being fed Nestlé Bear Brand Coffee Creamer as a breastmilk substitute and as a result suffered malnutrition and death. The product logo shows a bear holding her baby in a breastfeeding position which 50% of surveyed adults interpreted to mean the product was good for infants and children. The product also carried a warning sign of a baby bottle with a cross through it, but 50% did not understand its meaning. Only 1.6% of interviewees (who were more literate than average) believed it meant the product was dangerous.

Barennes H et al Misperceptions and misuse of Bear Brand coffee creamer as infant food: national cross sectional survey of consumers and paediatricians in Laos. BMJ 2008;337;a1379

most profitable companies in the world, claimed to be too poor to change a label. In 1999, high profile British comedian and activist Mark Thomas made a TV programme on the baby food issue.[22] Suddenly a command came from Switzerland, from Peter Brabeck, the Chief Executive of Nestlé, to change the labels. Orders were obeyed. The Malawi Ministry of Health noted the labels lacked graphics or warnings and asked for these to be added, but Brabek decreed that the labels should be launched as they were. He could then boast to Mark Thomas that Chichewa labels had been launched. Nestlé highlighted this noble gesture in its 'Code action sheet', sent around the world. All Nestlé's labels in Switzerland are in three languages.

Parents want their baby to be healthy and the picture of a gorgeous child on the tin of milk conveys the message that theirs will be equally thriving and happy: a suggestion which led to the Code's ban of these idealised images. Some companies removed the baby pictures but replaced them with equally seductive images. Teddy bears, giraffes, rabbits, ducks and other cutesy-wootsy images all give the impression of a benign and beneficial product. The terms 'maternalised' or 'humanised' are banned by the Code but companies defied these rules and invented idealising brand names such as 'Nurture', 'Gold', 'Bebelac' and 'Similac'. Skilled marketing psychologists are highly paid to create words and images which convey trust, security and motherliness.

7. Only scientific and factual information to be given to health workers. Health workers need to know exactly what is in a product and the companies have a duty to provide these facts as clearly as possible. It is difficult to find objective information about products and advertisements in health worker journals do not provide it. If you ask truthful editors why they accept advertisements, they never say, 'They are essential reading to improve professional practice', but 'We need their money and couldn't publish the journal in its current form without company payments for advertising space.'

Some advertisements are dressed up as 'science'. For example, an advertisement for a Cow & Gate infant formula headed "What every midwife should know" announces that babies fed this product had fewer infections than those fed a "placebo formula". A placebo is an inactive substance. As infant formula can keep a baby alive and provide nutrients, it cannot be considered a placebo. Any comparison must be with breastfeeding or breastmilk-feeding. Barely noticeable at the top left corner is a statement: "Breastmilk provides babies with the best source of nourishment." It does not mention the anti-infective properties of breastmilk or the synergy of protection against infection through breastfeeding. The advertisement refers to a research study which any reader would assume referred to this infant formula. In fact the study used two Aptamil fully-hydrolysed formulas, not the Cow & Gate formula.[21] No midwife has the time to probe the advertisement and may believe that what she reads is science because of the charts and language. She may then recommend this product to a mother. What is of concern is that the UK Royal College of Midwives (RCM), an internationally renowned organisation, has published misleading information, presumably for financial reward.*[23]

* The RCM has announced that it will no longer take advertisments for infant formula. Babyfeeding Law Group, January 2009.

Company information should warn of the risks of the variability of nutrient levels, the likelihood of intrinsic pathogens and that some additives used in artificial milks have not been (and can never be) tested for safety in newborns. In the 21st century promotional health claims, for nutrients still open to scientific scrutiny, persist. If anything is proven to be important for infant development then its inclusion as an ingredient should be made a Codex standard. The failure to implement this part of the Code highlights the constraints on ordinary health workers who may waste time reading promotional materials but have no access to accurate information about products.

8. Governments should ensure that objective and consistent information is provided on infant and young child feeding.
Governments, health bodies and breastfeeding support organisations spend energy and money designing information and disseminating it through various media, but all is wasted if contradictory messages come through product promotion. When Brazil evaluated their multi-million dollar breastfeeding campaigns during the 1980s, they learned that if artificial milk and bottle promotion continued, it cancelled out the effectiveness. This inspired those involved to get good Code legislation adopted and breastfeeding rates rose.[24]

In 2004, the UK Government's Department of Health (DOH) sent an attractive and accurate pack of infant feeding information to health workers who worked with mothers and babies. The pack included a well-written explanation of the reasons and evidence for the UK policy (based on WHO) recommending six months' exclusive breastfeeding. However, jars of pureed baby foods continued to be mislabelled four years later.[25] This inconsistency demonstrates the inertia or impotence of governments to fulfill their commitments made at World Health Assemblies.

9. All information on artificial feeding, including labels, should explain the benefits of breastfeeding and warn of the costs and hazards associated with artificial feeding.
Electrical goods carry instructions and warnings about the risks of improper use. Baby milks, bottles and teats can be just as dangerous, so the potential hazards of misuse must be clearly explained. Labels should warn that the baby who is artificially fed is at greater risk of diarrhoea, pneumonia and other infections, however hygenic the feed preparation. Labels must also warn of the economic hazards. In Haiti a month's supply of commercial infant formula costs a factory

worker's monthly wage.[26] An artificially fed baby requires more medical costs. The label and any other product information must warn the purchaser of these matters before they make the decision.

10. Unsuitable products should not be promoted for babies.

Throughout the debate of the 1970s, when companies claimed to be following their own ethical codes, they argued that advertising artificial milks was necessary because ignorant mothers would use inappropriate foods. At the same time they promoted products such as sweetened condensed milk and custard powder for babies, even putting infant feeding instructions on the labels presenting them as suitable breastmilk substitutes.

From the Code's beginning, companies have picked out loopholes and launched other products, such as sweetened teas, juices, follow-up milks and water in tiny feeding bottles. Sweetened teas damaged babies' emerging teeth eventually leading to lawsuits by parents in Europe.[27] These teas were the well-packaged equivalents of the sugar water that the companies criticised poor mothers for using.

The companies invented 'follow-on milks' (FOMs) to avoid marketing restrictions. Experts agree that a baby who is not breastfed (or breastmilk-fed) should continue to be fed standard infant formula until one year old. A WHO resolution has judged FOMs to be unnecessary products.[28] FOMs are aggressively advertised in many countries. A UK survey revealed that one in five women had introduced FOM (a health risk for babies under six months) before three months.[29] They are however still breastmilk substitutes because babies need to carry on breastfeeding for two years or beyond and anything which replaces the breastmilk component of the baby's diet is substituting breastmilk. The promotion of FOMs creates confusion with infant formula because the brand and packaging designs are so similar. And that is the point. The companies did not invent them because health workers begged them to produce a less-modified milk for older babies. They created these products as a means of promoting all their breastmilk substitutes and to expand their markets; it has been a successful strategy.

11. All products should be of a high quality and take account of the climatic and storage conditions of the country where they are to be used.

As journalists and the Chinese authorities tussle over the truths behind the 2008 Fonterra/Sanlu contaminated milk scandal, few have

Aptamil

Prebiotics are found in breast milk.
That's why we've put them in our follow-on milk.

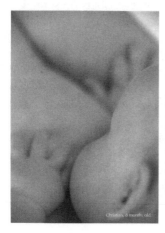

Breast milk and babies are designed for each other by nature. Every mother's breast milk is unique, created specially for her baby, to provide everything her baby needs, for healthy development.

It is well known that breast milk plays an important role in helping to build a baby's immune system. It contains a combination of protective factors including antibodies and prebiotics, helping to protect them from illnesses such as stomach upsets and ear infections. Prebiotics (also found naturally in some fruits and vegetables) are special nutrients that encourage the growth of friendly bacteria in the digestive system. In turn, supporting a baby's natural defences.

That's why Milupa Aptamil Forward contains prebiotics. To find out more about prebiotics you can call us or visit our website.

IMPORTANT NOTICE: Breast milk is best for your baby. Milupa Aptamil Forward Follow-on milk should only be used as part of a mixed diet and not as a breast milk substitute before 6 months.

Aptamil FORWARD

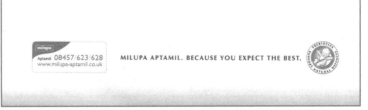

Aptamil 08457/623/628
www.milupa-aptamil.co.uk

MILUPA APTAMIL. BECAUSE YOU EXPECT THE BEST.

30 Companies deny that follow-on milks are breastmilk substitutes.

mentioned that if the Code were implemented this suffering would have been prevented.[30] Both government authorities and the manufacturers have the responsibility to set up monitoring and surveillance systems to ensure quality control. Human greed and corruption cannot be stamped out, but if Code implementation systems were functioning, dangerous products would be discovered earlier and their use prevented.

Most parents have taken it for granted, when they buy a tin of artificial milk, a bottle or a teat, that the contents are of high quality, but they are overly complacent. For decades there has been a worryingly high incidence of inadequate or substandard products, usually only discovered after babies became ill.

The possibility of faulty products being sold in poor countries is far greater. Consumer awareness and pressure may be weak and the expensive infrastructures for challenge non-existent. Transport, climate and storage problems make products more vulnerable. If laws do not exist to use sell-by dates, companies may not put them on the package.

If the Code were adhered to, the number of these accidents would be reduced. If companies stopped promotion, they could spend the money saved on better quality control. Suggest this and marketing managers admit that sales would fall without promotion, which belies their claim that they only sell artificial milk to fulfil a need.

12. Manufacturers and distributors should comply with the Code (and all subsequent WHA Resolutions on Infant Feeding) independently of any government action to implement it.

The basic concept of the Code was that all companies should follow the same ethical marketing practices. Some people believed that they might police each other. The big companies were actively involved in the drafting process. Were they entirely manipulative and cynical? It is possible that a few industry participants were sincerely seeking a functioning international Code, otherwise why had they contributed to the many compromises? Everyone knew that not all countries would have the infrastructures and political stability to establish and implement functioning rules and laws, so it was logical for the companies to agree that they would keep to the Code everywhere regardless of national situations. The experience of almost three decades has shown that companies will only keep to the whole Code if a government makes them do so. Despite repeated avowals at World Health Assemblies, many governments are still unable or unwilling to do this.

> *"Endorsement by association, manipulation by assistance."*
> Paediatrician Derrick Jelliffe (1921–1992) describing the relationship between the baby food companies and health workers

could the code work?

Even before the Code's adoption, one country, Papua New Guinea had legislated to control the use of feeding bottles and artificial milk, and as a result had dramatically reduced infant malnutrition and deaths. In 1976 a third of the children under two in the capital, Port Moresby, had been artificially fed and over two-thirds of these were malnourished. It was then made illegal to sell a bottle without a prescription, and a health worker had to prove it was in a baby's interests to be artificially-fed. Within two years, bottle-feeding had dropped from 35 to 12%, and malnutrition fell by a third. There was high awareness among health workers and the policies could be implemented fully because the companies had not yet established a big market in PNG. The authorities were resolved to make the policy work so at that time the companies did not attempt to sabotage it. The government and health workers were united in their efforts to implement the law.[32]

Then, during the 1990s, satellite TV started to beam advertising into the country, political will faded, and artificial-feeding began to increase.

The international action of the 1970s and 80s had motivated the companies to form an alliance, the International Council of Infant Food Industries (ICIFI). ICIFI was refused NGO status at WHO because of evidence that they had been undermining countries' efforts to implement the Code. Then in 1984, ICIFI transmuted into the International Association of Infant Feeding Manufacturers (IFM). Learning from WHO that it still might not be accepted, it joined an existing umbrella organisation, the International Society of Dietary Food Industries (ISDI) and in 1987, under ISDI's balmy shelter, IFM achieved its longed-for status within WHO. In 2008, IFM was directly funding Pan American Health Organisation (PAHO) projects. This contradicts WHO Guidelines on interactions with the private sector yet PAHO is the Office of WHO for the Americas. The current political climate is now one where the enduring marriage between doctors and baby food companies has spread into a veritable orgy of passion between big business, governments and the UN agencies. Whether they are all consenting adults I cannot tell.

the international health agencies' roles

It is a measure of the limitations of the international health agencies' influence that, in spite of their skill in drafting the Code in a compromise form to suit everyone, including the artificial milk and infant feeding product industry, they could not achieve the health advocacy to enable governments to resist the less acceptable influences of business interests. WHO and UNICEF have only ever had moral authority; they cannot prosecute a government or a company which ignores the Code. Member states create the consensus for WHO to formulate its policies, and what a health minister agrees to at the World Health Assembly often proves difficult to implement at home. With overburdened legislatures and political instability, public prosecutors have been reluctant to bring a case against a powerful foreign company when other problems were so pressing.

the rule of law and big daddy next door: guatemala versus gerber

The case of Guatemala's Code provided a vivid example of how a powerful company can undermine a country's resolve. Guatemala created a splendid Code by involving all the ministries – health, labour, education, economics and so on – in a multi-sectoral committee. There was real political will and cooperation. They appointed a full time person in the Ministry of Health to monitor the Code (commonly the task is tagged on to some overworked official's 'to do' list and gathers dust in their pending tray) and they made a law with real 'teeth'. Sanctions started with warnings and led up to fines and jail sentences. Within the first year over 100 cases were brought to law, real Code implementation was established and breastfeeding was increasing quite dramatically.

Then Gerber,[33] maker of squidgy foods in little jars, applied to register a new range of products. The Guatemalan Ministry of Health refused because it was now illegal to have baby faces on any infant food label and Gerber did. Gerber was outraged. If it really felt its products were essential for the well-being of little Guatemalans the company might have quietly removed the baby faces, but instead Gerber immediately turned to Big Daddy. Gerber claimed that the Guatemalan Code law violated the General Agreement on Tariffs and Trade (GATT) (it did not) and quickly got the US government to threaten withdrawal from the Generalised System of Preferences (GSP). Such action by the USA would have had devastating results for Guatemala's economy. Eventually, Guatemala's Supreme Court of Justice ruled in favour of Gerber by finding a wondrous ambiguity in the interpretation of Spanish. The phrase, "todo alimento, manufacturado o preparado localmente"' which meant "any food whether manufactured or locally prepared" was deemed to mean that their law only applied to locally prepared foods, not the imported Gerber.[34]

In my naïve youth I would have expected WHO to explain to the US government and Gerber, that the Guatemalan Code was vital to protect the health and lives of their babies and that its moral authority would have won the day. Sadly it does not work like that.

Developing countries desperate to keep their fragile economies cobbled together are at the mercy of transnational companies, the international moneylenders and the governments who back them. Poor countries cannot take truly effective stands against such issues as environmental pollution, let alone something as taken for granted as advertising and promotion. Besides, national governments are mostly dominated by men and any issue which affects the daily lives of women is of secondary importance to the 'serious' concerns of defence and trade.

17 power struggles

"Power concedes nothing without demand."
Frederick Douglass (1818–1895)
abolitionist, reformer and women's suffragist

There is a bitter irony that just as the Code was taking its first breath, one of its original parents (the USA) was deciding that it did not want this baby after all and was doing its best to strangle it at birth. The dominant political ideology of the 1980s, led by Ronald Reagan in the USA and Margaret Thatcher in the UK, was based on the economic philosophy of Milton Friedman (1912–2006), an economist famous for saying that there was no such thing as a free lunch.[1] Deregulation was the watchword. Apparently the fewer rules companies had to follow, the more they would thrive and the happier we would all be. If there were any regulations at all they must be voluntary. Most companies publically claimed that they want to behave ethically, yet they worked hard to prevent the enforcement of binding rules which might help them be ethical.

What if individuals behaved in the same way? Any man who thinks it is immoral to beat his wife will welcome laws against all domestic violence. I believe the same principle applies to companies. If companies are sincere about wanting to behave ethically, then they would welcome strong regulations. There is a world of difference between the 'red tape' of silly bureaucracy and the freedom to damage human health with impunity. Deregulation has permitted much of the latter yet has not removed so much of the former.

The Global Compact, launched in 2000 by UN Secretary General Kofi Annan and the President of the International Chamber of Commerce, Adnan Kassar, was supposed to encourage big business to behave ethically, yet its founding principles were that there should be no rules, no monitoring of behaviour and no sanctions.[2] Companies merely had to show intention to fulfil nine stated principles of human rights, labour and environment. No one was going to check up on them. These were such fundamental issues that it is shocking to think that in the 21st century so many companies were still flouting them. Issues such as abolishing child labour, avoiding complicity in human rights abuses and promoting greater environmental responsibility seem the most basic of business morals. Supposing we took this approach with street thugs: 'Now please no mugging old ladies, stabbing rival gangs or setting fire to cars; if you can just show us the intention to try and stop doing these things we'll be terribly pleased with you.'

The Global Compact's framework reflected the balance of power that had shifted so strongly in favour of big business since the concept of the Code was discussed at the time of the 1978 US Senate hearing. When Nestlé was able to join the Global Compact without challenge from the UN, then many observers realised how powerless the UN had become.

From the beginning, a truly international and functioning Code was being crushed as it struggled to stay alive. If it had not been for the tenacity of the International Baby Food Action Network (IBFAN), it might have been utterly forgotten. It seemed to be the hope of some sections of WHO that the Code would simply go away. As campaigners in the 1980s, my colleagues and I often found it difficult to obtain copies of the Code, even when we were paying for it. Once at a WHO international conference, there was a beautiful display of all published WHO booklets, except the Code. When I questioned this, the director of the conference gave me a meaningful look and said, "Don't fight losing battles."[3] It seemed obvious that the Code was supposed to die.

WHO's constitutional objective is "the attainment by all peoples of the highest possible level of health"; but this can "only be achieved to the extent permitted by the manpower and budgetary resources available".[4] Financial support is weighted and it has always been difficult for WHO to implement policies which offend the big paymasters. These have been governments who themselves have become beholden to big business for political and financial support. As former UN Senior Advisor Erskine Childers (1929–1996) wrote in 1993, the USA deliberately kept the UN on the brink of bankruptcy.[5] Any move by WHO to support Code implementation was like pulling the lion's tail. It was an impossible situation.

WHO employees spend their lives balancing on a rickety fence. Their task is to battle for health – and in the modern world much ill-health comes not only from nature or lack of knowledge, but from the effects of the international economic system and the might of transnational companies. This can apply to hunger caused by the appropriation of good land for export crops; the Bhopal disaster*; the role of junk food marketing and lack of breastfeeding in the obesity

---

* In 1984 the Union Carbide pesticide plant in Bhopal, Madhya Pradesh, India, released 42 tonnes of methyl cyanate gas killing 3,000 people immediately, 16,000 in the ensuing weeks and months and leaving thousands more disabled, including the children of mothers who were pregnant during the incident.

epidemic; or the promotional tactics of infant feeding product companies.

Towards the end of the 20th century, the old definitions of 'left' and 'right' became obscured. In the Former Soviet Union (FSU), communists were called 'conservatives' and in the UK, Margaret Thatcher's brand of conservativism was dubbed 'radical'. A government's stance is immaterial, for international trade is dominated by those who control the markets. The so-called 'free market' policies of both elected and non-elected governments came under the influence of big business more comprehensively than ever before. The developing nations have been at the mercy of the controllers of international trade and finance. Any moves to redress the balance of power can ricochet back on the poor. For example, when the oil-exporting nations invested their burgeoning wealth during the 1960s and 1970s, they did so within the international banking system which is dominated by the industrialised nations. The last thing any moneylender wants to do is pay out interest, and the financiers solved the problems of high deposits by flinging money in the form of loans into the poorest nations, thus creating the state of indebtedness which has crippled them. In 2008 people in rich countries now had direct experience of the effects of irresponsible lending, but it is the poor in those rich countries who are suffering most. It is ordinary workers, not the bankers who oversaw the profligacy, who find themselves homeless.

In the impoverished nations, the handicap of financial debt constrains independent decision-making for national policies. The evolution towards real democracy cannot happen if the policies that citizens vote for are crushed by outside forces. In the 1980s, the World Bank (WB) and the International Monetary Fund (IMF) bailed out indebted countries on condition that they 'adjusted' their entire economic and social infrastructures according to the paymasters' prescription. These financial cardinals demanded major cuts in internal investment in health systems. The WB openly advocated a two-tier system, with the state providing minimal healthcare for the poor, insisting on charges for services and leaving the rest to 'the market'. These 'Structural Adjustment' packages damaged the health of mothers and children; for example, in some countries, women stopped going to health facilities for ante-natal checks and childbirth because they could not afford to pay.[6] The industrialised world preached democracy, but its financial institutions assumed the right to interfere with internal policies.

It is important to state that by the 21st century the WB acknowledged that the inequality resulting from structural adjustment was bad for economic growth. They had failed in their own purpose. They also admitted that poverty is as much a political problem as an economic one.[7]

WHO did not challenge these health-damaging policies, perhaps for fear of offending the governments and other paymasters who backed these policies and on whose subscriptions WHO depended. UNICEF was a little bolder and in a publication titled Adjustment with a Human Face argued that "adjustment policies should safeguard the vital needs of a country's population and put human concerns at the centre of development."[8]

The world has now changed way beyond the terms of my somewhat simplistic analysis. Now it is almost impossible to distinguish the boundaries between governments and big business. There have always been interactions between UN agencies and business but now the cult of 'Public-Private Partnerships' between companies, governments, and some NGOs is preached with little debate. There is no agreed definition of a 'Public-Private Partnership' yet it is the buzz phrase of the 21st century. The proportions of money that governments pay to UN agencies, though still important, are less significant now that big business has gained so much power and influence. It seems that democratically elected leaders must engage with non-elected henchmen to promote their common interests. This might be good or bad. The process is not transparent and many of the actors involved are not accountable to measures for public scrutiny.[9]

UN Special Envoy, Stephen Lewis, is disturbed by the deals signed between the companies and the UN. Lewis says that "UN agencies seem willing to partner with any multinational, whether it be the maker of Agent Orange (Dow Chemical) or fast-food behemoths like McDonalds." He cites the deals with the pharmaceutical industry which contributes low cost drugs to fight the AIDS pandemic. It looks good, but what it really does is give legitimacy to 'Big Pharma'. This is a case of 'image transfer', sometimes called 'bluewashing' which makes the UN Global Compact so helpful to business interests.[10]

The experience of all those engaged in trying to achieve Code implementation (and they include a broad range of bodies, agencies and individuals) for the past 27 years is that the infant feeding product manufacturers have at best ignored and at worst sabotaged efforts to make the Code work. Where Government authority has established working rules, there is a constant attempt at erosion.

I do not have space to analyse the balancing act that WHO employees perform every day of their working lives, but I can give a personal anecdote. In 2000 I was attending a WHO/UNICEF meeting on infant feeding in WHO in Geneva. It had been officially agreed between both sides that representatives from neither NGOs nor the infant feeding product industry would be invited or permitted to attend. During the meeting my boss had to visit the Director General's office – and there discovered that representatives from the baby food industry were listening in on the meeting.[11]

the nature of the beast

The transnational enterprises integrate themselves with governments, because this is the best way of achieving their ends. Conflict with them is counter-productive to business advancement. This is why companies are so chameleon-like. If they can advertise on television in one country they will, if not allowed to in another they will not. They will boast of their innovative marketing in the one and of their ethical marketing in the other. Now, through the internet, they can evade national regulation.

Because PR departments are skilled at projecting a benign image, we forget that the primary purpose of companies is not to do good or even provide useful products. In the 1980s, a director of US Steel (later renamed US X) remarked that his company's purpose was not to make steel but to make money. In the 1990s ENRON manipulated energy supplies in California resulting in serious power cuts. Through depriving the population of energy ENRON increased its profits. Public health and well-being and the pursuit of profit can be conflicting goals. Enterprises which market less aggressively find themselves pushed out of the market place by their less squeamish competitors, so that it becomes more difficult for companies who want to behave well to do so.

History has shown repeatedly that without legal restraints companies will behave unethically, and when this happens others must follow suit or shut up shop. It is up to us to say when to stop, and if we really do live in democracies we must demand that our representatives, our governments, establish the checks. If international measures are ignored, then we must persuade our governments to fulfil them. If we find that the channels for protest and challenge are blocked, then democracy does not truly exist.

It is a waste of energy focusing on whether the director of a

> *"The distribution of breastmilk substitutes as humanitarian aid almost destroyed our breastfeeding programmes."*
> Dr Anahit Demirchyan, Baby Friendly Coordinator for Armenia, 1996

company is a 'nice person' or not. The participants in the transnational enterprise game (and most of us who use money are participants) are not evil beings plotting destruction, they are players (some willing and some not) in a system that is out of control. What we must be suspicious of are the protestations of companies that they are principally concerned with human welfare. That is not their role; the 'caring' image is simply part of marketing and has nothing to do with the realities of big business.

The US government has often criticised the human rights records of other countries. If the US had taken a moral stand on the infant feeding issue it could have led the world in implementing change for good. The companies would have had to reduce their markets in breastmilk substitutes, as tobacco companies are expected to do with cigarettes. Tax incentives could have been devised to help companies 'demarket' milks and to diversify into other products. The so-called 'free' market system is manipulated through fiscal measures by most governments, and many products are supported by both open and hidden subsidies. The US was one of the first governments to support 'demarketing' when it paid farmers not to produce certain crops because this was judged to be for the common good. Surely this was a far more draconian infringement of free market principles than setting guidelines for the marketing of a product which could kill children?*

Every baby in the world is an individual and has a right to the life and liberty that the US has claimed to be defending in many a military conflict, yet when it came to the commercial exploitation of babies, these rights are set aside. Now UN and government aid agencies (including USAID), urge poor women to breastfeed as though mothers themselves had established the sales and promotion of the products and the damaging medical customs. If the Code were fully implemented in the USA, it would be easier to implement it worldwide. The head of UNICEF is a US citizen, yet she is restricted by an unwritten code of practice from publicly criticising her government for its stance on this issue. Where is this freedom that the USA proudly claims to fight for? The US corporations have benefited from being

---

* In 2008 when the effects of deregulation started to hurt banks and bankers, governments suddenly forgot their religious devotion to the free market.

treated like individuals under the 'due process' clause of the 14th Amendment and yet are not accountable as individuals for any damage that they cause worldwide.

back to the boycott

After the 1981 adoption of the Code, each company wrote its own weakened version of the original. Nestlé continued its marketing practices, so the boycott continued. The company invested in a new PR system and its director persuaded the diehards within Nestlé that it was commercially expedient to make concessions. The company issued a statement saying it would keep to the Code. Its marketing practices and the boycott continued. Nestlé then brought out guidelines for its employees. It made an agreement with the International Nestlé Boycott Committee (INBC) to abide by the WHO/UNICEF Code and to concede to WHO's final decision in any dispute about the details of implementation. The boycott was suspended in 1984 at the INBC conference in Mexico City. After a six-month test period, when evidence in eight regions indicated reforms, the boycott was ended.

Not everyone was happy. Because of limited purchasing power and product availability, a boycott could not function effectively in poor countries, so citizens depended on activists in industrialised countries to make their protest felt. Health workers from developing countries worried that the ending of the boycott would place them at the mercy of industry once again. Nevertheless, Nestlé convinced the boycotters of its good intentions. The Vice President wrote to the European Boycott Coordinator stating that "the company favours strong national codes" and was willing "to make this position public".[12]

There was another matter, however. In the horse trading that happens in every conciliation meeting, Nestlé had resisted on one count. It refused to keep to the Code in Europe until the other companies agreed to do the same.

what about europe?

By 1986, in three separate sessions, the European Parliament had voted for the Code to be law in the European Community (EC).*[13] Each time, the European Commission (the European Civil Service) drafted a Code which echoed, almost to the letter, the weak baby food

* The European Union was formed in 1993.

industry codes. European commissioners deny company influence and from one aspect it is hardly necessary: both the Scientific Committee for Food which advises the European Commission, and the Codex Alimentarius Commission (CAC) which lays down food compositional standards, is made up mainly of individuals with food industry connections.

The European Commission's Code-drafting group included representatives from each European member state, most of whom knew little about breastfeeding or the Code. During the drafting period, the Commission received statements of concern from hundreds of health bodies, action groups and individuals involved in infant feeding issues. When the European Commission Directive on Infant Formulae and Follow-on Milks was finally adopted in 1991, it did not directly contradict the Code, but it omitted and weakened key points. Meanwhile Nestlé intensified promotion in Europe, revealing the mendacity of their statements to the INBC. A group of sincere activists had been duped by the sweet talk of a cynical PR exercise.

During the 1990s political changes led to the opening up of the Central and Eastern European markets. The baby food companies swooped in like children at a fun fair. In Poland, where breastfeeding had been the norm, mothers were bombarded with messages promoting artificial feeding and discouraging breastfeeding. These infiltrated the health system and all media. Breastfeeding declined. Poland had no functioning Code and it suffered some of the most aggressive marketing in the world. Just across the Baltic Sea in Sweden the companies would not have dared exploit and deceive women in the same way. An international study showed that Polish mothers and infants were victims of the lack of regulation and that without it, companies showed no restraint.[14]

But marketing does not consist only of advertising. In 1990, a relief agency, Médecins Sans Frontières (MSF) requested EC Aid for medical kits to distribute in Romania. EC Aid agreed to provide them, on condition that the agency distributed powdered milk, including branded infant formulas. MSF was reluctant and there was internal disagreement, but finally the urgent need for medical kits made it submit to the EC Aid conditions. The nutritionist in charge of the milk distribution was horrified by the Romanian situation; breastfeeding rates were low and the infant death rate the highest in Europe. She considered the milk distribution harmful, but felt powerless to defy her superiors.[15]

This was not an isolated event. During the 1990s branded infant formulas flowed into Russia and other former Soviet Bloc countries in the guise of humanitarian relief. As happens with aid, products leaked onto the open market. Nestlé's Nan infant formula, with the European flag stamped on the tin, was distributed in Russia and later found on sale in Estonia.[16] If manufacturers can manipulate a European Union body to act as a channel for unethical marketing, no wonder more vulnerable regions succumb to company pressures. The eastern bloc countries, where groups of dedicated and underpaid doctors work to protect breastfeeding, still suffer aggressive marketing.

European Union policies are both contentious and crucial: the first, because of the tension between the sovereignty of member states* and the 'rule from Brussels'; the second, because, as one of the world's largest trading bodies, it has a strong voice at international meetings such as that of the Codex Alimentarius Commission (CAC). In theory every European Union Directive has been agreed upon democratically by the member states. When people in France or the UK grumble about a European directive (as they do), they forget that their delegates have contributed to that agreement. In practice the European Commission, the civil service, has great power – not least because few citizens understand how it works. It is an unelected body, yet it drafts the rules that affect Europeans' lives. These rules can diverge from the European Parliament's intentions.

When it comes to the Code (called the European Directive) there is confusion. Many states believe they cannot implement regulations which go beyond the European Directive. This is not true. In 2001, the European Trade Commissioner, Pascal Lamy, who now heads the World Trade Organisation (WTO), was asked whether member states had the sovereign right to bring in and retain legislation which they believed necessary for human rights and health protection. Lamy answered, "Yes, if non-discriminatory and ultimately science-based."

Now please do not throw this book aside and switch on your computer or TV. I am sorry about civil servant language, it does make you fall asleep, but it is important. Pascal Lamy gave written answers which I will reference in full for the lawyers and pedants among you.[17] He did say he regretted Europe's slow progress towards the Code and subsequent WHA Resolutions, and would prefer it to move forward in 'metres' rather than 'inches'. He linked this slowness to strong US opposition to the Code in the past. Personally I think that is a bit of a cop-out. Publicly, Europe seems to pride itself on standing up to the USA in trade disputes, so why not on baby food marketing matters?

* By 2008 there were 27 member states of the EU.

Anyway, the USA had signed up to the Code in a 1994 WHA Resolution. But if anyone knew what went on behind the scenes, Pascal Lamy certainly would. You do not get to be European Trade Commissioner or head of WTO if you are naïve.

In 2002 the Legal Officer for UNICEF informed Central and Eastern European states who were applying for EU membership that the European Directive on Infant Formula and Follow-on Milks permitted member states to adopt more restrictive provisions. He had to do this because key policy makers in these states were being told behind the scenes that if they adopted the Code, it might jeopardise their chances of EU membership. There was no legal basis for these ideas.[18]

The issue for all European readers is to know that you are legally entitled to have as strong a Code as you want in your country, provided it is "science-based". The evidence for the necessity of controlling marketing to protect breastfeeding and safer artificial feeding is irrefutable, so the science is rock-solid. The Code makes this protection possible. The EU has produced a Blueprint for Action which is the European version of the WHO/UNICEF Global Strategy on Infant and Young Child Feeding which requests urgent Code implementation. The Blueprint was launched with some fanfare at the EU Conference on the Promotion of Breastfeeding in Europe in Dublin Castle, Ireland, in 2004 when the Irish held the Presidency of the EU. One of its recommendations is to "present exclusive breastfeeding for 6 months, and continued breastfeeding up to 2 years and beyond, as the normal way to feed infants and young children, in all written and visual materials relating to or making reference to Infant and Young Child Feeding and to the role of mothers."[19]

So go for it all you Europeans, educate your politicians and remind them of their duties. After all, you pay their wages.

18 dying for the code

*"From the moment of conception, though the pregnancy, birth
and beyond, a mother and her child represent
a valuable commercial opportuity."*
Hunter M Cashing in On the Fruits of Labour,
PR Week, 12 December 1997

the philippines' experience

Any country dependent on the political and economic patronage of
the USA would be reluctant to implement the Code and the
Philippines was an example. At first an ineffective industry-friendly
Code was adopted. The Marcos government (famous for Imelda
Marcos's vast shoe collection) would never have disturbed big
business. In 1983, the Swedish actress and UNICEF Ambassador Liv
Ullman visited the Philippines. She was astonished when told not to
mention breastfeeding on a TV chat show sponsored by Nestlé. Liv
Ullman had never been censored in her life and she told the press.
The embarrassed TV producers and the Marcos government feigned
shock. The Marcoses' daughter had just given birth and it was quickly
announced that she would breastfeed, but there was no mention of
withdrawing Nestlé's TV sponsorship. Liv Ullman had stumbled across
the free market in action and found it involved curtailment of other
freedoms to function.[1]

After the Marcos downfall, the Aquino government made the
Philippines Milk Code law in 1986. It banned free milk supplies, but
had the major weakness of allowing advertisements if approved by a
government committee. The companies found a way round the free
supplies ban: they invoiced the hospitals for the milk but never
collected payment. Advertising continued, but with a mention of
breastfeeding.

Then matters slowly improved. Highly aware people in the
Department of Health and citizens' groups – such as IBFAN –
monitored the code violations and threatened companies with legal
action. In 1989, IBFAN held an International Forum in Manila and
representatives from 162 countries applauded the country's
commitment to making its Code work. In 1992, the Breastfeeding and
Rooming-in Law was brought in as a back-up to the blossoming Baby
Friendly Hospital Initiative (BFHI). The baby food companies

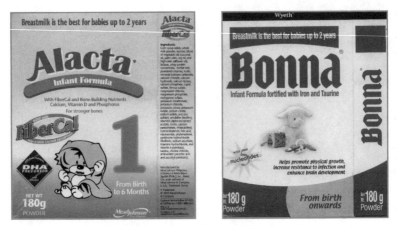

31 Philippines product labels with misleading
health claims and idealising images 2006

challenged the law, claiming that rooming-in was dangerous and increased infection. A worried doctor in the Philippines Senate contacted the Institute of Child Health (ICH) in London and Baby Milk Action (UK IBFAN). Industry's claims contradicted medical evidence, yet lack of access to good information (no internet access at that time) made this doctor feel unable to prove the case. The evidence was faxed and the law went through.[2]

By 2002 breastfeeding promotion and support was flourishing and the Philippines could boast of 1,047 Baby Friendly hospitals. However, the baby food industry increasingly flouted the rules. The government committee proved a toothless watchdog and promotion became more blatant. Visiting Manila in 1997, I saw TV advertising banned in many other regions (including Europe). An SMA advertisement showed a mother bottle-feeding her baby. As the music faded a monotone voiceover gabbled the mantra that breastfeeding was best. If it had any effect it was to associate the product with breastfeeding.

A 2007 UNICEF film Formula for Disaster shows parents echoing TV promotional claims that infant formula is best for your baby and will make your child more intelligent. A mother says she uses the formula her doctor recommended. A salesperson explains how they provide doctors with fares and accommodation at conferences, sponsored parties and donated gifts. Health centre staff earn 500 pesos (US$10) for every 10 infants they convert to using a particular brand. Midwives receive incentives for distributing samples and discharge packs. The companies spend US$100 million a year on advertising breastmilk substitutes in the Philippines. Powdered milk sales outstrip any other consumer product. 30% of the population live on less than US$1 a day. The official minimum wage is 382 pesos (US$7) per day, but the informal daily wage is between 100 and 200 pesos (US$2 to 4). A can of infant formula may cost 300 pesos (US$6). Just 16% of Filipino babies under 5 months are exclusively breastfed.[3]

In 2006 the Philippines Department of Health had issued implemention rules for the Code. They prohibited all promotion of infant formula for children up to two years of age, free samples, gifts for health workers and company contact with mothers. In short, 25 years after its adoption the Philippines had a Code up to the standard of the International Code, just as the World Health Assembly had intended. It is worth mentioning that in 2002 the newly adopted WHO/UNICEF Global Strategy on Infant and Young Child Feeding had emphasised Code implementation as a matter of urgency. The Philippines was fulfilling its commitments along with all the other nations at that 2002 WHA which included the USA.

The representatives of the baby food industry, the Pharmaceutical and Healthcare Association of the Philippines (PHAP), immediately filed a plea to the Philippines Supreme Court for a restraining order on the implementation rules. It was rejected. The Supreme Court concluded that: "The framers of the constitution were well aware that trade must be subjected to some form of regulation for the public good. Public interest must be upheld over business interests." Both WHO and UNICEF welcomed the decision, but, once again Big Daddy put his head round the door. Thomas Donahue, President of the US Chamber of Commerce, which represents three million businesses, wrote to President Gloria Arroyo warning her of "the risk to the reputation of the Philippines as a stable and viable destination for investment" if she did not "re-examine this regulatory decision". Four days later the Supreme Court imposed the restraining order. So much for a legislature separate from government, a value enshrined in both the US and the Philippines constitutions.

There was public protest, including a 'bare breast' demonstration outside the Supreme Court, and support from campaigners overseas. UNICEF and WHO representatives in the Philippines expressed approval of the rules and regretted the restraining order, as they had to; support for their agencies' policies was part of their job descriptions. Suddenly, both representatives were 'promoted' to their agencies' offices in other countries.

The Philippines Department of Health then asked a senior government lawyer, Nestor J. Ballocillo, to contest the restraining order. In December 2006, Ballocillo and his 21 year-old son were shot dead in the street near their home. The former Philippines Solicitor General suggested that the case might be connected. President Arroyo offered a 1 million peso (US$20,000) reward for information. Ballocillo was working on other contentious issues at that time. The killer has not been found.[4]

In early 2007 PHAP ran a series of print ads in major newspapers, showing concern for women unable to breastfeed. The UN's former special rapporteur Jean Ziegler described them as "misleading, deceptive and malicious in intent". He claimed that they manipulated "data emanating from UN specialized agencies such as WHO and UNICEF . . . with the sole purpose to protect the milk companies' huge profits, regardless of the best interest of Filipino mothers and children."[5]

The Filipino government was fighting in its own courts to implement its own law. Its action was based on repeated and urgent recommendations by the UN to implement the Code. The Philippines is a sovereign nation, yet foreign-based companies with the backing of a US-based business federation were openly blocking implementation of a universally agreed health measure.

In October 2007 the Government finally won its case and became legally entitled to implement the Code. As a former WHO Technical Officer says, "The challenge now is for the Department of Health to implement despite the pressure from the industry."[6]

another country: no room for whistle blowers

In 1990, a British TV team visited Pakistan and was shocked by what it found. Five million babies were born each year of whom half a million died. Almost half of that half million died from diarrhoea – unlikely if they had been exclusively breastfed in their first six months of life. Most Pakistani babies were, and still are, mixed-fed. In 1990 only 12% of women had access to contraception and with such disrupted breastfeeding, birth rates and short birth intervals were (and still are) unacceptably high, jeopardising the health and survival of Pakistani women as well as their babies. In 1990, just half the population had access to safe water and less than a quarter to sanitation. Female illiteracy was 80%, 30% of people lived below the absolute poverty level,* and a tin of baby milk cost the average daily wage of about US$3.

These conditions did not inhibit the companies. Abbott-Ross, American Home Products (Wyeth), Boots (Farleys), Mead Johnson,

---

* Defined as being unable to afford a nutritionally adequate diet.

Meiji (the market leader), Morinaga, Nestlé, Nutricia and its subsidiary Cow & Gate, and Snow Brand together enjoyed a doubling of sales during the 1980s. In 1987 an estimated 9 to 18 million US dollars worth of baby milk was sold and 4.5 million feeding bottles imported. The film team met company reps in hospitals who boasted: "My job is to promote my product," as they produced free samples. A doctor responsible for a large newborn unit enthused about follow-on milks as the rep showed her a promotional brochure. There were company posters in the wards, and in the streets billboards advertising follow-on milks and bottles.

The film team followed babies dying of diarrhoea into the emergency rooms and discovered a complicating factor. Many had been given Imodium (Loperamide hydrochloride), an anti-diarrhoeal drug made by Janssen (a subsidiary of Johnson & Johnson) sold over the counter in the form of paediatric drops unavailable in Europe or North America. Imodium immobilises the gut, making death more likely for children. It was as though the jackals had followed the vultures for any leftovers. However, within days of the film's transmission, Johnson & Johnson announced the withdrawal of its paediatric formulation.

The milk and bottle companies whose products triggered the initial diarrhoea did not follow Johnson & Johnson's example. In 1991, the US company Abbot-Ross was promoting Similac as 'comparable to the nutritional characteristics of breastmilk fat'. The Japanese firm Meiji advertised its follow-on milk 'Meiji Fu' on TV as 'the secret of health'. Cannon, a British bottle and teat manufacturer, claimed on billboards that they had had 'mothers' confidence for 50 years'. Free supplies from eight main companies were found in Pakistani maternity hospitals in 1991.[7]

the salesman's story

In 1994, 24 year-old Syad Aamir Raza celebrated getting the job of his dreams, as a 'Medical Delegate' with Nestlé Pakistan. His job was to promote infant feeding products and increase sales. He had to arrange baby shows, contact health workers and charm everyone. He had no training in the International Code and was unaware of its provisions. He was trained to say 'breast is best' quickly before launching into his sales pitch. He gave free Cerelac samples to mothers and then struck up a conversation about the milks. He provided gifts for doctors, usually lunches or air tickets, and lipstick or perfume for nurses. He had an allowance for these expenses, but had to ask his Group Brand Manager at National HQ for permission to give larger gifts. One doctor asked for an air conditioner and the manager wrote: "Aamir OK. But Nan and AL100 sales should go up." Nan and AL100 are two types of infant formula. It was taken for granted by both sales personnel and health workers that gifts were to increase sales. There was a performance incentive scheme and sales targets, both banned by the Code in relation to infant feeding products.

In late 1996 Nestlé circulated their 'Charter', a weakened version of the Code, and Aamir received his copy. He was astonished and confused. The 'Charter' stated that Nestlé did not give gifts to doctors, contact mothers or use sales incentives schemes.

Just a few months later, Aamir was waiting in a doctor's office, the only one on his circuit who refused all gifts. The doctor came in, having just dealt with breaking the news to parents that their three-month-old baby had died. "Why did this child die?" Aamir asked, "Because of people like you," replied the doctor. Aamir was stunned. As he left the office he saw the grieving parents.

Aamir returned home to his wife and two-year-old son and thought. Not long afterwards he resigned from his well-paid, prestigious job and returned the motorbike that went with it. He kept copies of all the documents that proved the truth of the working practices. His next step was one of great courage and great naïvety. With his father's help, he wrote a Legal Notice and sent it to Nestlé with eighty pages of his damning evidence. The Legal Notice asked Nestlé to "withdraw all its infant products from the Pakistan market" and "to terminate service of staff involved in non-professional and unethical practices within 15 days".

Every time I read these words I want to cry. It reminds me of those wildlife films where a gazelle trots over to drink from the pool where the crocodiles are waiting. What would you have done? Many modern Davids just slink away from modern Goliaths.

Aamir wrote to WHO Pakistan to inform it about the Code violations. WHO wrote back, saying it could do nothing as its role was only advisory. WHO passed on his letter to the District Health Officer without Aamir's permission and Nestlé soon had access to it. Once again Aamir was stunned.

He did have the moral support of the Pakistan IBFAN group, The Network. He contributed to their 1998 publication Feeding Fiasco which documented the pervasive marketing tactics throughout Pakistan.

Aamir had a family to support, however, and life was getting difficult. He received death threats and shots were fired at his house. He wrote to Nestlé, asking them to condemn the attack. Nestlé did not reply, but circulated a report stating that the attack had never happened.

Aamir had to flee the country. He went abroad as a refugee and was separated from his family for seven years. His parents died while he was in exile. Eventually his wife and children were able to join him.[8]

US babies can die too

Aggressive marketing tactics are not unique to poor countries, nor is government inertia and nor is infant death. During the 1980s in the USA, while 200,000 babies a year were hospitalised for diarrhoea, infant feeding product promotion intensified. A later analysis of 1988 data found that one in five of the US babies who died at between seven days and 12 months of age did so because they were not breastfed. In the absence of the Code or any regulations, the AAP and the companies had for years kept a 'gentlemen's agreement' to forgo public advertising. This was maintained until the mid-1980s when Nestlé bought the Carnation Company and initiated TV advertising of infant formula. Bristol Myers/Mead Johnson and Gerber followed suit. Sales rose and within five years there was a 24% decline in infants being breastfed at six months. The 'gentlemen' in the AAP were impotent.[9]

In 1991, IBFAN monitoring discovered more Code violations by Nestlé than any other company, partly because it was the biggest. It has remained the leader in baby foods for over 130 years and has the lion's share (around 40%) of the market. It is now the largest milk processor in the world with a dairy turnover of €4.3 billion in 2006.[10] Despite its public commitment to the boycotters during the 1980s, it continued to distribute free supplies in 55 countries. Nestlé knew the effect of these donations – for having ignored the experts' consensus at the 1986 World Health Assembly, in 1988 it had embarked on its own research.

the mexico exposé

During the first boycott, Nestlé had set up the 'independent' Nestle Infant Formula Auditing Committee (NIFAC) in Washington D.C., chaired by the venerable US Senator Edward Muskie. Several years of inaction became untenable, so they hired a team of reputable researchers to investigate infant feeding in Mexico. The study results were damning. Most mothers went into hospital planning to breastfeed. Almost all had their babies snatched away to suffer the barbaric and useless medical ritual of gastric lavage. They were put into nurseries and routinely bottle-fed with free supplies provided, for the most part, by Nestlé, but also by the Mexican state food company Conasupo. Mothers went home with free tins of artificial milk. By three months, 45% of mothers were artificially feeding and 55% were mixed feeding. Just one mother exclusively breastfed. Mothers who had received free samples were significantly more likely to be using infant formula by two weeks.[11]

Nestlé closed NIFAC down before the study was published. When asked why, a Nestlé UK Executive, Ron Hendey, said, "Well, they were all getting on a bit".[12]

the second boycott

I must emphasise that almost every manufacturer of artificial milks, infant foods, drinks, bottles, teats and dummies, violates the Code. Campaigners have focused on Nestlé because, as the market leader, it affects the lives of more babies than any other company. It also sets the tone of what is acceptable for the rest of the baby food industry.

When the companies carried on promoting with free supplies unchecked, the action groups relaunched the boycott against Nestlé in 1988. At first they also targeted Wyeth, the second largest company, but this action faded. Any marketing expert knows that a double campaign fails, you must focus on one issue. Also, Wyeth was a drug company and it is harder to boycott pharmaceuticals than coffee and processed food.

The second Nestlé boycott spread from the USA to the UK and other European countries. By 1991 Australia was the 14th country to join.* That year the Church of England (C of E), known for its caution and conservatism, endorsed the boycott and attracted wide media coverage. UK Nescafé sales dropped by 3%. The UK Methodist Church then joined, as did the Women's Institute (WI), the largest women's organisation in the UK and the social backbone of rural England. The WI was founded in the early 20th century by a Canadian woman concerned about rural babies dying from artificial feeding.

Nestlé was caught off-guard by the challenge from these pillars of

* By 2009, 19 countries had joined the boycott.

respectability, and it cranked its PR machine into high gear. It distributed carefully worded publications. One claimed that "Throughout the Third World, Nestlé abides by every dot and comma of the WHO Code and by the undertakings it has given. Where a country has adopted its own stricter code, Nestlé adheres to the stricter of the two." In the same booklet it admitted donations of free supplies to hospitals.[13]

When the General Synod (the C of E parliament) met in 1994, top Nestlé executives flew in from around the world. They hired, carpeted and furnished a room, put up glossy displays and distributed food and drink. The General Synod had rarely experienced such glamour. Its members narrowly voted to suspend the boycott, but decided to commission independent research to investigate IBFAN's claims. This went ahead and in 1997 an academic team, with no connection to IBFAN, reported that the Code was widely flouted and that Nestlé was among the top violators along with Gerber, Milco, Nutricia and Wyeth. The researchers concluded that companies violated the Code in a systemic manner and that breastfeeding "remains under threat from the marketing activities of manufacturers and distributors of breastmilk substitutes".[14]

At the 1997 General Synod in York (UK), top Nestlé executives flew in with staff from developing countries. The company pledged to keep to the Code and all subsequent WHA Resolutions. The C of E dropped the boycott completely. That year Nestlé gave £100,000 to the York Council of Churches. IBFAN's 1998 monitoring report, covering 39 countries, showed that Nestlé's promotion of infant feeding products had not changed.[15]

nestlé monitors itself

Despite its triumph over the bishops, Nestlé still had PR problems. The UK Advertising Standards Authority (ASA) had condemned Nestlé advertisements claiming Code compliance because it could find no evidence for its claims. Nestlé appealed and lost. The case had lasted almost three years. In January 1999, the magazine Marketing Week described the ASA decision as "a damning verdict on Nestlé, which effectively brands the global corporation a liar, insofar as it claimed to have marketed infant formula products ethically". It featured Nestlé on its front cover with a cartoon of a skinny black woman suckling a fat white baby with Nestlé written across its bulging stomach.[16]

That same year Nestlé published a wondrously dignified tome.

Bound in navy-blue buckram, A4 size and with those handy little cut-out indentations for easy page turning, it bore, in gold engraved letters, the splendid title: "Nestlé implementation of the WHO Code, (International Code of Marketing of Breastmilk Substitutes), Official Response of Governments". Lower down its noble frontage was Report to the Director-General World Health Organisation, July 1999. Inside it announced "a new monitoring process which Nestlé instituted with governments beginning in 1998" and which included "official responses from 54 governments (or designated monitoring bodies) that verify Nestlé compliance with the International (WHO) Code of Marketing of Breast-milk Substitutes." The report was a response to the World Health Assembly's 1998 request that companies strengthen monitoring of their practices. Inside were tables of countries, remarks of responding officials and copies of their original letters with translations into English.[17]

It looked beautiful, but the contents were rather less than was needed. There are 194 countries in the world, if you include Taiwan,* which Nestlé did.** Why it had published barely a third of country responses is not clear, but the company wrote that the process was continuing and "current discussions with other governments [were being] brought to completion and additional governments being approached."

Could we rejoice that Nestlé was at last fulfilling its duties under the Code? Closer scrutiny was disappointing. The report did not list the countries that had been approached, nor who had refused. For example, China's Ministry of Health had declined to issue a certificate of Code compliance, yet this was not mentioned. South Africa stated that "The Nutrition Directorate does not have the capacity to monitor transgressions of the Code." Some countries complained about modified translations. Several other countries made non-committal statements. For example, Denmark simply replied that "the ongoing food control system is currently supervising that the law is being respected" and not that Nestlé complied with it. Twenty-two countries out of the 54 had not given Nestlé a "certificate of Code compliance." Nor could they. The Code requires that governments and manufacturers use distinct and separate monitoring systems and few replies were based on independent, systematic monitoring. Many of the

---

* Taiwan is not a member of the UN so therefore has no official status at the World Health Assembly. Nevertheless it takes WHA decisions seriously.

**Extraordinary to think that a company which represents no body of human beings has official status at WHA whereas a democratically-elected government cannot represent its people.

letters implied that no violations had been brought to the governments' attention, not that the governments had systematically looked for them.

What about the governments who gave Nestlé a clean bill of health? The Philippines Secretary of Health claimed to conduct spot checks and investigations and that "few violations [were] reported to this Office". It was a nice letter and Nestlé could show it with pride.[17] That same year Nestlé's PR company, OgilvyOne, won a prize for its "Nestlé loyalty campaign" in the Philippines. In a Business World magazine article OgilvyOne's managing director in Manila boasted that, "When we designed Nestlé's infant nutrition program, we made full use of direct marketing insights and breakthroughs that are now reshaping the way we market brands as well as the relationship between consumers and brands." The article explained that "the key to the effectiveness of OgilvyOne's winning program was building a relationship with the customer by communicating with mothers – through direct mail packs – in all different stages of motherhood". Any such contact is a violation of the Code.[18]

UNICEF's response to Nestlé's Report stated that there was still a long way to go in achieving full implementation of the International Code and subsequent relevant WHA Resolutions.[19]

why not just do it?

There was a story around in the 1970s that the famous advertising agency J Walter Thompson had advised Nestlé to pull out of the infant feeding market because it damaged its image. I asked a friend in advertising why, having paid for expert advice, Nestlé rejected it. He told me that the client often thought he knew better than the professional advertiser. To me it would seem so much easier for Nestlé just to keep to the Code. Its stance reminds me of a schoolboy who puts so much time and energy into making excuses for not doing his homework, that you wonder why he does not just sit down and do it. Just imagine the PR outcome if it decided to market artificial milk ethically. What a cure for global cynicism.

Nestlé has sometimes claimed that it was not in the baby food business for the money: "infant formula in developing countries is now less than 1 percent of our consolidated sales. It would be very easy simply to drop this matter, be rid of the controversy. Why don't we do it? Because we believe we fulfil a need." So said Nestlé PR man Francois Perroud in 1988.[20] It could easily replace this market with other acquisitions; it just stayed in the business out of concern for babies. A glance at the profits from baby food sales made me ponder this claim. The fact is that twenty years later they have not pulled out of the market, it has expanded in the developing world and its profits have soared.

As happened before in critical times, Nestlé hired a new PR agency and was advised to "aggressively advertise its links with charities and good causes." Which it did most assiduously. However, these links did not always help the good causes. After accepting £250,000 from Nestlé, the British Red Cross commissioned independent analysis of the effects of a Nestlé gift to a charity. It was found to be a reputation risk, especially when the projects involved children or development.[21]

shame and success

In 2005 Nestlé's Nidina formulas were found to be contaminated with printing ink fixative but it did not immediately recall the products. Later, Italian police seized over two million litres. Nestlé was also fined €3.3 million by the Italian authorities for price fixing in collusion with other companies.[22] In May 2006 the US Food and Drug Administration (FDA) turned down Nestlé's application to put a claim on its product Good Start Supreme infant formula, implying that it reduced the risk of food allergy. Good Start's credentials had relied on the Nestlé-funded research of Dr Ranjit Chandra of Memorial University, Newfoundland. Dr Chandra suddenly retired and went abroad, and later in 2006 a Canadian Broadcasting Corporation (CBC) three-part TV documentary exposed Chandra's work as fraudulent.[23]

Whatever shame Nestlé might have to shrug off, financially it has been successful. Nestlé Nutrition (which is approximately 7% of its overall turnover) doubled its sales between 2005 and 2007 to over CHF10 billion (€6.1 billion) with almost three-quarters of revenue coming from 'infant nutrition'. Between 2006 and 2008, sales of infant foods rose from CHF4.8 billion to CHF8.0 billion. This was partly due to Nestlé's acquisition of Gerber in 2007. Nestlé now has 79% of the US complementary foods market.[24]

Consider those huge profits: the bulk come from the suppression of knowledge and good support for breastfeeding. All that marketing is paid for by families who buy the product. Most are not wealthy. Article 24 of the Convention on the Rights of the Child (CRC) recognises "the right of the child to the enjoyment of the highest attainable standard of health" and recommends "that all segments of society, in particular parents and children, are informed, have access to education and are supported in the basic knowledge of child nutrition, the advantages of breastfeeding." (see Appendix 4).

When knowledge comes from company promotion and ill-trained or corrupted health workers, parents and children are deprived of these rights. This misinformation contributes substantially to the profits of the infant feeding companies. Those knowledgeable and supported families who are aware that breastfeeding is normal, that artificial feeding carries risks and that cheaper, safer complementary foods can be made from locally available foods, end up healthier and less poor. The Code states that governments are responsible for ensuring that objective and consistent information on infant and young child feeding is provided. However, it is hopeless investing public money in providing such information if it is eclipsed by promotional untruths.

Nestlé's Director of Public Affairs writes:

"Outside research has shown that no global company matches Nestlé in terms of the public rating of the company in social responsibility, in the developing world as well as globally." He does not cite the source of this "outside research". He goes on to quote two other business analysts, saying, "If . . . corporations were to analyze their prospects for core business choices, they would discover that CSR [Corporate Social Responsibility] can be much more than a cost, a constraint, or a charitable deed – it can be a source of opportunity, innovation, and competitive advantage."[25]

The boycott continues.

the big picture?

In 2007, the world baby milk market was evaluated at 907,000 tons (921,560.6 tonnes) accounting for between US$9 billion and US$11 billion. Worldwide, baby foods and artificial milk sales are set to reach US$20.2 billion by 2010. This means more ill-health, short- and long-term, more obesity, more breast cancer, more diversion of medical resources, more environmental degradation and more infant death. The Asian market is the largest (54%), partly because of sheer population size, but also because of 'economic growth'. The more breastfeeding decreases and the more sales of breastmilk substitutes go up, the better the economic figures. Something is gravely wrong with our accounting systems when human ill-health makes the economy healthier. Global Industry Analysts Inc. report cheerfully that "manufacturers are currently focusing their efforts on India and China." In the margin of its report online are offers of free baby food samples from Bebvita, low-priced infant formula, an invitation to join Hipp baby club, and recipes for food for babies of four to six months; all are potentially harmful to babies and violate the Code.

Industry salivates over Asian babies; there are just so many of them. Roughly half the Asian market is in China where around 16 million babies are born each year and the "baby formula consumer group" of under-fives is over 80 million. A 2005 article in the Shanghai Star describes the efforts of Danish-based International Nutrition Co Ltd (INC), which markets Dumex, to double its share of the 'premium baby formula market'. Managing director Alejandro Rivas complains that only 4% of this group is using baby formula, which is seventeen times lower than in Malaysia.[26]

Well hooray! Many Chinese families are aware that breastfeeding is good for their precious only child. In 1991, the government launched an energetic Baby Friendly Hospital Initiative (BFHI) and by the mid 1990s China had more BFHI-awarded hospitals than any other country in the world. China also had a political culture of provision of maternity leave and breastfeeding in the workplace, but transnational company working styles have undermined this progress. UNICEF data for 2000 to 2006 indicated that 51% of Chinese mothers exclusively breastfed for six months, but I suspect the government might present polished figures to UNICEF. Despite having some provisions as law, the Code is now ignored.[27] Chinese parents are buckling under an onslaught of marketing. Besides the big foreigners such as Nestlé, Wyeth and Mead Johnson, Japanese Morinaga and the New Zealand Dairy Board, there were over 15 Chinese companies all scrambling to relieve families of their hard-earned cash. These included the now notorious Sanlu company, offshoot of the New Zealand based dairy company Fonterra. Sanlu aggressively advertised its melamine contaminated milks on TV and elsewhere.[28] The Chinese artifical milk manufacturers have now almost collapsed and the foreign companies are benefitting. Mead Johnson infant formula costs a third of a blue-collar worker's wage. The market for all milks expanded during the period of economic growth which earned China so much admiration from the Washington financial pundits. The corruption of Sanlu and its parent company Fonterra has caused illness in 300,000 babies and six deaths.[29] That it could happen illustrates that greed is more powerful a force than concern for infant welfare; it also masks the ignorance about breastfeeding and the complacency that artificial feeding is harmless. China has a good health system and it has been mopping up the problems of artificial feeding for years, just as we do in the west.

I lived in China from 1997 to 1999 and found all manner of inappropriate labels, products and promotions. Besides the usual suspects, I was able to buy Wandashan Brand infant formula ("when breastmilk is not enough to feed the infant") which claimed to contain bovine colostrum which would "enhance the infant's immuno-competence". What could be more dangerous than giving a newborn an alien species' colostrum?

Well, one thing far more dangerous is giving a baby 'fake milk'. This story has been eclipsed by the Sanlu scandal. This rapid amnesia indicates systematic neglect of infant welfare. Bee Wilson summed up the story in her book Swindled.

In 2004 in Anhui Province hundreds of babies became seriously ill, and thirteen died, because they were fed breastmilk substitutes made of sugar and starch with a minute amount of essential nutrients. The victims were the babies of low-paid Chinese workers. It turned out that 45 types of substandard powder were being manufactured in 141 factories across China. It was of course cheaper than the standard infant formula. Premier Wen Jiabao announced an investigation and over 100,000 bags of the powder were seized. Forty-seven suspects were publically shamed, 40 formally charged and 97 local Communist party officials punished. As Bee Wilson points out: "This is the sort of fraud which flourishes when an unbridled market economy in food coincides with the wrong type of government". She compares this incident to those of the contaminated cows' milks of the laissez-faire governments of industrial Britain in the 1820s and New York in the 1860s.[30] In her exposé of food cheats she does not mention Néstle's promotion as infant food of its sweetened condensed milk without vitamins A and D in the early 20th century; nor the long silence about the intrinsic pathogenic contamination of infant formula in the late 20th century that led to deaths in Europe and the USA before official action was taken. Even then, this action did not cure the problem, but simply led to revision of the hygiene rules for artificial feed preparation, putting the burden on parents and carers to counteract the intrinsic dangers of the products.

There are aspects to the Chinese fraud that the news reports did not pick up. For instance, the New York Times (NYT) reported that

"In the USA, between 1999 and 2004, mass media advertising of infant formula and bottle-feeding products went up significantly, with TV ads increasing from 7,000 to 10,000 per year, totalling 40,000 in that time period. Annual formula company expenditure for TV, print and radio ads grew from approximately US$29 million to US$46 million in the same period. Hospital staff gave formula samples or offers to 80% of women who wished to breastfeed exclusively, and 47% of their infants were supplemented in hospital."
Still Selling Out Mothers and Babies by Marsha Walker
National Alliance for Breastfeeding Advocacy, 2007

when Liu Li gave birth to a daughter, she was unable to produce enough breastmilk to feed her baby. However, the reporter did not ask why, in a country so committed to the BFHI, no health worker or mother support group had helped Liu Li to increase her breastmilk supply. No one has found out what happened just after the birth. Evidently breastfeeding knowledge was not disseminated in Anhui province. If Liu Li really had insufficient breastmilk, using any artificial milk would have prevented her baby from increasing her supply. Any Baby Friendly Hospital should have prepared Liu Li with the knowledge and skills to increase her breastmilk or to get help outside the hospital for any breastfeeding problem. Both Liu Li and the NYT reporter were so ignorant, they assumed a breastmilk substitute was needed. The normalisation of artificial feeding created by the transnational marketing machine made it easier for the fraudsters to peddle their contaminated artificial milks to the vulnerable.[31]

The NYT report focused on 'protein-short formula'. This misses the point. Correctly designed infant formula must be low in protein, just as breastmilk is. Indeed because of long-term ill-effects such as obesity and diabetes, scientists are trying to find ways to reduce the protein in standard infant formula.[32] The whole point about breastmilk is that it is the balance of nutrients (and lots of other factors) that makes it work so perfectly. Besides low protein, these Chinese sub-standard milks had insufficient fats, minerals and vitamins which are all important. Take any one nutrient out of an infant formula and babies get damaged. The same year 15 Israeli babies fell seriously ill because they were fed on Humana's Remedia Super Soy that lacked thiamine (vitamin B1). Humana allegedly paid out between US$16 million and US$22 million in compensation. As far as I know the

Chinese families got no compensation. One hundred and eighty four people were punished but it seems that lessons were not learned. The Chinese authorities apparently established no effective systems to check artificial milk quality nor to address the problem of widespread artificial feeding. The Sanlu scandal followed just at the time when one would expect public scrutiny to be at its most rigorous.

This sad situation is summed up by Cai Shouqiu, head of the Chinese Academy of Environmental Law: "Making and selling food is so lucrative and so rampant that we don't have the means to control it. Everyone just wants to make money."[33]

the wet-diapered philanthropists

The USA has led the world in promoting the philosophy of free market economics with accompanying reduction of government funding of public welfare systems. However, when it comes to subsidising artificial feeding the US government is a hotbed of socialism. It seems that US politicians cannot sleep easy in their beds unless US tax payers' money is streaming into the bank accounts of infant formula manufacturers. The North American market is approximately the same as that of Europe. As roughly twice as many babies are born in Europe than in North America (because of population size not because of a higher birth rate), this means that on average European babies get far more breastmilk than do US babies. (I will leave out Canada because there are far fewer babies and more breastfeeding than in the USA.) Two companies, Abbot-Ross and Mead Johnson, dominate and, according to business reporting and other sources, one-third to a half of the market is supported by US government programmes.[34]

The United States Department of Agriculture (USDA) Special Supplemental Nutrition Program for Women, Infants and Children (WIC) provides 'nutrition services' to 1.9 million infants, approximately half the babies in the USA. WIC was created in the 1960s to help poor mothers provide better nutrition for their children, and infant formula distribution was a cornerstone of the policy. WIC has probably contributed as much to breastfeeding decline among poor US women as bad hospital practices. Breastfeeding is now promoted in the WIC programme, but it is under-funded. The financial support for the provision of free infant formula, however, is like a well-oiled juggernaut. The WIC progamme purchases half of all the infant formula used in the USA. The food package given to·a mother who artificially feeds is three times the value of the package the breastfeeding mother receives. WIC dieticians sometimes give out infant formula vouchers in maternity wards.

The WIC system is a strong incentive not to breastfeed, even if mothers want to. This is backed up by the 1996 Welfare Reform Act which mandates that mothers on welfare are required to engage in work activities even when their babies are very young.[35] The USA has no national maternity leave policy. Breastfeeding while returning early to work outside the home needs organisation and support, especially from the employer. In Robert Greenwald's 2005 film Walmart: The High Cost of Low Price, an exhausted and underpaid Walmart employee explains how she can just about feed her children because her low wages entitle her to WIC infant foods. Her work schedule makes breastfeeding almost impossible. One group of researchers calculated that if the 1996 Act had not been passed, US breastfeeding at six months would have been 5.5% higher in 2000.[36]

To try and control costs, the US Federal government requires the state governments to conduct competitive bidding from the infant formula companies. To compete, the manufacturers offer rebates on each can of infant formula bought by WIC. Yes, it is complicated I know, but please stay awake. The companies might repay to state WIC progammes between 85 and 98% of the wholesale value of their products. In 2002 rebates totalled US$1.48 billion. I will not even attempt to investigate tax benefits for the companies. The issue is, why would a company give such an enormous cash-back on a product? How could they still make a profit?

I was baffled until the redoubtable Marsha Walker of the US National Alliance for Breastfeeding Advocacy (NABA) explained matters. WIC is yet another marketing channel. If one manufacturer gets its brand contracted to WIC in a region, then that brand has a higher price in the shops, so the non-WIC parents pay more. As Marsha explains, some US taxpayers pay the manufacturers twice, once through their federal income taxes and a second time when they buy WIC formula. They also help to subsidise the owners of Walmart and other companies with similar low-wage policies, because WIC provision helps maintain the low pay.

Many mothers might be in the WIC programme for their first baby, but off WIC benefits when they have their second and third children. However, they tend to use the same brand with subsequent babies. WIC brands get more space and eye-level placement on retail store shelves. Physicians recommend the WIC brand so as not to differentiate between WIC and non-WIC mothers. Some hospitals provide the WIC brand in hospital so that mothers do not have to change their babies' milk when they go home. There is now a trend to use 'non-contract' formula, often newer, more expensive milks. The companies love this because they do not have to give a rebate; in the end the Federal government will always pick up the tab. The terms 'WIC approved' or 'WIC eligible' are used misleadingly in advertising materials even when inappropriate. There are many more methods of companies utilising WIC to promote their brands. It is the largest single infant formula market in the world and a money-spinner.

What shocked me in learning about this system is how much WIC contributes to the early establishment of artificial feeding. When there is no free formula, even mothers who do not want to breastfeed might do so for a few days which could have a positive impact on their babies' immune systems. We also know that the closeness of breastfeeding promotes bonding, and often this virtuous circle prompts mothers to change their minds: women who had planned to artificially feed end up enjoying breastfeeding and stick with it.

Twenty-seven per cent (around a million) of US babies do not even get their mothers' colostrum. Even removing 2% of that 27% to allow for orphans, abandoned babies, drug-dependent mothers, babies of HIV-infected mothers who are told not to breastfeed, mothers with breast cancer and babies with a rare medical problem, this still means that a quarter of all US babies are artificially fed from birth for no good reason. Why?

Considering the amount of breastfeeding knowledge and support skills in the country, there must be only one reason: US taxpayers keep shelling out the money. They must keep supporting those manufacturers in the manner to which they have become accustomed.

The US taxpayers' generosity continues beyond the provision of federally funded artificial milk. Most WIC mothers depend on federal government-funded Medicaid to pay for the treatment of the infections and illnesses their children inevitably get from being deprived of breastfeeding.[37]

A hundred years ago most US babies were breastfed and most artificial feeding was done by rich women, or their servants. Now the class pattern is reversed. Hospital birth, company promotion and WIC have contributed much to this change. It is not just the avoidable sickness of US babies that is so tragic. The USA is collapsing under an obesity epidemic, diabetes is rising, and cardio-vascular disease (CVD) remains a big problem. The world-famous US Centre for Disease

Control (CDC) states that the only two cost-effective strategies to deal with the childhood obesity epidemic are decreased TV viewing and breastfeeding promotion.[38] I am no expert on how to decrease TV viewing, but I feel confident to say that breastfeeding promotion is not going to work if government-funded support for the companies continues. They certainly do not tolerate effective and truthful breastfeeding promotion. The 2004 federally-funded media campaign 'Babies were born to be breastfed' was scuppered because of company pressure.[39]

Infant formula, baby food and bottle companies are thriving. Next time you see a poor mother popping a bottle of infant formula into her newborn's mouth do not sigh, just think how much that little one is contributing to the health of Wyeth, Abbott-Ross, Mead Johnson, Nestlé and other baby food and bottle manufacturers. Both the wet-diapered philanthropists and the generous US taxpayer have those companies' interests at heart.

19 documents and declarations

*"So all my best is dressing old words new,
spending again what is already spent."*
William Shakespeare, Sonnet 76

For those of you who are parents of new babies, or work in health and infant feeding, I need not describe the chutzpah of the companies' marketing tactics any more. However, the promotion is so well targeted that many policy makers are unaware. "I myself was shocked to see a re-emergence of these promotional tactics," said a leading UNICEF decision-maker in reaction to an IBFAN presentation at the launch of the renewed Innocenti Declaration in 2005 (see Appendix 2).[1] He was unaware that the promotion had never stopped, but then he probably did not read pregnancy and baby care magazines, visit the baby food shelves in supermarkets and pharmacies, watch TV, surf the net for babycare advice or visit maternity wards or paediatricians' clinics. He was too important and too busy.

Since the Code was adopted in 1981, a steady stream of policy documents has emerged. They have been produced with much sweat and tears and most of their contents are impeccable. In 1989 WHO and UNICEF had launched an official joint statement, Protecting, Promoting and Supporting Breastfeeding, the Special Role of the Maternity Services, which presented the Ten Steps to Successful Breastfeeding, the gold standard for maternity care.[2] Then, in 1990, 30 governments and 10 UN Agencies developed and adopted the Innocenti Declaration (ID)* which called for a radical approach to policies in order to create a global breastfeeding culture. Society had to change if women's right to breastfeed their babies was to be fulfilled. The ID set four targets: every country should have a breastfeeding coordinator with authority to do the job; every maternity facility should practice the Ten Steps to Successful Breastfeeding; the Code and Resolutions should be fully implemented; and legislation to protect working women should be enacted. These were to be achieved by 1995. They were not. Too many commercial interests, too much political inertia and the overwhelming conservatism of the medical profession got in the way.

* So called because it was adopted at the UNICEF Innocenti Research Centre in Florence.

> *"We will have time to reach the Millennium Development Goals –
> worldwide and in most, or even all, individual countries – but only
> if we break with business as usual."*
> UN Secretary General Ban Ki-moon, 2008, www.un.org/millenniumgoals

However, that did not mean it was a waste of effort. The ID's simple language and brevity presented a vision of a sane world and was adopted as a WHA Resolution.

Shortly after, the Convention on the Rights of the Child (CRC) included "knowledge of breastfeeding" as part of the child's right to the highest attainable standard of health. Every nation in the world – except the USA and Somalia – has ratified the CRC.[3]

In 1991 the leading breastfeeding support organisations formed the World Alliance for Breastfeeding Action (WABA) to coordinate their efforts. WABA initiated World Breastfeeding Week to provide an annual focus for action. That same year, UNICEF launched The Baby Friendly Hospital Initiative (BFHI) to motivate maternity facilities to implement the Ten Steps and stop the mistreatment of mothers and babies worldwide. In 2000, an International Labour Organisation (ILO) Convention, together with ILO Recommendations, set international standards for maternity leave and breastfeeding breaks in the workplace.[4] Discussion of these issues reminded people of the 1979 Convention on the Elimination of all Forms of Discrimination against Women (CEDAW) which calls for everything in its title.

Ten years later the WHO/UNICEF Global Strategy for Infant and Young Child Feeding was launched. Its purpose was to "revitalize world attention to the impact that feeding practices have on the nutritional status, growth, development, health, and thus the very survival of infants and young children." Designed as a Guideline for Action, it was built on the Code, the ID and the BFHI. It coordinated with other international policies on nutrition and HIV/AIDS. It emphasised the needs of mothers and babies in exceptionally difficult circumstances and spoke of the urgent need for action. The Global Strategy was also adopted as a WHA Resolution.

In 2000, the UN Millennium Summit agreed on the Millennium Development Goals to overcome poverty, hunger and child mortality (see Appendix 5). If Ban Ki-Moon really means breaking with business as usual then he is an exceptional UN Secretary General. The goals to reduce child mortality and improve maternal health cannot be achieved if all these noble declarations and policies are ignored.

Should we lapse into cynicism about all these fine documents? I do not think so. All these 'instruments', as the politicians and international civil servants call them, are carefully worked out and written. They hold some of the keys to justice and sanity. They should be used. We must remind our politicians that they exist and that they approved them.

In 2005 many of the original creators of the 1990 ID, together with new supporters, met in Florence, Italy. What had been achieved in 15 years? About 80 countries had some form of national breastfeeding authority and some form of Code regulations. Nineteen thousand hospitals in 150 countries had been awarded Baby-Friendly status. Fifty-nine countries had ratified at least one maternity protection convention. Within 10 years of the adoption of the ID, declining breastfeeding rates had reversed. In the developing world, exclusive breastfeeding increased by 15%.[5] In 28 countries over half of infants were exclusively breastfed for six months. These included societies as diverse and different as Guatemala, Ghana and Chile, but they had all achieved a U-turn in trends. Without the inspiration and direction of the ID and the resulting nationwide coordination, this would have been impossible.

In the developing world, 76% were breastfeeding at one year, but only 40% at two years. The latter is a serious deficit because breastfeeding into the second year and beyond protects against hunger, disease and death. Nevertheless considering the damaging spillover effect of HIV infant feeding policies (see Chapter 8) it is remarkable that breastfeeding has been sustained. Less than 60% of children get nutritious complementary foods when they should.[6] Continued breastfeeding together with better access to the best bits of locally available foods is needed for health and survival. Many families cannot afford to buy nutritious foods and in times of scarcity they can be unavailable.

It has been harder to gather information from Europe and the former Soviet Bloc countries because data are collected so haphazardly. It is shameful how the industrialised countries show glaring blank spaces where breastfeeding information should be in UNICEF's State of the World's Children's data columns. The message to the poor world is that breastfeeding does not matter to the rich. Exclusive breastfeeding for six months is still unusual, but rates of any breastfeeding have risen in almost every country. Almost 80% of Austrian and 70% of Norwegian babies are exclusively breastfeeding at three months and 46% of Austrian mothers are exclusively breastfeeding at six months. 36% of Norwegian babies are still suckling at a year old. In contrast, only 15% of babies in France and 28% in the UK are getting any breastfeeding at all at three and four months respectively.[7]

The former Soviet Bloc countries tended to have higher breastfeeding rates than western Europe but almost no exclusive breastfeeding. For example, in the Central Asian Republic of Uzbekistan, 90% of babies were breastfeeding at six months, but almost all had been given teas and other foods at an early age. In Georgia in 1998, any breastfeeding was 65% at three months and then dropped dramatically to 5% at six months.[8] In the USA breastfeeding initiation fell by 4% between 2002 and 2003, but rallied to 72.9% in 2005. However, exclusive breastfeeding fell from 62.5% in 2003 to 59.4% in 2005. Only one state, Oregon, achieved exclusive breastfeeding of 25% until six months. Nationally, any breastfeeding at six months rose from 36% to 39% in those same two years.[9]

The original 1990 ID had an influence beyond statistics. It influenced the scientific and medical culture. More academics and health programmers began to take breastfeeding seriously, and the definition and detail of infant feeding patterns had to be included in scientific articles. When the well-known medical journal The Lancet published its watershed article on child survival in 2003, it showed that improving breastfeeding practices could prevent the deaths of 1.5 million children a year and more people woke up.[10] Politicians and public figures stopped raising their eyebrows at the mention of breastfeeding. Without the influence of the ID many of the scientists would not have started to look at breastfeeding practices in detail.

Back in the 1980s a trade union leader in the UK described a colleague and myself as "you two women with your heads in the clouds" when we raised the subject of maternity leave and breastfeeding breaks. Nowadays British trade unions tackle the subject themselves. Previously, very few health workers thought they needed to learn anything about breastfeeding, but now the need is accepted even if institutions are slow to change. Pre-service training is still inadequate but there are plenty of educational courses and materials. WHO and UNICEF courses are widely available and used.

Maternity leave and breastfeeding breaks are still woefully neglected in many countries, particularly in the informal sector and especially in the USA, but the trend is progressive. The Code is not honoured as it should be, but some governments are on the defensive. Almost every nation has groups, both official and unofficial, who strive for the Innocenti vision. Before the ID there was almost no coordination between the different groups; national policies, if they existed, varied widely. Now there is more consistency of language and in training. Without the ID, none of this progress would have happened.

learning from brazil

In 1975 the Brazilian art of breastfeeding was dying along with the babies deprived of it. The median duration of breastfeeding was two months and 136/1000 children (compare the 1970 UK figure of 23/1000) did not reach their fifth birthday.

This huge, vibrant and complex country looked into its soul and decided something had to be done. Brazilians have been through periods of real political pain and repression. Brazil has extremes of wealth and poverty; it has corruption, especially regarding the destruction of the Amazon rainforest and the allocation of land to cattle and soya farmers; it has a vast diversity of cultures and peoples. But Brazil changes, and it is the people who push for action. We could all learn lessons from Brazil.

Artificial milk company promotion in Brazilian magazines and scientific journals started as early as 1916. Nestlé had already arrived with imported milks and by the 1930s it was manufacturing its products from local cows' milk.[11] Artificial feeding spread steadily. By the 1970s the companies had infiltrated the medical and health training institutions and seduced students and professors alike. The government provided free powdered milk from birth. Brazilian infant death rates were a disgrace and something had to be done.

In 1974, in Pernambuco State, the Health Secretary, Professor Fernando Figueira, banned the distribution of bottles and infant formula in all maternity facilities. He also translated The Baby Killer into Portuguese. His main teaching hospital, Instituto Materno Infantil Pernambuco (IMIP), went on to become the first Baby Friendly Hospital in Brazil. Professor Figueira was a key figure in the original drafting of the International Code and in Brazil's Instituto Nacional de Alimentação e Nutrição (INAN).

Brazilians were unable to coordinate a national boycott against Nestlé, it was a dangerous time for activists, but the international boycott alerted people to the issue. From both within and outside the country, more and more Brazilians were learning the value of breastfeeding and about the damage caused by the companies' stranglehold on health workers. How systemised this was can be illustrated by paediatrician Dr Mirian Silveira's experience. She had her first two children in 1976 and 1978 while a medical student. Nestlé sent free infant formula for the whole first year of both her babies' lives, plus ten free jars of desserts and soups every month. Nestlé did this for both medical students and paediatricians. In 1981, when the International Code was adopted, Mirian, now a practising paediatrician, had her third baby. Nestlé did not send her free supplies.[12] Brazil was changing.

By now, a core body of Brazilian health workers had high awareness, substantial knowledge and international contacts. They applied to the Pan American Health Organisation (PAHO) for funding to create audiovisual education materials. Their targets were politicians, health authorities, mass media, community and church leaders. How wise these Brazilians were. Breastfeeding campaigns are often first directed at mothers who have the least power to change hospital and marketing practices. Pregnant and newly-delivered women should not be burdened with fighting battles that are the responsibility of a whole society.

The health workers focused first on politicians. During this era of economic crises, scarce foreign currency was being squandered on imported milks. There is nothing like a public cost saving to bring a politician on board. Brazil created a nationwide communication programme. It was coordinated, inclusive of all sectors of society and used multi-media. The message was simple, 'Breastfeed for at least the first six months'. Almost 100 TV channels beamed out messages seen by millions of viewers. Popular soap operas, called 'telenovellas', carried breastfeeding themes. Around 600 radio stations broadcast the message and 17 songs with pro-breastfeeding lyrics were written. Bank statements, utility bills and lottery tickets all carried the message. Famous film stars posed for breastfeeding posters. A champion basketball player was filmed breastfeeding her baby just before a game. The pictures and words in posters, films and songs were gorgeous, witty and emotional. Nowadays this campaign may sound clichéd, but in the early 1980s this was innovative and glamorous. This media blitz was sustained for six weeks.

Breastfeeding duration started to rise slowly but steadily. There were constraints. Breastfeeding support varied according to individual approaches; advice and practices were inconsistent. International guidelines and training courses were not yet well established. There were no coordinated policies for hospital protocols. Many health worker training schools were still teaching the same outdated

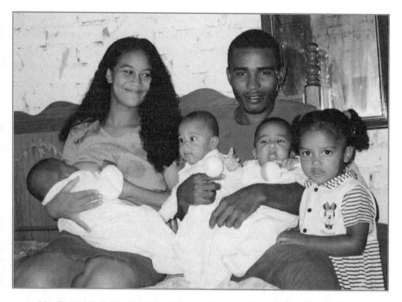

32 Proud Brazilian parents Rozenilda and Janailson with daughter Beatrice and triplets, Matheus, Marcos and Thiago. (Photo Mike Brady 2001)

nonsense. This was all before the ID and the launch of the BFHI. Infant feeding company promotion had continued during the media campaign. The one lesson that everyone can learn from Brazil's experience, is that breastfeeding promotion gets diluted if it runs alongside product promotion. Indeed it can be worse, the companies can hijack the breastfeeding message to promote their products.

IBFAN Brazil was formed in 1983. Its members launched training and monitoring of company behaviour. They joined the national Code committee which included a range of government, non-governmental and industry organisations. The Code was made law in 1988. Real implementation began and much of the worst marketing ended. In 1989, the Ten Steps were introduced nationally, two years ahead of the global launch of the BFHI. Brazil was leading the world in progressive practice. The Code was redrafted with stronger provisions and now encompassed all foods for children up to three, feeding bottles, teats, dummies and nipple shields. Brazil took the Gerber baby face off the jars and, unlike with Guatemala, the USA did not start bullying.

During the 1980s campaigns, human milk banks became established. They had existed sporadically in one or two hospitals, but now these were systemised. They are unique in the world in that they function as both collecting and distribution points for donated breastmilk as well as centres of breastfeeding support. By 2008, Brazil's 190 human milk banks were half the world's. One imaginative idea was to use firemen to collect breastmilk from women's homes; another was to provide basic training for postmen so they could advise women with breastfeeding difficulties and direct them to support organisations. Mother-to-mother support groups flourished. National legislation was developed to protect maternity leave; breastfeeding rights for women in the workplace were developed. Employers had to provide facilities and time for breastfeeding or expressing breastmilk. By 2007 maternity leave was extended to six months and paternity leave was introduced.

In 1996, the Brazilian version of WHO's Breastfeeding Counselling: a Training Course had been launched. More health workers were now getting good training and the system began to cascade. It was between 1996 and 2000 that breastfeeding rates soared. Trainers, IBFAN, mother support groups, health workers, community leaders all worked together, sometimes with quarrels and often with financial problems. Brazil has some of the most talented people I have met, but what has struck me more than their great intellects and their energy, is their emotional investment. These people have engineered a revolution in child health, one that is continuing.

Professor Fernando Figueira died in 2003. He never stopped promoting breastfeeding. He had every reason to die a proud and happy man. In three decades, he saw the median duration of breastfeeding rise from two to ten months. He saw under-five mortality drop from 136 to 20 per thousand (UK 6/1000). Brazil has achieved one of the most sustained records in progress in child survival in the world and breastfeeding has played a key role. IMIP is now re-named Instituto Materno Infantil Professor Fernando Figueira.[13]

Afterword: In 2004, President 'Lula' introduced his Zero Hunger campaign in which he collaborated with Nestlé to provide processed foods and powdered milk to poor families. The chicken was inviting the fox into the coop. In April 2007 Nestlé invested US$19 million in a new 'breastmilk centre' at the Federal University of Pernambuco Hospital and provided 1.5 million units of 'special milks'.[14] Fernando Figueira must be spinning in his grave.

the enduring attraction

Once again we return to the old love affair. During May to July 2008, an advertisement for the 'Nestlé Nutrition Centre' headed the Table of Contents email from the AAP journal, Pediatrics. It blends with the text, giving the impression that it is AAP endorsed. Eight infant formulas are advertised without any mention of the benefits and superiority of breastfeeding. This is the same company that claimed to "keep to every dot and comma of the Code". Indeed two milks are "ideal for use from birth as a supplement to or transition from breastmilk".[15] This makes it clear that their milks are directed at mothers who can breastfeed and not for infants of HIV-infected mothers or orphans. Has the AAP investigated and analysed all eight milks and deemed them superior to all other brands? As the majority of infants in the USA are artificially fed, surely it is important that the AAP, of all institutions, has a system of ongoing scrutiny and testing of all artificial milks on the market? AAP policy endorses the protection, promotion and support of breastfeeding in all sectors in the USA.[16] Why then does AAP not insist that advertisers mention the superiority and benefits of breastfeeding in any company information? If advertising of one brand makes no difference to AAP's members' practices why does Nestlé pay to advertise in Pediatrics? It is known that doctors' practices are strongly influenced by company marketing.[17]

An important proportion of medical and nutritional research is financed by the baby milk companies. The professional health bodies (who have the responsibility of reporting Code violations) frequently receive funding for salaries, grants and conferences from manufacturers. Research is prestigious, but it is costly and researchers' careers depend on the generosity of their funders. Both companies and researchers earnestly claim that there are no strings attached to the funding, but coincidentally the same recipients of company money are often those most silent about the unethical marketing and its effects. But, I hear many researchers cry, they never influenced my research. Here is money, say the companies, and do what you like, we are only too happy to support open research. Good, if this is true let it be publicised. I have yet to meet a researcher with infant feeding product industry funding who publicly challenges unethical practices.

Often company influence is so subtle it is almost subconscious. Once IBFAN offered its materials for a resource centre. The doctor who ran the centre said, "Oh, I can't take that because we're supported with Nestlé money." There had been no conditions with the Nestlé donation; if asked it would have denied any wish to censor this doctor's materials. The doctor changed his mind and used the IBFAN materials, because he was so startled by his own spontaneous complicity with the company. It is a natural human reaction to feel bound by generosity, no one wants to bite the hand that feeds them. Scientists pride themselves on objectivity, doctors dedicate themselves to the prevention and cure of disease, but both set boundaries to their thinking. Like all of us, they have their price, they are dedicated to their work and the threat of having it taken away is powerful. He who pays the piper calls the tune. Reseachers may think they are free pipers, but intuitively they stop playing anything the paymaster dislikes, for in their hearts they know that if the tune offends his ears, he will give the pipe to another player.

20 work, economics and the value of mothering

"Equality for women demands a change in the human psyche
more profound than anything Marx dreamed of.
It means valuing parenthood as much as we value banking."
Polly Toynbee The Guardian 19 January 1987

the first breastfeeding economists

Back in the 1970s, a well-known nutritionist, Alan Berg, calculated the market value of breastmilk by comparing the costs of equivalent nutrients in commercial artificial milks. He found that the decline in breastfeeding in the Philippines was equivalent to a loss of US$33 million (equivalent to US$191.2 million in 2006).[1] Around the same time the World Food Conference rejected a Norwegian proposal that human milk be included in world food production statistics.[2]

Then breastfeeding advocates Derrick and Patrice Jelliffe estimated that it would take a herd of 114 million lactating cows to replace Indian women's breastmilk.[3] In 1982, John Eliot Rohde valued breastmilk in the Indonesian economy. Indonesian mothers produced over a billion litres a year with a conservatively estimated market value of over US$400 million (US$836 million 2006). Savings in healthcare costs and fertility-reduction added a further US$120 million (US$251 million 2006) to the economy. 'Mother milk', as he called it, was one of Indonesia's most precious natural resources, exceeding tin and coffee in gross monetary value and approaching that of rubber. Breastmilk was worth more than double the national health budget and equalled the cost of imported rice, of which Indonesia was the world's largest buyer. This resource was renewable, equitably distributed, benefited consumer and producer alike and provided far-ranging advantages to society.[4] Other researchers calculated values for Ghana, Ivory Coast, Tanzania and parts of the Caribbean, and each time showed huge economic savings. It seemed that at last women's unique contribution to their countries' economies was being acknowledged.

feminism and breastfeeding

As a 21st century reader you might assume that these facts enriched the growing feminist movement, providing some stunning arguments for women's physical prowess and their contribution to the economy and human welfare. But they had the opposite effect. Feminist Fran P. Hosken in the Women's International Network News was disgusted by Alan Berg's calculations: "The obvious obscenity of such an equation points out dramatically the basis of the reasoning that was pursued by all the groups who, by all means, promoted breastfeeding".[5]

The women's liberation movements of the 1970s accelerated and publicised a centuries-old struggle for justice and economic equality. Rights that many readers (but certainly not all) take for granted today were absent in many countries, both rich and poor. Voting, education and employment rights; the freedom to travel without a male relative's permission and the removal of other indignities, have been achieved through the pressure of brave and persistent women. Now in the 21st century, people forget that French women could not vote until 1948, the same year that Britain's Cambridge University finally let women receive degrees. Swiss women had no national vote until 1971 and one canton held out until 1990.[6] In the late 1960s, 98% of companies recruiting at my university baldly stated 'no women' in their interview information. Now laws forbid such discrimination; it still happens, but it can be legally challenged.

There has been a cultural shift in many nations. The much-mocked feminist rebellions and writings helped change the consciousness of a generation and entitled young women today to an equality with men which they assume is normal . . . as they should. Globally there is still a great deal to do, as the third UN Millennium Development Goal to achieve gender equality demonstrates (see Appendix 5). The world is still run predominantly by men, and women still suffer discrimination. Nevertheless, the standards which most governments pretend to respect exist because of those mass movements of women around the world.

However, some 1970s feminists had ambivalent attitudes to their bodies and reproduction. In the striving for equality, some women came to scorn birth and breastfeeding. Much energy in the women's movement came from the USA, where childbirth and infant feeding had been made a humiliating, disempowering experience. At that time most US babies were delivered by doctors and most US doctors were male. Instead of being supported to achieve this supreme act of human strength and to rejoice in their bodies' power to breastfeed, women were coerced into passivity and made obedient, drugged and incompetent.[7] I do not want to glorify all birth in other societies, there have been risks and horrors, as there still are. My point is that in many different cultures, birth and breastfeeding are experiences where women can support each other and feel pride in their achievements. Midwifery remained a dominant and respected profession in Europe, Japan and elsewhere, and even when the system was at its most rigid, there survived an understanding and a way of care that contrasted with the medicalised, supine, stirrup-bound births of 20th century USA.

British feminist Ann Oakley has claimed that the way childbirth is managed affects the position of women in society.[8] It also influences how women feel about themselves. One radical US feminist, Shulamith Firestone, saw reproduction as the cause of women's oppression and had a vision of a day when all new humans would be reproduced and reared in laboratories and nurseries.[9] Presumably she rejoiced in routine artificial feeding as long as women didn't have to do it.

mother-to-mother support

Just before the explosion of feminism in the USA, a blossoming mother-to-mother support movement was reclaiming breastfeeding as a loving act rooted firmly in supposedly traditional family life where the man was the breadwinner and the woman the homemaker. The book The Womanly Art of Breastfeeding was first published in 1958 by La Leche League (LLL), an organisation founded by a group of women who wanted to breastfeed and challenged the artificial feeding culture of the time. LLL broke new ground in the USA because it dared to put the welfare of the child at the centre. Until then, although motherhood was sentimentalised, a woman's main job was to serve and support her husband and run the home. A baby's needs came second. Even if not slavishly obeying their husbands, most mothers obeyed the paediatrician and most knew little about breastfeeding. LLL acknowledged and celebrated the fact that a baby needed close, physical contact with a loving mother, and that breastfeeding was the ideal way to provide this. It gave confidence and practical support to women whose own mothers had lost breastfeeding skills. The book also conveyed a world where a regular income was the norm and the man would provide it – but at that time so did most other literature directed at women. Single and/or lesbian mothers were not mentioned. Supposedly the name 'La Leche League' ('la leche' means 'the milk' in Spanish) was necessary because the word 'breastfeeding' was taboo in US society. As use of language reflects culture, this says much about attitudes at that time.

LLL's values provided a light in societies where unwitting cruelty to infants had become acceptable. It played a major part in the rescue of breastfeeding from near extinction in the USA. The volunteers who carried on the work helped, along with the numerous mother-to-mother support groups which sprang up around the world, to bring back the skills that commerce and doctors had almost destroyed. The moves to revive breastfeeding in the 1970s industrialised world did not come from health workers but from mothers who were ahead of them in their motivation, knowledge and skills. To this day, women helping other women is the most effective form of breastfeeding support.[10]

Somehow, breastfeeding came to be regarded in some circles as anti-feminist and there was a polarisation of attitudes.[11] This was more prevalent in North America than in northern Europe. In Scandinavia, where women were successfully gaining equal rights, motherhood and feminism were not seen as contradictory. Nevertheless some feminists viewed breastfeeding as inextricably linked with domestic oppression and even associated it with the 'Kinder, Küche, Kirche'* anti-feminist policies of Nazi Germany where women were expected to conform to a doctrinaire model of domesticity.[12] In the mid-1980s IBFAN campaigners approached Auschwitz-survivor and highly-respected French politician Simone Veil (b. 1927) for support for the European Code. She described breastfeeding as "un pas retrograde" (a backward step), reflecting the views at that time of many leading women thinkers and champions of progress. She later changed her views as did other leading feminists.

was the left any better?

The 1954 film, Herbert Biberman's The Salt of the Earth, about a zinc mine workers' strike, showed the strikers' wives, imprisoned for their part in the action, demanding 'formula' for a baby. My heart sank when I saw this classic political film, a sensitive examination of the relationships between employers and workers and men and women.

The main character does breastfeed, but the camera conveys this as an act of poverty and pathos. In the prison scene, the baby is being bottle-fed with 'milk that makes him sick'. The women decide he needs 'formula' and start shouting 'We want formula'. Finally, the

* German for 'Children, Kitchen, Church.'

warder gives in and gets it, presumably from the company store. It is a scene of triumph.

The real strikers and their wives were involved in the film making, so I presume the story is true. It illustrates how widespread was the belief in the superiority of a commercial product, even among radicals who were aware of the exploitative nature of commerce. The women and the film makers were evidently unaware of how to increase breastmilk and keep the baby alive without manufactured products. Ignorance is so powerful it can restructure political demands. Consider the other prison situation, the Japanese internment camp where all the British women fed their babies. They did not have to demand 'formula' because they had Cicely Williams's knowledge that breastfeeding was possible in the worst of circumstances.

The record of the socialist countries in protecting breastfeeding was in some ways better than those of the free market economies, principally because maternity provision was a right and there was no aggressive promotion of commercial baby foods. The Former Soviet Union's (FSU) legislation forbade employment discrimination against a pregnant or breastfeeding woman. The statutory 112 days' maternity leave was fully paid and could extend to a year with partial payment. Breastfeeding breaks were a right. Most socialist bloc countries had similar provision.

However, the destructive ignorance of western medicine seemed to cross all political boundaries, and legislative support is useless if breastfeeding is sabotaged by other means. In the FSU and surrounding regions babies were separated at birth, fed to a routine and tightly swaddled, making suckling difficult. The strict hospital protocols were enshrined in law so that when, in the 1990s, these countries started their BFHI reforms some had to revoke legislation. Free or cheap artificial milk had been provided by the state and health workers handed it out as a panacea for breastfeeding problems or to anyone who wanted it.

In 1994 I went to North Korea, then the most politically and culturally isolated nation in the world. Even there they had managed to absorb the rigid western systems that made breastfeeding so difficult.

is women's lot better now?

In the 21st century, women are under pressure to be simultaneously engaged in a workplace and be ideal mothers. Most workplaces do not make this easy and the topic is ignored in the big gatherings of silverback males where the powerful decide what is good for us. Many women in that world can be reluctant to push for issues associated with women's rights in case they are sidelined by the dominant males. The WHO/UNICEF Global Strategy for Infant and Young Child Feeding emphasises the health-promoting and life-saving ideal of breastfeeding for two years or beyond. Governments, health agencies and a range of media, bombard parents with information about the right and wrong ways to care for children. With the exception of a few enlightened societies, the details of how a woman earns her living while mothering, or how she mothers her children while she works is viewed as a private matter, of little concern to the big planners. Meanwhile the economic cardinals pressure governments to curtail social and financial support for mothers.

Maternity leave and breastfeeding breaks have expanded for the formally employed in many countries, but the great majority of women work in casual 'hire and fire' employment and cannot, or dare not, demand their rights. Women make up half of the world's informal work sector, and up to 90% in some countries. Eighty-five per cent of home-based workers in sub-contracted or unpaid family businesses are women. So too are 75% of street vendors and 30% of casual or seasonal agricultural workers. In India 40% of construction workers are women. In the cities, where extremes of poverty and wealth exist side by side, women pick through waste to extract saleable products; there are 25,000 women waste pickers in Mumbai, India, alone. Domestic workers, fisherwomen, waitresses, bar girls, sex workers and many more work unrecorded and unprotected by any official bodies.[13] While politicians sing the hymn of family values, no global system records the numbers of young children separated from their mothers. An exception is a UNICEF paper which has estimated that 1.5 million children are left behind when the 1.45 million Filipina mothers work overseas.[14] That is just one calculation for one country yet we know that many others, eg Indonesia, encourage thousands of women to seek jobs abroad.

In most developing countries, poor women breastfeed for longer than rich women, but they may resort to early substitute feeds because poverty drives them back to informal employment (or unpaid subsistence tasks) too soon. The 2000 ILO Maternity Protection Convention (C183) specifically includes all women in atypical work, but a let-out clause enables countries to postpone or evade full implementation.

Such unregulated employment is not just an unfortunate by-product of a developing country's economic transformation. Deregulation* has been a sacrament of our economic religion. Women in the USA and parts of Europe also endure lives of unremitting toil and insecurity.[15] When fathers renege on parental responsibilities, many governments see pushing a mother into underpaid work as the solution. Who looks after the baby while a mother works when she cannot afford the luxury of a one-to-one mother substitute? Few employers of casual labour know or care whether employees have children. The lack of support for mothers who are separated from family networks can be devastating for any woman in any country. Immigrants whose bureaucratic status is undefined are especially exploited.

janipher's story

Thirteen years old, orphaned and raped by her employer, Ugandan Janipher Maseko was helped to escape to the UK in 2002. Refusing to believe her age, the authorities curtailed her right to stay and she entered the baffling bureaucratic world of legal hearings and appeals. She managed to enrol in a college course. There she met her boyfriend and, ignorant about sex and babies, she gave birth to her daughter Chantell and then quickly became pregnant again. The boyfriend left. She was just eighteen, alone with her one-year-old daughter and due to give birth when she was evicted from where she was living and her benefits cut. When she tried to get help, a social services manager shouted at her, "You are an illegal immigrant, an asylum seeker. We're not going to help you."[16]

She slept on the pavement with her daughter outside Hillingdon Hospital in London. Allowed in to give birth, she was soon back on the streets with a sick Chantell and her new son Colin. She ended up in a police cell with her children removed. Still bleeding from the birth, her breasts engorged with milk, Janipher was desperate for her baby son and daughter. She cried for two weeks. She was given paracetamol and anti-depressants but not allowed to see her children. Both were ill and neglected when they were eventually returned to her.

All three were taken to Yarl's Wood, a prison for people who have been born in the wrong place and failed the bureaucratic tests. One woman there helped her send a fax to the Black Women's Rape Action Project. There was an explosion of action and networking. Well-known people got involved and the Minister for Immigration was challenged.

---

* Or a changing of the regulations to protect the interests of companies over and above those of the employees.

A flurry of emails between women supporters discussed how to help Janipher re-establish breastfeeding Colin. Eventually she was released, housed in a small flat and allowed to care for her children while awaiting the decision on her deportation.[17]

This story shames me as a British citizen. The UK government has endorsed the WHO/UNICEF Global Strategy on Infant and Young Child Feeding which makes support for mothers in exceptionally difficult circumstances its cornerstone. It also makes public statements about teaching parenting skills and supporting breastfeeding mothers. But if you are abused, black, ill-informed and foreign, woe betide you if you think you and your children have equal rights with those who got born in the right place. Article 19 of the Convention on the Rights of the Child (CRC) states that "every effort should be made to prevent the separation of children from their families". The UK has ratified the CRC (see Appendix 4).

who does the work?

The 'boom years' of the late 20th and early 21st centuries have been based on a hidden slavery. Much of the admired economic growth in developing countries has depended on the compliant and low-waged labour of women who produce the abundant low-priced goods sold in the rich nations. The big supermarket chain Walmart does not just profit through exploitation of its US workers, but also benefits from the low wages, long hours and curtailed maternity rights in factories in the poor world.[18]

As for the better-paid managerial jobs, any equalisation of men's and women's work and pay does not mean a significant proportion of men taking career breaks to raise children, or even a real revolution in the division of domestic labour. With some notable exceptions, middle class couples in many countries buy in labour because they find it difficult to negotiate task sharing. All those lovely possessions have to be cleaned, all those clothes laundered, all those children's toys tidied. All the 'stuff' we amass and discard must be sorted.

Poor mothers care for the children of rich mothers, often at the price of separation from their own. A Filipina domestic worker who had left her two-month-old baby in the care of a relative said, "The first two years I felt I was going crazy. You have to believe me when I say it was like I was having intense psychological problems. I would catch myself gazing at nothing, thinking about my child." Deprived of closeness to their own babies, nannies often redirect their maternal love onto the baby in their care: "The only thing you can do is to give all your love to the child [in your care]. In my absence from my children, the most I could do with my situation was to give all my love to that child," said a Filipina nanny.[19]

Jealousy of a nanny's skills can be a problem. I met a successful Malaysian businesswoman who employed an Indonesian nanny. On returning from work, she asked for her baby who was sleeping soundly on the nanny's back. The nanny suggested waiting a little until he woke up. She was sacked. The mother told me the story herself and added, "I didn't like it that my son was getting too close and perhaps preferring her smell to mine." Though well-educated she was oblivious to the fact that the abrupt change of mother figure could harm her child.

In many countries, including Indonesia, Sri Lanka and the Philippines, female migrant labour is encouraged because it solves unemployment problems and enriches the economy through the remittances the women send. Marriages crumble and mother-child relationships are strained, but this is all 'good for the economy'. Thus the economic machine punishes all children: those of the migrant labourer deprived of their mothers, and those of the privileged women, who may suffer emotional damage when mother substitutes are changed according to the whims and circumstances of parental career progress or petty disputes with the nanny such as the one I described above. I am not suggesting that all women should stay at home. What is missing is the economic, social and cultural prioritising of a small child's needs. This requires flexibility, imagination and innovation: all the qualities business gurus claim to love. They exist in a few progressive companies, but these are the exception. Most women feel grateful for, not entitled to, good treatment. That grieving Filipina mother could have brought her two-month-old with her to the USA and still carried out domestic tasks in a flexible way. Then two people would have suffered less. Would the state immigration bureaucracy or the employer have permitted this?

who is the economy for?

When a mother uses a breastmilk substitute, money goes from a mother's pocket into that of the manufacturer. Even the artificial milk industry acknowledges the superiority of breastmilk and its method of delivery, so why are the producers of this product not better off than the manufacturers of the inferior product? Carolyn Campbell summarised the denial of the economic value of breastmilk aptly:

"The discussion of whether or not breastmilk is the ideal infant food is like asking whether or not the kidneys are the ideal means to eliminate wastes from the body and suggesting that dialysis machines ought to replace human kidneys. Human breastmilk is controversial because it is a highly valued product produced by the family for family consumption, and at least up to now has been totally removed from capitalist market control. Subsistence production is contrary to the needs of capital which, to be effective, must incorporate into the market as many goods necessary for or 'desired' by humans. Without commodity production and distribution via the market, there is no surplus value extraction, i.e. no profit."[20]

Economic dogma disregards time for mothering. From the employers who dictate women's reproductive lives, through threat of dismissal, to the World Bank and IMF pressures on countries' internal systems, mothering is not only unsupported, it is punished. In 1997, the World Bank (WB) offered a US$20 million loan to the small Balkan country of Macedonia to reform its primary health care system on the condition that maternity leave would be reduced from nine to three months. Thanks to UNICEF advocacy, the WB was persuaded to change its policy and the condition was dropped. The original pretext had been 'fiscal responsibility', but the WB does not punish countries for government spending on roads, police forces or military expenditure because they are 'for the public good'. The WB does not count mothers caring for their own babies as an investment even if it saves a country millions in healthcare and social costs.[21]

So in a money-obsessed world, I am all for economic evaluations of breastfeeding because that is a language the powerful understand. As Australian economists Julie Smith and Lindy Ingham explain: "While some may find putting a price on mothers' milk offensive, putting no price on it suggests that it has no value".[22] It is amazing how hospital managers, politicians and other decision makers' eyes glaze over when the subject of breastfeeding comes up; mention cost savings and the sparkle returns and they pay attention. No less an entity than the US Department of Agriculture calculated that if breastfeeding in the USA reached the US Surgeon General's* modest targets of 75% at birth and 50% at six months, then cost savings of treatment for just three childhood illnesses would amount to US$3.6 billion.[23] Some illnesses are particularly costly. Necrotising enterocolitis (NEC),

---

* The chief authority of public health. In another country she or he might be called the Chief Medical Officer.

prevalent in low birth weight babies, costs more than US$200,000 for each survivor.[24] Breastmilk feeding and breastfeeding protect against NEC. If all British babies were breastfed for three months, the UK National Health Service would save £50 million a year on the treatment of one childhood disease – gastroenteritis.[25] If all British mothers breastfed for three months or longer, 400 deaths from breast cancer might be prevented.[26] The evidence for wide health cost saving is overwhelming.

Though I feel ambivalent about this as a principle goal, I must point out that breastfeeding benefits business. Besides the reduced costs of medical treatment, Marsha Walker calculates that if half of the 4 million babies born in the USA are not breastfed, a 5 point per baby deficit in Intelligence Quotient (IQ) may result in a lost 10 million IQ points. This loss is valued at US$145 billion because more intelligent people make more money.[27] When the CIGNA insurance company established its 'Corporate Lactation Program', researchers from the University of California, Los Angeles (UCLA) investigated the results. Breastfeeding duration rates of 72% at 6 months and 36% at 12 months were double the US averages. The company saved US$240,000 in healthcare costs with 62% fewer prescriptions for breastfed children. There were 74% fewer absences saving the company US$60,000 a year.[28] Despite this laudable support for its employees, CIGNA, like many other US health insurance companies, does not routinely reimburse for breastfeeding counselling despite its proven effectiveness and cost-saving. Why not?

an existing monetary evaluation: human milk banks

Screened and processed donated human milk has a monetary value despite the fact that, though superior to artificial milk, it is inferior to a mother's own milk which matches her baby's needs, needs no pasteurisation or freezing and therefore retains all its immunological properties. Sometimes the existence of human milk banks diverts health workers from helping mothers to express their own milk for a sick or premature newborn. It may be quicker and easier for staff to feed donated milk than support a mother's lactation. Nevertheless donated human milk saves lives and protects the development of premature or sick newborns whose mothers cannot or do not provide their own breastmilk. Often small quantities of donated milk provide interim feeding while a mother is establishing her own milk supply.

In some countries women who donate their milk are paid a small sum of money to cover the expenses (sterilisation of utensils, fuel, water, etc) but altruism is important to maintain quality. Breastmilk donation requires trust between donor and receiver. If a mother expresses her milk for money, then she may be tempted not to tell the milk bank that, for example, she occasionally smokes or that she has had a course of antibiotics. Just as with blood or organ donation, financial incentives can do harm.[29] Many people want to help others. There has never been a shortage of women eager to donate their milk when they know it will save the lives of sick or premature babies. Perhaps this is 'the hormone of love', oxytocin, at work again.

Human milk banks must be well run and well regulated. The milk must be collected from the donors, tested, pasteurised, documented and stored, all within a limited time. This costs money. In the UK this is covered by a hospital's budget but, because currently only 17 UK hospitals have milk banks, when they supply other hospitals there is a 'handling charge' to cover costs. In 2008 this was approximately £100 (US$200) per litre of human milk supplied. In the USA larger human milk banks have more efficient economies of scale and the costs to other hospitals range from US$106 to US$176 per litre (US$3 to 5 per ounce).[30] In 2005 the Human Milk Banking Association of North America (HMBANA) distributed 21,130 litres (745,329 ounces) from their 11 centres to 80 cities in the USA and Canada.[31]

The expense of running a human milk bank is ultimately cost saving. As I mentioned above, premature babies who do not get breastmilk are at high risk of NEC. One 2002 analysis from the USA found that non-surgical treatment for NEC cost an additional US$138,000 per infant and surgical treatment an additional US$238,000 per infant. The author estimated that in one US state (Texas), where in one year 189 babies suffered NEC, an additional US$32,682,000 was spent because of inadequate use of mother's own milk and donated human milk.[32]

Putting a monetary valuation on a measure of breastmilk as a life-saving medical commodity and treatment is easy to calculate. It is rather like costing a drug treatment. Breastfeeding as a long-term commitment is a far-reaching comprehensive preventative public health strategy, yet its value is mostly ignored in the measurement of health expenditure. Healthy women tend to have healthy babies. It may be that some of those mothers who delivered sick or premature babies would have borne full-term and healthier babies if they themselves had been breastfed. Who is paying the price of their early deprivation?[33]

rightful earnings

National economic evaluation is just as vital in poor countries. A 21st century analysis in eight west African countries of the monetary value of human milk shows that mothers contributed an estimated billion litres of human milk to their nations' food supplies. Replacement with artificial milk would cost US$412 per infant. As a majority of families in that region live on less than US$1 a day, artificial feeding would be impossible merely on monetary grounds.[34] The health costs alone would cripple their economies. Market development is commonly viewed as the answer to a nation's poverty. Here is a primary resource. If the financial cardinals persuaded governments (and such persuasion is their business) to provide some form of payment for a mother's public health contribution then a woman could re-circulate that money into the general economy. This also might help achieve the Third Millennium Development Goal to promote gender equality and empower women.

Cash transfers work. In Ethiopia, the Productive Safety Nets Programme (PSNP) provide 7.2 million people with 30 Birr (US$3.50) per head per month.[35] Mothers spend the money on food, soap, clothes and access to health services. In general, women use money more wisely than men do. Analyses of micro-credit systems, whereby banks and governments have provided small loans for poor women to set up modest income-generating enterprises, have been remarkably successful, benefiting families. These women have repaid loans more reliably than conventional businessmen. Bangladeshi banker Muhammad Yunus and the Grameen Bank, who launched micro-credit schemes for women, won the Nobel Peace Prize in 2006, yet micro-credit for poor women has still not become universally used.[36]

biased economics

When I first wrote this book, I was unaware that at the same time a remarkable woman was writing the very book I needed to read. In If Women Counted,[37] economist Marilyn Waring described how international accounting systems ignored women's major contribution to the global economy. The UN System of National Accounts (UNSNA), the established worldwide method of assessing the 'health' of economies, discounted lots of important productive activity that makes the world a better place. Home food production, protection of the environment, caring for children, aged, sick or disabled relatives, home-making, helping neighbours, and all the other myriad tasks that mostly women do, counted for nothing in the UNSNA system. Weapons manufacture, polluting the environment (we now have 'carbon trading') and even the earnings of a pimp (national systems may include circulating money from the 'hidden economy') count. Every officially recorded activity which damages the planet is considered to benefit the 'health' of the economy. These values applied to the government-controlled economies of communist countries who damaged their environments just as much as the 'free market' nations.

However, it is the big corporate appropriation and control of land, forests and water systems which get the giant economic rewards and damage the planet the most. For example, when the Amazon rainforest is cleared for logging, cattle or soya production by companies fully engaged in 'the market', this makes Brazil's economy look good; protecting the irreplaceable bounty of that forest makes the economy look bad in terms of the UNSNA system. According to dominant economic doctrines, if the Amazon is entirely 'developed' then Brazil's economy will be the envy of the world. But it will be a world where humans cannot live.

maria's life does not count

Maria and her husband José live in their earth-floored, two-roomed wooden house in a remote region of Guatemala. It is set in a third of a hectare (0.8 acres) of land, about five hours' hard walking from the nearest rough road. They have an outside tap with water piped from a spring and a well-maintained latrine. They have brought up eight healthy children (the eldest is 27), all born at home with only José's help, and all breastfed for two or more years. They feed their family entirely from their own labour with maize and beans from the communal cultivation area. Around their house they produce vegetables, fruit, chickens, turkeys, a pig, fish in a little pond and two coffee bushes. They gather wild foods such as river snails and keep a semi-wild beehive in a log suspended on an outside wall. The local cash crop for export is cardamom. When world prices go up, cash income does too. Their expenditure is for sugar, soap, candles, clothes and, when possible, their children's education. In monetary values they are very poor, but the family has not gone hungry.

In her forties and illiterate, Maria was chosen by her community to take the government-sponsored training course to become a birth attendant. She has since supported 19 women through birth. In her community, exclusive breastfeeding is the norm and problems are unknown. All 19 mothers and babies did well except for one baby who died three weeks after being flown with his mother to the nearest hospital. The only emergency transport is a light aircraft owned by the local 'narco baron'.

Maria and José are respected by their community. Maria's skills and knowledge make her one of the most productive women I have ever met, and certainly one with a 'zero-carbon footprint'. Yet her outstanding contribution to society is invisible. Everything she does is not counted. A US citizen owns the land their community cultivates. If he decides to reclaim it for cattle-rearing, which is viewed as the profitable thing to do, the whole village would be dependent on food aid or go hungry. Local water sources would become polluted (cattle cause water contamination and disease), tree clearance for grazing would damage the micro-climate, provoking flooding and landslides. Yet any milk and meat sold would be viewed as economic progress in Guatemala's national accounts.

Maria works hard but she is an unstressed, calm woman. During the evening after supper in the candlelit house, she cuddles her six-year-old son (her youngest and last child) until he falls asleep. We converse from time to time, but all is peaceful. During her twenty years of pregnancy and breastfeeding she never needed a cushion, a breast pump, a book or a video, and she worked at her daily tasks without any sense that she was doing anything special. Though she does not know it, she is at low risk of breast and ovarian cancer and hip fractures. Her children are polite and intelligent and take part cheerfully in the family subsistence duties: shutting up the pig and piglets at night, catching fish in the pond, shelling beans, making tortillas for every meal. Maria's and José's lives are hard-working, dignified and a great contribution to the health and ecology of their community and country, yet these lives do not count. Only their monetary share in cardamom sales (or if José does some paid labour) and cash spent on candles, sugar or soap, mean anything to economists. If the economy 'improves', the small local shop will sell more soft drinks and processed foods which will add nothing to public health.

Meanwhile the local 'narco baron' who lives in a mansion over the mountain keeps cattle, employs staff and buys furniture and luxuries; his contribution is counted.

a market analysis of breastfeeding in australia

Back in my own urbanised world, breastfeeding remains as economically invisible as Maria's productivity. Economists Julie Smith and Lindy Ingham show the economic stupidity of excluding breastfeeding from national accounting systems by examining their own country Australia.[38] In 1993, the UNSNA international accounting guidelines were revised, partly to try and reflect subsistence production like Maria's. The new parts are called UN System of National Accounting 93 (SNA93). Not all countries have taken SNA93 on board, but Australia has. One national accountant commented that ignoring unpaid household activities was not a matter of economic principle but a practical convenience. In other words it was just too much bother to work it all out. I feel much the same about my tax returns, but punishment awaits me if I neglect them. It seems that governments sometimes just dump the difficult bits. Apparently a significant body of economists have been pointing out the limitations of the UNSNA system for many decades, but as one great economist wrote about our system in general: "…what is convenient to believe is greatly preferred."[39]

Anyway, the revised SNA93 guidelines (if used by a government) reflect some unpaid work in households. Now in Australia the value of home-grown fruit, vegetables, meat, eggs, beer and wine are included in the Gross Domestic Product (GDP) which is the measured sum of the national income. In 1997 all this home production amounted to A$1 billion. National income is not just about production of goods but also services. Turning fresh food into 'added value' products in a factory is an economic activity (that makes Nestlé very rich), but so too is serving food in a restaurant. Now, apparently, economists are recommending that the value of unpaid service work, such as childcare, domestic chores and voluntary work, should be taken into account. The way to do this (economists must have a tidy system, even if it baffles the rest of us) is to pop these value-assessments into the so-called 'satellite accounts'. These are separate from the core national accounts, which record all the market transactions (commercial sales and services), but are still consistent with them. Now I am not sure I quite understand, but I see it like this: 'We have a clever bank account system, but you are not quite important enough to use it. But we can value the coins in your piggy bank and we will count them regularly and acknowledge they exist.' So it is a step in the right direction.

But environmental and human capital assets are not yet included in national balance sheets. The value of reproductive work – that is, giving birth, breastfeeding and providing the consistent responsiveness that all babies need – is still ignored by accountants. Governments and commercial companies will 'invest' billions in expensive new technology – roads, bridges, airports, dams or power generation plants – 'for the good of society'. They may even 'invest' in schools and hospitals, but the crucial primary investment in the emotional, physical and mental health of all humans, which breastfeeding and mothering provide, is invisible. Most of the studies I quoted at the start of this chapter, calculated the value of breastfeeding by comparing it with artificial milk, but that is a poor comparison. It is as though you suggested a mahogany forest could be replaced by ranks of potted petunias and the value would be the same.

These bold Australian women economists (I can imagine the ribald remarks from their male colleagues when they designed this research) have explored different methods of valuing breastfeeding in economic terms, but the one which I find most understandable is that of the estimate of a nation's capital assets. Just think of a diamond or gold mine, a thousand highly qualified engineers or a telecommunications company. These all make a country rich. Well, these economists calculate the capitalised value of breastfeeding in Australia to be around A$37 billion. This is comparable with the value of Telstra, the big Australian telecommunications company which was valued at A$30 billion at the time of the paper's publication. It far exceeds the value of livestock (A$17.9 billion) and plantation forests (A$4.5 billion). If Australian women were supported to practise the WHO/UNICEF recommendations, ie six months' exclusive breastfeeding and continued breastfeeding for two years and beyond, then the value of breastfeeding and human milk production would be A$100 billion, three times its current level and three times the value of Telstra. The folly of the current accounting system is that when breastfeeding declined over the decades, this contributed to Australia appearing richer. Whenever breastfeeding increases and infant formula and bottle sales go down, the accounts show this as a decline in economic output.* This is ridiculous.

---

* I am indebted to Julie Smith for her guidance in this section. Any errors of interpretation are due to my failure to unravel the tangled knitting wool of economic terms.

what are we afraid of?

The case for acknowledging breastfeeding as an economic asset is convincing, but it can still make us feel uncomfortable. Is it a good or a bad thing? If it is a national asset, who controls it? Would monetary evaluation of breastfeeding be associated with state interference in our private lives? Would economic acknowledgement lead to commercialisation of donated expressed breastmilk and wet nursing? Already one US company is marketing breastmilk, something which does equate women with dairy cows.[40] It also undermines the intrinsic altruism which motivates many wet nurses and donors.[41] What about the tiny percentage of women who cannot breastfeed? What about women who do not want to breastfeed?

All these issues and others need to be pondered. Somewhere I suspect deep down in the minds of planners (if they have thought about this at all) is the haunting fear that if we make breastfeeding and mothering pleasant, prestigious, economically rewarded and a marker of a nation's wealth, women might start giving birth like gerbils.

The evidence proves otherwise. Official payment does not influence whether a woman breastfeeds, or indeed whether she decides to have children. When Quebec, Canada, raised the subsidy for breastfeeding, it did not have a dramatic effect on breastfeeding rates.[42] In the Scandinavian countries birth rates did not soar as family-friendly benefits were brought in. They just created healthier, more equitable and more cohesive societies.[43]

For decades, France's pro-natalist benefit system had little effect on French women's chosen family size. In my own country, the UK, the universally entitled child benefit helped me through lean times and, importantly, boosted my sense of value as a mother. I still had half the number of children my mother had and she had a harder life.

Most women know how many children they can cope with. They have more children than is good for their own and their children's health for several reasons. A lack of control over their lives fosters early marriage and/or coerced sex and fatalism about conception. This often goes with an entrenched acceptance of male indifference or irresponsibility. Decisions about too many women's lives are made by other people. Access to family planning services is still woefully inadequate. In the least-developed countries only 30% of women use contraception; in west and central Africa it is just 17%. If breastfeeding practices improved, there would be fewer closely-spaced births. This would save women's as well as children's lives.[44] Contrary to many

> *"One international advertising executive is alleged to have stated that women should not be appointed to senior roles because they might 'wimp out, go home and suckle something'."*
> Kate Hilpern citing Caroline Gatrell in 'Well, why haven't my shirts been ironed', Guardian, 2 February 2008.

assumptions, less-educated women are just as eager to space and limit their families when they know they can. In Bangladesh, the average size of a family halved in a generation because of good family planning services.[45] I am not looking at this issue from a demographic point of view but as a question of women's rights.

Most importantly, family size is related to female education and equality. When women are confident that they will have the opportunity to participate in worthwhile and valued occupations, they are motivated to take control of their reproductive lives. The aim of the Third Millennium Development Goal is to increase female participation in education, the labour market and politics. Quite right too. What must be addressed is whether women's inclusion in the labour market, without well-planned and financially-supported provision for breastfeeding and mothering, will lead to more separation for babies, less breastfeeding and more exploitation of an underclass of poorly-paid child carers.

who benefits from benefits?

Most women have little choice about their lives. Keeping poverty at bay separates women from their babies in poor and rich countries. The privileged minority who have the luxury of choice can be confused about the conundrum of meeting the needs of their babies and maintaining their lives beyond motherhood. Some are frankly scornful. British journalist Lowri Turner, mother of three children, has denounced stay-at-home mums as "intellectually stunted, spaghetti-brained morons" for choosing to look after their children themselves.[46] Does she hire one of these 'spaghetti-brained morons' to care for her own children?

In 2008, Nicola Brewer, head of the UK Equalities and Human Rights Commission warned that 'generous' maternity leave might sabotage women's careers and make them unattractive to employers. Her solution was to increase paternity leave.[47] Firstly, I challenge her basic argument. In countries with financial and social support for breastfeeding and mothering, women have become more equal and more powerful. Scandinavian nations are the shining examples. The argument has to be turned on its head. These societies have become more economically stable because women's talents and skills are incorporated into every aspect of society while, at the same time, a period of close physical contact between a mother and her child is politically supported. These countries have quotas for women in parliament.* Their systems were not devised because of a sentimental nostalgia for mum with her apron, but because secure early childhoods are as vital for prosperity as a clean water supply.

Secondly, Nicola Brewer's solution is illogical. Paternity leave is taken around the birth (or the time of adoption) and is usually about two weeks. This is mostly enjoyed by couples in formal employment in some richer countries. Even if extended to a couple of months, paternity leave would not affect women's participation in the workplace because this is the time when all women need to recuperate from childbirth. The purpose of paternity leave is for the father to bond with his new baby, care for other children, support his partner emotionally and do the household tasks. For some parents this phase is called a 'babymoon', a time when a couple can relish the joy of unrestricted time with their new baby. Some men hang about the house, feeling – and sometimes being – incompetent at meeting the needs of a mother and her newborn. Many men are wonderfully supportive, while a few feel resentment at the woman's focus on the baby. A few might undermine a mother's confidence by being too expert. New mothers sometimes overwork because their culture obliges them to look after the man, and sometimes his extended family. Some women secretly long for their partners to return to work and prefer the support of female relatives or friends. The needs of new mothers vary greatly according to character, culture and partners' personalities, but they all need support. The time when paternity leave is vital is often when older children need care. In Scandinavia there has been provision for either parent to take periods of leave throughout childhood according to need, for example during an illness.

Men have children too, but employers do not refuse employment to a man in case he has children and attends to their needs. They tend to assume he will not. When, in 1997, the British parliament significantly increased its proportion of women MPs, there was discussion of how the parliamentary schedules must be made more 'woman friendly'. The phrase should have been 'parent friendly'. After

* In Norway the law stipulates that all executive boards must be 40% female.

all, women without children had no need to change a schedule that had suited generations of MPs. For decades, male politicians had accepted a system which prevented them from putting their children to bed, bathing them, reading them stories, rushing out of work when they were ill. Throughout those years, there was never a campaign for fathers' rights to change parliamentary work hours to accommodate more physical, loving contact with their offspring. And this is probably true for most seats of government around the world. Why not?

Women will only have equality when large numbers of men demand a saner system so that they can be better fathers. David Landes, professor emeritus of history and economics at Harvard University, states: "The economic implications of gender discrimination are most serious. To deny women is to deprive a country of labour and talent, but – even worse – to undermine the drive to achieve by boys and men."[48] David Landes does not elaborate on what these achievements might be. I hope he does not just mean money-making.

Whatever systems are devised to meet the needs of both small humans and economic structures (and there is no limit to human imagination and creativity), it is essential to consistently love and care for small children if we want adult humans to be mentally and physically healthy and resilient. What is material prosperity beyond food and shelter for if people are still miserable? As economist Richard Layard points out, for much of the industrialised world, living standards have risen dramatically since the 1950s, yet people are no happier.[49] Parents may work long hours to buy numerous clothes, equipment and toys for a child who actually only needs her mother's breast, a lullaby and the sense that her parents delight in her smile. These treasures cost nothing. In our increasingly extended lifetimes, this brief period of close parental contact takes up a fraction of our lives.

If breastfeeding and mothering were economically valued, then mothers might feel more confident and less ambivalent about breastfeeding. If the lies of the commercial marketing of infant feeding products were stopped and health workers properly trained, then breastfeeding misery experiences would fade away. Of course women do not want to breastfeed when human ineptitude turns a pleasure into a pain. Are Norwegian women suffering agonies because they all breastfeed? In fact they are the richest and most powerful women in the world. They choose to breastfeed because they are confident, well informed and well supported. Moreover, they are not excluded from the spheres of power and influence when they do so.

entitlement

Professor Amartya Sen won the Nobel Prize for economics in 1998. His groundbreaking book Poverty and Famines[50] introduced the simple and convincing concept that people do not starve from lack of food but from lack of entitlement to food. During the 19th-century Irish famines, grains were exported to England. The Irish died because they depended on potatoes (which became blighted) and had no entitlement to the grain-crops which they grew as rent for the English landowners. So too with 20th-century famines in Asia and Africa; people with land, money or some other form of entitlement have not starved. Sen's theory has proved robust. In 1997 I bought Ethiopian lentils in the UK. That year the Atlanta-based Carter Center proudly announced that Ethiopia had become a food exporter for the first time.[51] The World Bank had demanded economic reforms which included the export of grain reserves to repay debt. In 1998 another famine began – but both the rulers and foreign advisers working in Ethiopia maintained their usual bodyweight. You may notice that journalists or politicians in famine zones do not faint with hunger before the TV cameras. They have entitlement to food.

So too with breastfeeding. There is no shortage of breastmilk. If all existing, supportive policies were fully implemented, breastfeeding rates could be doubled within a short time. No other production process is so easy to switch on and off. Women who stop breastfeeding because their confidence has been crushed through misinformation and inept care, or because they are denied access to their babies, have had their entitlement destroyed. Constraints in health systems, ignorance, commercial misinformation and greed, inhumane and unimaginative working systems, distorted cultural values and political blindness all come together to destroy the entitlement of women to sustain their children's health and lives, and protect their own bodies. All over the world there are breastfeeding famines and they are not caused by nature but by a loss of entitlement.

childcare is not housework

The linking of the two tasks of domestic labour and childcare has marginalised both activities. Why is housework linked with childcare when being a business executive is not linked with office cleaning? Often a woman who relinquishes a paid job to 'stay at home' with her baby engages in domestic tasks which have nothing to do with her baby. Vacuuming the carpet or preparing adults' food does nothing for the baby, but it is assumed to be a mother's task. Even the debate over maternity leave confuses the two issues: "Maybe it would be kinder to teach our daughters to sew, play the piano and cook to help them enjoy their home-making careers," a journalist writes.[52] All these tasks and their equivalents are fine occupations, but they have nothing to do with mothering. Indeed the ridiculous idea that a mother must be a domestic goddess is contrary to good childcare. Many of my generation were quelled into routine feeding, left in prams or playpens and ignored as much as possible so that homes could be kept 'spotless' and husbands' shirts ironed. In the 20th century household tasks actually increased for women as standards of living rose.[53] Some women and some men enjoy housework. More people could do their share of cleaning up after themselves without damage to body or dignity. If everyone reduced the purchase of unnecessary products there would be far less tidying and cleaning to do. 'Homemaking' is a fine occupation, but it has little do with suckling, massaging or talking to a baby. The chief executive may be a dab hand at curtain or sandwich making, but he or she does not usually find it part of the job description. In traditional societies, women were often relieved of their household and food processing tasks for several months when they had a baby.

The private arrangement that many women make with the baby's father makes them dependent on a man's economic survival in the market place and also on his personal favour. Thousands of mothers find themselves poor and destitute simply because their children's fathers abandon paternal economic responsibility. Every health and development report bemoans the problem of the number of households 'headed by women', as though the very femaleness of the breadwinner is the cause of the problem. The problem is that most economic production, employment and reward is weighted against women. In most traditional societies, women are the main food producers. Often they and their children would be better nourished if good land had not been appropriated for cash crops, which in the majority of cases are controlled by men. Modern production methods do not take a baby into account. Breastfeeding does not work like a machine, like 'clockwork', and the attempt to restrict it has damaged the process.

who holds the baby?

Even in societies such as Sweden, where equal share of parental care has been encouraged, most couples decide that the baby needs her mother more and most women choose to be the principal nurturer. Many men, however, can be sensitive, responsive and loving carers of babies. As psychologist Penelope Leach says: "We must dig out the old idea that no man can take full care of a child and that every woman can." However, she goes on to say:

"Even when they are freely made, [such] choices about children are never truly equitable because carrying, delivering and nurturing a baby is an integral part of most women's self-fulfilment and cannot be of men's. That is the crux of the gender difference. As long as it is assumed that society will continue to be organised by men, according to a *distinctively male model to which every individual aspires*, it will remain too dangerous a differentiation for women to acknowledge. But is that not the assumption itself that needs rethinking?" (my emphasis).[54]

There is no reason why a mother could not give birth and breastfeed, and her male partner could perform all the remaining attendant tasks and be the main child-carer for the rest of the child's growing life. A few rare couples may do this, but most do not. One reason is that childcare is low-paid and lacks kudos.

Neurological evidence now backs up psychological theory that affection shapes a baby's brain[55] and that the attention a baby receives impacts her brain structure. Research has shown that full-time nurseries are bad for small babies, who can only cope with about ten hours a week of day-care before it affects their emotional development and their 'social brain'. Sue Gerhardt writes:

"These findings are not what working parents want to hear, nor what a government dedicated to getting single parents back to work wants to hear. Unfortunately the most likely scenario for such single parents is the worst-case one: having to put their babies into poor quality, full-time nursery care before the age of six months. It is their children whose emotional and social development could be compromised, not those of better-off parents who can afford to work part-time or buy in the highest quality care. This is not a solution which benefits society in the long term."[56]

All babies need to be loved, which means the same few people consistently and sensitively responding to their needs as they arise. These needs may differ and 'high needs' babies may be especially vulnerable. You need to know a baby well to be able to respond. Mothers who have bonded with their babies know them intimately. Once a paediatrician told me, "Baby Friendly protocols help my work. When mothers are with their babies all the time they notice small changes in behaviour or feeding that I might not pick up in a clinical examination, yet their observations often turn out to be predictors of some clinical problem."[57] This intimacy comes from physical closeness. In the past, when babies were whisked away and only brought for routine feeds, some mothers found it took weeks to bond. Sometimes it never happened and many women found motherhood a dreary round of dutiful chores. Now bonding is encouraged, yet many women are under pressure (both economic and social) to delegate that babycare to anyone else as soon as possible. Sometimes, where maternity leave is poor, women decide not to breastfeed at all, in anticipation of returning to work. This may be because they are not helped to combine breastfeeding and work outside the home; it may also be because a woman cannot face the pain of bonding and then separation. It may be easier to be a 'detached' mother, but it is not good for a baby. Babies need good emotional attachment just as much as they need good physical attachment at the breast. The two forms of attachment go together very well.

Many governments, particularly in Europe and North America, express concern about alienated youth who care little about their society and rush into anti-social behaviour or criminality. Our early years shape our whole lives, yet 'welfare' policies send a message to a poor mother that she is doing more good stacking shelves in Walmart or Tesco than suckling, cuddling, talking or singing to her baby. Employers in these temples of modern consumption do not permit a woman to carry her baby on her back while she works, or to take a break whenever her baby needs to breastfeed. If her baby's care is inadequate, her employers carry no sense of shared responsibility, but if her baby comes to harm, society may blame her for not making better arrangements.

The assumption that all childcare must take place in the home has led to the exploitation of women in a new way that reverses the effects of factory organisation, without regaining the flexibility and communality of traditional household production. During the deregulation policies of the 1980s, both transnational and local companies increasingly turned to home-based labour by women to reduce the costs and responsibilities of worker welfare. This increased the exploitation of women as low pay, lack of insurance and health and safety provision became accepted, even in rich countries. Dangerous machines and chemicals are used in conditions which escape the inspection of any official eye, whether government or trade union. In India 80 million women do such home-based work.[58] This change spread almost unnoticed because it affected women more than men, and both management and unions have neglected to investigate home-based women's work. This happens in both industrialised and developing countries. The 19th-century myth of the 'hearth and home' still puts women and their children at risk.[59]

a model soon to be lost: the baka

Until fairly recently there were human societies where there was fairness in relations between men and women, and children were cherished by both. The Baka Pygmy people of the Cameroon Rainforest treated children with a wisdom and sensitivity that made any psychology book redundant. A 1987 film[60] showed a wise and gentle father being utterly involved in supporting his small son through the experience of the arrival of a new sibling. The mother was as completely involved in the communal hunting procedures as her husband was with his child's physical and psychological welfare. There was no conflict between earning their livings and being responsive parents. Naturally, children were breastfed for several years in this society, but women were engaged in the processes of production and had equal status with men.

Since that film was made, however, the Baka way of life has been eroded. There are an estimated 75,000 Baka spread throughout the rainforest, but their environment is under siege and they are now mixing and intermarrying with their Bantu neighbours. By Baka tradition the woman is head of the family. A woman chooses her spouse and provides the family shelter, and the men follow the women wherever they choose to live. Now Baka women suffer violence, sexual harassment and economic exploitation by adjacent Bantus. They have no legal documents and therefore cannot claim their rights to land or justice. In 2003, the aid agency Plan initiated The Pygmy Rights and Dignity Project and witnesses were spellbound by the Baka women's powerful presentation of their woes,[61] but I fear for the survival of their way of life. The industrialised world has much to learn from these dwindling societies who live in balance with their environment.

21 ecology, waste and greed

"Almost unconsciously, we begin to think of justice for the rich and human rights for the poor. Justice for the corporate world, human rights for its victims."
Arundhati Roy Speech on her acceptance of the City of Sydney 2004 Peace Prize

When I told a colleague how I valued the ecological contribution of breastfeeding, her reaction was, "Oh no, you're not using green issues to pressure women to breastfeed." It had not crossed my mind. I just saw facts. But her words made me aware that whenever I present a fact about breastfeeding, someone thinks I am trying to 'make' women do it.

Every woman has the right to make decisions about her body. Any coercion to breastfeed is not just morally unacceptable, it is impractical; in the end only a woman and her baby can make breastfeeding happen. A woman has the right not to breastfeed, but she must be fully informed of the effects on her child and herself. And of course in many places not breastfeeding can mean death. Every woman has the right to that knowledge and to be supported to breastfeed. This is enshrined in the conventions and declarations I described in Chapter 19.[1] If governments tolerate commercial misinformation, neglect the reform of health professional training or ignore a woman's right to earn her living and breastfeed, they are breaking their commitments to human rights. Cynics might say, 'what else do you expect?' My response is that cynicism gains nothing but a bitter smugness for the cynic. The 20th century engendered some of the worst human rights violations and the best human rights commitments. The latter were produced through the learning, experience and skills of the best women and men dedicated to the improvement of society. The former were produced through the uncontrolled impulses and manipulations of the worst human beings. Why not take advantage of the best? We own those human rights commitments and we need to pressure our governments to implement them.

When it comes to breastfeeding as an environmental issue, I feel as passionate about this as when I wrote about it in 1987. Since then Penny Stanway, Andrew Radford and others have explored the topic further. I will only present examples, but since it has become fashionable to work out the carbon footprint of human activity, I propose that readers look at their own lives and discover the difference breastfeeding makes to the conservation of energy. For comparison take the example of a 1.9 litre (1/2 US gallon) carton of orange juice which takes greenhouse gases equivalent to 1.7kg (3.75 lbs) of carbon dioxide to produce. The bulk of this comes from production costs such as fertilizer, transport and fuel. In contrast a woman can produce hundreds of litres of the super-fluid breastmilk for a zero 'carbon footprint'. A well-nourished woman utilising her body fat stores needs no extra food, and for some women the body's metabolic adjustments (possibly through oxytocin) might make her an even more efficient user of food energy and nutrients.[2]

Long before the concept of 'carbon footprint' was devised, wise health planners were confronting the environmental costs of artificial feeding. Way back in 1982, the Mozambican Ministry of Health calculated that a 20% rise in artificial feeding over two years would cost this poor and indebted country US$10 million, a price which excluded fuel, distribution or health costs. The fuel just for boiling the water would use up their biggest forestry project.[3] For every million artificially-fed babies, 150 million tins are used, made from 23,706 tonnes (23,333 tons) of metal. The paper labels amount to 341 tonnes (336 tons) and the wasted paper materials of the promotional nonsense go way beyond that figure. There is an increasing use of 'tetrapak' cartons which are neither biodegradable nor recyclable.[4] Millions of plastic feeding bottles contain bisphenol-A (BPA), a chemical which makes plastic last longer and leaches into the environment.[5] A director of bottle, teat and pump manufacturer Avent boasted that its UK factory distributed 20 million bottles a year, exporting 80% to 70 countries overseas.[6] This is a fraction of the infant feeding equipment sold and distributed around the world. Both manufacturing processes and disposal problems make much infant feeding equipment environmentally harmful. This might be justified if the products improved infant health, but they do not.

Exclusively breastfeeding women do not menstruate, and continued breastfeeding extends this benefit. The average breastfeeding woman will not have a period until her baby is at least 14 months old, but if periods do return during continued breastfeeding, they are lighter than in the non-lactating woman. Not menstruating (amennorhoea) is good both for women's health and the environment.[7] Sanitary towels and tampons get flushed through sewage disposal systems and pollute the seas, a serious problem, even in countries with good regulations.[8]

The measure of 'food miles', a term created by British food policy expert Tim Lang,[9] addresses another aspect of the environmental impact of what we eat. For example, shellfish (langoustines) caught in Scotland are flown to Thailand for shelling and returned to Europe for consumption. This 21,000km (30,000 mile) trip and similar astonishing journeys of other products make the way we eat a key contributor to climate change.[10] Cows' milk is transported from farm to factory for processing into powdered milk, itself an energy intensive process. It then goes to another processing plant to be made into artificial milk for infants. This is marketed globally and transported over thousands of miles. For example Wyeth, Abbott and Nutricia milks are manufactured in Ireland and their combined output accounts for 15% of the world's powdered infant formula.[11] If there were an award for the food that used the least food miles it would have to go to breastfeeding.

Cows' milk, along with red meat, is the most emissions-intensive food. The two are connected because many beef products are made from dead dairy cows or their unwanted male calves. Livestock account for 18% of human-caused greenhouse emissions: 9% of all carbon dioxide, 35 to 40% of methane and 65% of nitrous oxide. Because of their ruminant digestive systems, cows produce methane.[12] Cattle rearing is linked with water contamination and soil erosion. Cattle feed products are also transported across the world. For example, soya is exported from Brazil to Europe.

I know these calculations pale into insignificance beside the polluting effects of the weapons or aircraft industries and the needless use of fuel-profligate vehicles. The globalised world trade system is geared towards carrying goods back and forth across the world with scant regard for environmental costs. I do not want any parent or carer who artificially feeds to suffer guilt over this giant global problem. The issue is recognition. Inventors of fuel-saving cars are rewarded, so why not energy-sparing women? If a non-polluting factory can earn carbon emission points from a polluting one (which just transfers the problem), why not reward a breastfeeding woman for her contribution to environmental protection?

protecting, promoting and supporting the dairy industry

If cows' milk were not so protected, artificial milks would not be so profitable and the motive to push their use would lessen. Cows' milk comes at a price that has less to do with the 'invisible hand' of the market than the invisible hand of government subsidy. In the USA, cows' milk has been a state-subsidised product for over 70 years.[13] So too in much of Europe since the Second World War. New Zealand subsidised dairy production until the 1980s, and Australia until 2000. Does this mean that the US and European administrations endorse an idyllic world of happy dairy farmers, calling their cows by name as they amble peacefully from sunlit fields to milking sheds? No, on the contrary, small dairy farmers are a disappearing breed and they have not been the main beneficiaries of subsidies. In the USA in 1980 there were 350,000 farms with an average of thirty cows; by 2003, 58,000 farms with an average of 105 cows. In the UK the 35,000 dairy farms that existed in 1997 halved within a decade. The pattern is the same across the European Union. This does not mean less milk production. On the contrary, agribusiness methods, which include the routine use of hormones, antibiotics and intensive feeding, have increased milk yields per cow by an annual 2.1% since 1980. A cow need only produce 10 litres a day to feed her calf. Intensively bred and fed cows produce over 70 litres a day. They are usually killed after three or four lactations, whereas in the past they would live through ten. Some stay indoors their whole lives. Their milk is not as nutritious as organically produced milk.[14]

Despite World Trade Organisation (WTO) rules designed to restrain subsidies, US$4 billion a year of US taxpayers' money goes mostly to big rich corporations.[15] Every US dairy cow is subsidised by US$700.00 per year, an amount greater than the income of half the world's population.[16] Since 1985, much has been in the form of export subsidies mainly for powdered milk. A system of Federal Milk Marketing Orders is aimed at "equalizing competition between proprietary handlers and producers and promoting a greater degree of stability in marketing relationships".[17]

The European Union has a similar system. Most subsidies go to manufacturers and processors who control the dairy farmers. Processed dairy products have become concentrated in the hands of a few powerful corporations. At the end of the 20th century the subsidies paid across all the OECD countries (i.e. the rich and powerful) amounted to half the value of the milk. The European Union paid €1.4 billion in export refunds to processors and exporters in 2004. The top 20 global dairy corporations' turnover increased by 60% between 1992 and 2000.[18] Nestlé is the largest, with a dairy turnover of €14.3 billion in 2006. In 2005 Nestlé had received more than £30 million in subsidies over two years.[19]

I must resist the temptation to tell you more and more about the system whereby your money is used to finance milk-marketing corporations. The point is that the industry would not be putting so much money and effort into promoting ever-diversified processed milk products if taxpayers were not helping to finance production. In the USA and some other countries taxpayers pay once again for artificial milk for the infants of poor mothers, the very children who are most at risk from not breastfeeding. Should taxes contribute to the profits of already profitable dairy companies? Free market doctrine says not, but the recent orgy of publically funded generosity towards collapsing financial institutions has been like discovering vegetarians enjoying an ox roast. It has revealed that the sacred free market never truly existed. The revolving door of government and company service means that the very tax breaks which make companies rich have been engendered by corporate influence.[20] Companies invest millions to push the products they have made out of subsidised raw materials and blatantly ignore the Code. Perhaps this could be defended if there were a 'level playing field' of influence. However censorship of the truth of corporate power is widespread in the 'free' world. When the Canadian-based organisation Adbusters wanted to air (and pay for) a counter-consumerism advertisement for 'Buy Nothing Day', the US stations NBC, CBS and ABC refused to broadcast it.[21]

Who are these kindly and mysterious taxpayers who prop up the milk business? They are certainly not wealthy companies and individuals. The rich are far too skilled at tax avoidance. If all the money kept in 'tax havens' went into the public purse it would raise US$225 billion, enough to finance the millennium development goals five times over.   In the UK, Her Majesty's Revenue and Customs estimate that companies avoid £13.7 billion worth of taxes. As Polly Toynbee writes: "'Corporate social responsibility' becomes an oxymoron when top companies who avoid so much tax parade policy documents adorned with pictures of wind turbines, smiling black faces and laughing children labelled 'sustainability', 'diversity' and 'community'."[23] In most countries the bulk of tax is paid by the mass of ordinary middle or low paid people.

While gathering information about the USA , an informant told me that mothers "are not able to stay home for a year and dreamily breastfeed their days away". She explained: "We have a tough reality here – no paid maternity leave, employers who couldn't care less about breastfeeding, crushing commercial pressure to formula-feed. Many of our low income mothers must work as they have no other choice."[24] How often have 'welfare mums' been presented as the great sponges of public finance when all the time taxpayers were providing welfare cheques for dairy company executives or their wives 'to stay home for a year and dreamily breastfeed their days away'.

Why not 'protectionism' for breastfeeding? Why subsidise one product, cows' milk, so comprehensively when more important products are ignored? When we live under the global theocracy of the religion of the free market, this hypocrisy stings. Poor countries get their wrists slapped if they dare subsidise any food production, yet decades after shortages had disappeared, rich countries fed the dairy industry with taxpayers' money, despite pious statements at world trade talks. These cunning ploys damage poor countries because the import of subsidised cows' milk undercuts small local farmers and distorts trade balances.[25]

Am I against cows' milk? No. I am against its overproduction and overuse. Switching from the average North American diet (high dairy, high meat) to a plant-food dominated diet could cut greenhouse emissions by 1.5 tonnes carbon dioxide equivalent per person. This would free up land for much needed plant crops and reduce destructive farming methods, land misuse and food shortages. This could ease global hunger and reduce diseases of affluence such as cardiovascular disease, diabetes and cancer.[26] Small amounts of dairy products are useful in a varied diet, but the applauded nutrients are abundant in plant foods. Seeds, nuts and vegetables can easily provide as much or more calcium than milk. Small children who have stopped breastfeeding do need some animal products in their diet, but no adult needs the vast quantities that have come to be considered normal in rich societies.

The overproduction and over-consumption of dairy products has more to do with maintaining the health of the dairy industries than that of human beings. What is important is a sense of proportion. A plant-based diet with a small quantity of animal products is the key to the health of humans and the planet. The reverse pattern has evolved because of the power of the producers who bankrolled politicians and distorted national health messages. In her book Food Politics, Professor of Nutrition, Marion Nestle (no connection with the company) shows how US public health nutrition policy was manipulated out of shape in the interests of corporations. The US dairy industry has given large sums of money to political campaigns whatever the party and it has been a successful strategy.[27]

what are we paying for?

There is a consensus that poverty is the great enemy of child health. On every level from governments to the household, from bank accounts to the meal table, women are worse off than men. Women who care for children are usually poorer than women who do not. If every mother were entitled to proper economic reward, this would facilitate a redistribution of resources that could benefit any society on every level.

The first obstacle, usually from politicians and economic gurus, is the cry of, 'we can't afford it.' Governments have always found the resources to do what the powerful consider important. Between 1945 and 1999, US $4 trillion was spent on nuclear weapons production, enough weaponry to kill every person on earth 12 times over.[28] Military defence experts have pointed out that nuclear weapons do not assist military goals yet spending continued.[29] Global military expenditure exceeds US$1,000 billion a year, about US$166 for every human being on the planet, more than the annual income of millions. These costs do not include the peripheral services, administration and research which cushion the arms industry. The UK, France and the USA are the largest exporters of arms. Despite free market ideology, taxpayers foot this giant bill for killing. In 2003, half of all US government discretionary expenditure was used for military purposes. At the end of the 20th century South Africa spent US$5 billion on weapons 'for peacekeeping'.[30] As JK Galbraith wrote, "Arms expenditure does not occur after detached analysis by the public sector. Much is at the initiative of the arms industry and its political voice, the private sector."[31]

The justification for profit-seeking is that 'growth' leads to prosperity and improved human welfare. This is evidently untrue, though it has kept a minority of the world's population comfortable. As Cambridge economist Noreena Hertz explains: "Wealth does not always trickle down. There are limits to growth. The state will not protect us. A society guided only by the invisible hand of the market is not only imperfect, but also unjust."[32] The redistribution to mothers of money diverted from the pockets of artificial milk and bottle manufacturers could change the direction of the economy not depress it. Women spend money on food, seeds and other commodities which really do improve health and the quality of life as shown when NGOs have established such support systems.[33] Worldwide, most women put their children's welfare first. Sadly there is evidence that men often do not.[34]

One historical example of redistribution being more effective than wealth is shown by the effect of national policies during the Second World War in Britain. The country's resources were severely limited, yet health and nutrition improved because they were fairly distributed and women controlled the spending. Child welfare was given priority, and women were involved in decision-making and national economic production. Interestingly, public breastfeeding, which had virtually disappeared during the early twentieth century, became socially acceptable during the Second World War.[35] Women were supported to combine mothering and paid work outside the home.

The term 'children' in any fundraising appeal has an immediate emotive effect and people give generously when confronted with the images of suffering children, yet the question must be asked: what sort of world allows there to be 'children in need'? Why are there not fundraising appeals for weapons development, royal family weddings, presidential expenses or nuclear reactors?

Our current economic system is based in part on the philosophy of Thomas Hobbes (1588–1679) famous for his statement that for most people life is 'poor, nasty, brutish and short'. He believed that humans act on their appetites, mostly a desire for power, and their aversions, mostly fear of others. Our economic system grew out of his theories. It is based on the assumption that all human behaviour is motivated by material self-interest and that economically the individual is absolved of moral responsibility.[36] Perhaps if people had felt morally obliged to be aware of what their money was being used for, the recent financial collapses might have been prevented. Though much of what Hobbes described is true, he and modern economists chose to ignore the vast evidence for human kindness and altruism. Nowhere is this more evident than in the way most parents love their children; this cannot just be contributed to the theory of 'the selfish gene'[37] because adopting parents also love their children. Breastfeeding represents this altruism and the fact that it has endured unrewarded throughout the most materialistic era of human existence counteracts Hobbes' ideas.

The goal of ever increasing money-making has come to mean the destruction of our most precious capital. We are not just selling off the family silver, we are crushing it into dust. The pillage of the earth's resources is leading to the destruction of the source of all our wealth. We could turn to our most neglected and abundant resource, people. The levels of communication, knowledge and organisational skills that we have attained through the experience of industrial development can be diverted and utilised to build a truly productive society where waste is not the god but the devil. Most of the world's women do not benefit from wealth creation; it trickles past them rather than to them. Women use up fewer resources than men; they are biologically more energy sparing and yet most women are disadvantaged economically simply for being female.

the brave new world

When Shulamith Firestone demanded that technology should take over all reproductive functions, she opened a Pandora's box.[38] Almost four decades later, biotechnological science is hurtling towards this end. Biotech companies already harvest the pharmacological contents of human milk for profit. Who gets the money? One profit-making company, Prolacta Bioscience, markets human milk fortifier made of 100% human milk.[39] Reading the website, I feel convinced by the statements about the quality of the product, but I am uncomfortable with other aspects of this enterprise. Firstly my understanding is that commercial human milk fortifier should be used rarely and only after testing an individual mother's milk.[40] What troubles me is the fact that the company states that it does not provide donors with financial compensation. How are they compensated? The company justifies its for-profit status because it has invested over US$10 million. When this is paid back to the investors will it then become a non-profit enterprise? Should the women who donate take out a patent on their breastmilk? Should there be recompense for all the milk handed over to scientists and companies for research? In fact I do not want to propose that donors should be paid because it has been shown that altruism is a protection against poor quality of breastmilk, blood or organs, and is therefore safer. It is the exploitation of that oxytocin-driven altruism that troubles me. While the products of women's bodies are being cleverly utilised, it remains problematic for women to suckle (or provide breastmilk for) their own children. Kangaroo mother care is still not the norm for stablilised babies in the high tech units around the world, yet it is known to facilitate more effective breastfeeding. Why is the least costly and as effective method spurned? Does the profit motive suppress innovation? In his 1932 science fiction novel Brave New World, Aldous Huxley depicted a world where humans were reared in laboratories. In 1958, towards the end of his life, he expressed dread that his fantasy might be coming true.[42]

The zeal to solve the problems of nature has created more problems, and women have lost a power that their ancestors took for granted. The errors and the sabotage created the acceptance of the normality of a prosthetic instrument, the bottle, and of a third-class substitute for an amazing fluid that our own bodies miraculously produce. It is as if crutches intended for those with damaged legs were issued to everyone, in case their legs ached a bit after a long walk. When muscle wasting follows, everyone actually needs crutches and normal walking becomes impossible. People who dare to run freely are viewed with dismay or ridicule by those who are afraid to try, and especially by the crutch makers whose livelihoods depend on their use.

a world fit for whom?

In the industrialised world our capacity to feed our children was almost destroyed by the interaction of medical ignorance and authoritarianism with commercial interests. In her book The Commercialisation of Intimate Life, Arlie Russell Hochschild shows that the more that child care and family life is made into a bundle of commodities and services to be bought and sold, the more the mother image is glorified – "hypersymbolisation", she calls it. She writes that this is "partly a response to the destabilisation of the cultural as well as economic ground on which the family rests. As a highly dynamic system, capitalism destabilises both the economy and the family."[43] The divide between privileged and poor women has widened both within and between countries. Because the modern ruling structures originated from a male-dominated world, there is resistance to the acknowledgment of intimate childcare as a human right and need. Despite progress in some cultures, many men are still not able to fulfill the supportive roles that would make fatherhood such a positive experience for the child, the man and the whole family.

The 'working woman' is the woman who earns money. The 'non-working' woman may in fact work harder than the woman in waged employment, often because she is poorer. People outside the formal labour market work extremely hard. They have many skills – surviving on minimum income; dealing with irrational bureaucracy; wasting hours of time with the agents of welfare, if they exist; finding ways of supplementing income without being punished; foraging for cheaper necessities in the marginal economy of charity, discarded goods and food; and learning to tolerate hunger, cold, scorn and boredom.

Mothers who do not delegate their childcare and do not have paid employment are officially unemployed, but they can avoid the miseries if they arrange one vital factor. They must somehow manage to get someone to support themselves and their child or children. The common assumption is that the father of the child should do this. Many do not, and even within the conventional father-supported family, women and children are often deprived because resources are withheld by the man. Economist Sylvia Chant has challenged the stereotyped victimhood of female headed households. She shows through research in The Gambia, Costa Rica and the Philippines that women in male-headed households may be poorer. When women do earn money they may be expected to top up the man's spending money. Men are less likely to make sacrifices to support their children and wage-earning women without a husband may be able to use more money for their children's benefit.[44]

Women who live in societies and within a class where fathers are able and willing to provide financial, practical and emotional support may enjoy the time when they can intimately care for their young children. In Europe, state and employer supported maternity leave has improved life for the formally employed, but those outside the system can lose out. If a woman leaves paid employment because she, and maybe her partner, have certain ideals about 'good' childcare she risks losing her place on the ladder of prestige and economic security. She is a dependant; economically she changes from an adult into a child and sometimes her self-esteem and her partner's attitude to her change. A woman has to be supremely self-confident to survive this backward step in social status, which will affect her standing for ever. Her period of childcare will never contribute to the value of her curriculum vitae or gain her increments in her salary. No wonder that some women reject this humiliating episode and delegate their childcare in order to stay in the swim. For poor women there is not even the choice.

While health agencies urge breastfeeding, they rarely challenge the cultural systems which make it difficult. Expressing breastmilk is silently accepted as the only way for elite women to function. I hope I am wrong, but I have only once known a woman suckle her baby at the World Health Assembly and she was a member of IBFAN. I have friends in poor countries who are astonished to learn that some industrialised countries have brought in laws to permit breastfeeding in public. It is as though there had to be a law to permit smiling. Though attitudes have softened in recent years, in many 'advanced' countries there is an apartheid of those who care for their young children and those who do not. Many women who have control over their fertility still want to bear children, and this is increasingly becoming a momentous decision. The prestigious worlds of business, academia and politics have let women put one foot in the door on condition that they hide their reproductive functions. I have even met this in agencies concerned with mother and child health. Correct rules might be in place but the atmosphere for a woman who wants to breastfeed at work might be distinctly chilly.

When New Zealand biochemist Sylvia Rumball decided to have children she said to her professor, "I am going to have children and I want to reduce and change my timetable to suit my changed situation. I also want to keep my tenure and to get my deserved promotion; this is perfectly reasonable; I have two jobs to do and there will be no reduction in the quality of my work. You could equally arrange this contract to someone who wanted to run a farm as well as be an academic." Sylvia could claim her rights because she was a highly respected scientist and had the self-esteem to demand justice, but what she was demanding should be the right of all women. It is up to women with some measure of power to push for these rights. Sylvia led the way for many young women today. Motherhood is much more accepted now amongst assertive, educated women, but the less privileged still suffer.[45]

Every mother who is breastfeeding is caring for a child in the best possible way. She is nurturing and forming a future member of society. She is saving finite resources beyond valuation and billions of dollars' worth of healthcare costs. But the way our society is organised means that those who control and use up the earth's resources are the richest and the most revered. Waste is favoured because it produces what is defined to be wealth. The production of the perfect food delivered in the ideal way actually benefits a child and his mother, but this production and service does not make money for any company; in the economic terms of our world, it does not 'create wealth'.

There is nothing intrinsically wrong with production. It is the methods and scale of production that cause the problems. It is the fact that we are eating up at an exponential rate all the non-renewable resources, producing many goods that are at best useless and at worst harmful. The injustice is that the really useful products never reach a large proportion of humanity. To keep this system going we destroy intrinsically useful products and processes.

During the 20th century a vast array of means were used to

interfere with breastfeeding. Women and babies have been separated for many reasons: for custom, for labour, for sexual and other services to men, but most of all because people got in the habit of doing this and forgot why it was done. The production and aggressive promotion of commercial artificial milks took power away from women and gave it to industry. Industry got richer and women got poorer. Artificial milks will certainly be needed for the near future. The money that is squandered on marketing should be diverted into improved manufacture and quality control. There is an urgent need to implement impartial and transparent systems for effective and regular inspection of products. Production mishaps or contamination should not only be brought to light by the illness or death of infants. If health is the priority, then long-term planning for reducing output while making the product safer should be discussed at global level. The manufacturers run economies of scale, they must lure the great mass of women away from breastfeeding to keep their products profitable. It may be more ethical to view artificial milk as a non-profit product and take it out of the market altogether.

the growth factor

The hardest thing about writing this book has been coping with my own despair as I confront the facts of human 'progress'. It is not simply breastfeeding that is destroyed before it has even begun to flow, but the oxygen-giving, climate-maintaining forests, the food-abundant sea and the fertile earth. All the wealth, beauty and resilience that nature has provided for so long is being damaged irretrievably. As I check one fact with a biologist he casually uses the throwaway line 'with this endgame' as he refers to the state of affairs in the contemporary world. I admire him for being able to work so well while his consciousness of reality is so brutal. His words paralyse me for days. Another biologist offers me the image of a wave breaking to illustrate the crisis that is upon us and she convinces me that there is no hope. I cannot turn away from their considered judgments, but my only response is a denial of passivity. If the solidarity of Hadza women can keep the violence of their menfolk at bay, why cannot the solidarity of those who care about the world keep the violence of the economic system from causing so much human suffering and from destroying life itself? Even if global warming turned out to be a mistaken concept, the world and human society would be more at ease with each other if our current priorities of greed and destruction were reduced. If wealth were distributed more equitably, there would be less misery and less conflict.

I started out with the idea that breastmilk and breastfeeding was of such economic value that it should be recognised and valued in these terms. I find myself in a dilemma, for I now realise that 'economics' has become a religion that has been deliberately kept obscure so that the ordinary person does not rumble the truth. In medieval Europe, the Christian church controlled the people through a set of ideas which few dared to doubt or challenge. The threat of excommunication kept millions subdued, although they could not understand the language, Latin, in which the threat was made. The concept of condemning their immortal souls to hell kept them subject to a social order that benefited the powerful. In the modern world millions of the poor are kept down by the religion of economics whose priests use an equally obscure language and who threaten whole communities with excommunication if they do not obey their commandments. Like the medieval priests, many modern economists have (until recently) sincerely believed in their own religious edicts and have accepted the suffering of the poor as part of the overall plan. Perhaps even I could accept it if I thought there was some long-term good, but I see none.

The word 'growth' is apt to describe the aims of modern economists because it is also used for a tumour that eats away at the body. The principle of economic growth is like a tumour. The sources of thousands of beneficial products, the forests, are obliterated to provide hamburgers that contribute to ill-health, served in cartons that pollute the earth. The producers say it is 'uneconomic' to stop this production. The sea and land are poisoned with radioactive waste and chemicals designed to resist the healing cycle of nature and contaminate all living tissue. Women are led to believe that breastfeeding is not possible, or that it demeans them or is a trivial function, yet cows must consume poor people's food crops to produce expensive milk so that more women can participate in this relentless growth. More power stations must be built so 'production' and 'growth' will expand even faster. The tumour must be fed.

But, say the economists, we need this wealth to invest for our future. Where is this investment? I do not see the wealthy investing in good. I see enormous sums spent on drugs such as alcohol, tranquillisers, tobacco, cocaine and heroin, because people desperately need to escape from themselves, their pain and reality. I see salaries paid to bureaucrats, to police and military forces who are needed as agents of control, as 'development' accelerates social breakdown. Contrasts of poverty and wealth, more horrifying than any of those which precipitated the French Revolution (1789), widen across the world. Technology means that the poor can watch the rich at play on TV screens and computer monitors, while the wealthy can watch the poor starve. Rich, powerful men spend millions on entertainment, on the sexual exploitation of those who have only their bodies to sell. Money goes to the purveyors of pornography on the internet, in films, magazines and live shows so that a man can be stimulated for long enough for him to have sex with a stranger so that he can feel alive for ten seconds. Money is 'invested' in conspicuous consumption that makes up in opulence and extravagance for the empty soul of the owner. There have always been greedy people, and who can prove what causes the emptiness in someone's heart that compels them to seek out more than is needed for life and harmony? It is only with this flowering of industrialised capitalism that it has become a duty to maintain a system that depends on the greed and infinite consumption of the few and the stoicism and infinite degradation of the many. Greed has always been with us, but it has never had such ideological support. When Ghengis Khan brutally conquered half the world, few of the crushed peasants actually cheered. Now the transnational companies who are laying waste the world and enslaving the people boast about their conquests in TV and internet commercials, and worldwide people innocently display their badges.

A detective novel by Michael Gilbert, Fear to Tread (1953), describes a company that sells a charlatan cure for skin trouble. The 'cure' uses two products. The first is applied to the diseased skin and the user is told that this "draws out the toxins"; the second is the balm that soothes the inflammation. The first product is merely itching powder that causes irritation. Industrialised capitalism works on the same principle: many of its products are designed to sooth the itching it has itself caused.

There are other ways to solve problems. For example, cassava, a vital food crop in Africa, was being ravaged by a mealy bug, but the same blight was not happening in South America where cassava had originated. An entomologist researched for two years and discovered a predator wasp. This was introduced to Africa, colonised and kept the cassava pest under control.[46] But who will get rich from a solution that distributes itself and only benefits the poor household consumer? Where is the extracted value? Who has the incentive to pay for more research of this beneficial nature? It is the same with breastfeeding; it would save millions of lives and drugs and drips, but how would the artificial milk and bottle manufacturers stay rich if it were truly endorsed by the social and economic system? With the free market there must be the 'incentive', which is not the drive to make the world a pleasant harmonious place for everyone, only using technology when it is appropriate and beneficial. Rather the motivation must be the desire to do better than your fellows; competition to destruction. A 12-year-old boy I knew said, "I don't understand socialism because surely the whole point of working is to get richer and have more than your mates, to have a bigger car, better clothes and more toys." The world is run by little boys who think like this, only they are twice the size of the twelve-year-old and their toys are sophisticated weapons and factories that create as many poisons as useful products.

The infant feeding companies and many misguided individuals spent a century telling women that their own milk was not there or was not good enough. Now many women have lost faith in their own bodies, the milk has gone and they believe they 'need' these products to keep their children alive. Nestlé is now the world's largest bottled water company and it has been extracting and demineralising water so as to sell it, against the policy and wishes of the people in the state of Minas Gerais, Brazil.[47] Doubtless it will be among the first to find some way of marketing clean air if there is any left to sell. Other companies are no different. They started by destroying our milk and making us believe their cocktail of coconut and cow juice was better. They will end by destroying our planet and making us believe their wasteland is what we want.

epilogue

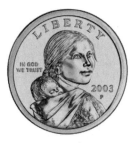

33 Golden Dollar Observe
(© 1999 US Mint)

This coin embodies much of what I have tried to say in this book. Issued to celebrate the start of the 21st century, this golden dollar represents the world's obsession with one kind of wealth: money. The engraved image of Sacagawea and her son represents another sort of wealth.

Sacagawea and her baby were crucial to the appropriation of the western territories of the USA. A skilled tracker, she accompanied Captains Lewis and Clark during their years of exploration in the early 19th century. She helped them survive in the wilderness, recognising and gathering the roots, berries and plants they used for food and medicine. She acted as interpreter and was known for her calmness under duress. Lewis and Clark could approach hostile villages because a woman with a baby was trusted: 'She was a living white flag, a sign of peace.' All this time she carried, fed and cared for her son, Pompey, 'the little dancing boy', who grew up to be a skilled explorer.[1]

Unwittingly, Sacagawea was a founding mother of what came to be the most powerful nation on earth. She was everything that is now despised. She was illiterate, poor, a teenage mother and a Native American (probably Shoshone); a member of the peoples who are the most damaged, scorned and ignored in modern North America. And she was a breastfeeding mother.

Now in the 21st century, a professor from the International Society of Research on Human Milk and Lactation boasts of "an impressive amount of publications on breastfeeding now; there are at least 50 or 60 relevant papers coming out every month."[2] These papers make no difference to the great majority of modern Sacagaweas whose talents are crushed before they are developed. Those Chinese mothers who fed their babies contaminated milk could have breastfed and used their various skills, but their human potential was sacrificed, along with their babies, to commercial greed. Economists still over-value products and processes that are leading to the destruction of the earth, yet when women breastfeed, it is not even registered as a productive activity. All the breastfeeding promotion in the world will be a waste of effort if this contradiction continues.

Sacagawea's husband got $500 and 320 acres* of land in recompense for her work. The revered and romanticised figure on the US coin never profited from her contribution to the Europeans' takeover.[3] Nevertheless, she and the European explorers took it for granted that a baby must be close to his mother for breastfeeding and care. Neither saw mothering, and work beyond mothering, as contradictory. Sacagawea was both exploited and respected. With the exception of a few advanced societies, such as Norway, in most of the world only a minority of women have a choice in their decisions about mothering, economic survival and participation in society. It doesn't have to be like this.

A creature from another planet visiting the Earth might ask, "If women are the ones that keep the human race going, why do they get the rough deal?" We need to answer that question, environmentally, economically and politically. And we can. There are so many huge and complex problems to tackle, but breastfeeding is one of the simpler ones.

* 129.5 hectares.

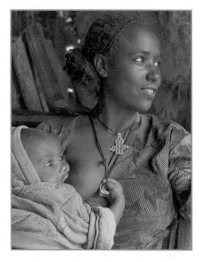

34 Ethiopian mother and her baby.
(Photo Frederic Courbet, courtesy
of Save the Children, UK)

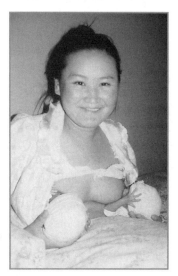

35 Mother suckling her premature twins
in special care unit, Ulaan Baatar,
Mongolia. (Photo Gabrielle Palmer)

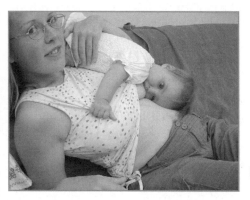

36 Mother and baby
breastfeed their own way.
(Photo Lucy Nicholls)

visit
www.thepoliticsofbreastfeeding.com
for news and links

acknowledgments

Great thanks to Lois Carter, Lorna Hartwell, Alison Jones, Lida Lhotska, Dennis O'Connell-Baker, Rachel O'Leary, Patti Rundall and Magda Sachs. They have all provided much skilled and generous support and without them this book would not be written.

Special thanks to my writers' group: Shelley Bovey, Janet Laurence, Maggie Makepeace and Georgina Newbery who have kept me going.

I also thank: Sue Ashmore, Maryse Avendt, Helen Ball, Annalisa Barbieri, Carol Bartle, Genevieve Becker, Nina Berry, Helen Bilton, Alison Blenkinsop, Mike Brady, Sandy Cairncross, Janet Calvert, Geoffrey Cannon, Adreano Catteano, David Clark, Clodagh Corcoran, Jan Cornfoot, Carmel Duffy, Fiona Dykes, Irene Elia, Tom Eve, Chloe Fisher, Peter Greaves, Karleen Gribble, Tom Hale, Sarah Hanson, Sophie Hinsliff, Elizabeth Hormann, Alessandro Iellamo, Sally Inch, Trudy Katzer, Julie Kavanagh, Sandra Lang, Sebastian Lucas, Sue Lucas, Miriam Labbock, Alison Linnecar, Ali McClaine, Marie McGrath, Tessa Martyn, Michael Mahsetky, Cally Matthews, Anthea Miller, Rachel Myr, Jim Paterson, Chris Perera, Abigail Perry, Belinda Phipps, Andrew Radford, Gill Rapley, Marina Rea, Flora Rees, Mary Renfrew, Judith Richter, Sue Saunders, Felicity Savage, Claire Schofield, Vilneide Serva, Mary Smale, Julie Smith, Betty Sterken, Teresa Toma, Elise Van Rooyen, Marsha Walker, Isabel Warren, Jenny Warren, Carolyn Westcott, Carol Williams, Gillian Weaver and James and Lisa Woodburn.

Amongst all my sources I feel most indebted to the work of Rima Apple, Andy Chetley, Valerie Fildes and Felicity Lawrence. They provided me with a gold-mine of facts and I am grateful for all the research they published.

I thank my husband John; our children Nathaniel and Frances, their spouses Maria and Robert and my siblings Kevin, Glynis, Michael, Any and Marianne for all their help and kindness. I thank my grandson Benjamin for reminding me just how delightful a baby can be and what a brief phase babyhood is.

I warmly thank Martin Wagner and Maria Pinter who cured me of cynicism about publishers and Anne Campbell for proposing they publish this book. I also thank Mark Le Fanu and his colleagues at The Society of Authors who steered me through a sticky situation with great patience. I thank producer Tony Laryea for permission to use the title of the 1984 BBC Open Spaces programme, 'When Breasts are Bad for Business', which was Patti Rundall's idea. Lastly I thank Sheila Kitzinger who, in 1986, asked me to write the first edition of The Politics of Breastfeeding.

abbreviations and explanation of terms

1. Abbreviations (organisations)

Codex	Codex Alimentarius Commission
EU	European Union
FAO	Food and Agriculture Organisation of the United Nations
FDA	US Food and Drug Administration
IBFAN	International Baby Food Action Network
IBLCE	International Board of Lactation Consultant Examiners
ICDC	International Code Documentation Centre
ICIFI	International Council of Infant Food Industries
ILCA	International Lactation Consultant Association
ILO	International Labour Organisation
IMF	International Monetary Fund
OECD	Organisation for Economic Co-operation and Development
UN	United Nations
UNICEF	United Nations Children's Fund
UNHCR	United Nations High Commission for Refugees
WABA	World Alliance for Breastfeeding Action
WB	World Bank
WHA	World Health Assembly
WHO	World Health Organisation
WTO	World Trade Organisation

2. Abbreviations (general)

AFASS	Acceptable, feasible, affordable, sustainable, safe
ARV	Anti-retroviral (drugs)
BFHI	Baby Friendly Hospital Initiative (in UK called BFI)
BMS	Breastmilk substitute
The Code	The International Code of Marketing of Breastmilk Substitutes
CRC	Convention on the Rights of the Child
C-section	Caesarean section
EBM	Expressed breastmilk
FOF	Follow-on formula
FOM	Follow-on milk
GSIYCF	Global Strategy for Infant and Young Child Feeding
HIV/AIDS	Human immunodeficiency virus/ acquired immunodeficiency syndrome
IBCLC	International Board Certified Lactation Consultant
LBW	Low birth weight
MDGs	UN Millennium Development Goals

MTCT	Mother to child transmission
NGO	Non-governmental Organisation
PIF	Powdered infant formula
POPs	Persistent Organic Pollutants
SIF	Soya infant formula

3. General terms

Big business: the large transnational commercial companies with considerable power and influence; also called multinational companies. I also use the terms corporation, industry (as in 'infant feeding industry') and manufacturers.

Developing countries/regions/world: the newest terms for the regions where most people live in poverty are 'the majority world' or 'the south'. I also use 'poor' and 'impoverished' countries/regions'.

Developed countries/regions/world/societies: I use 'industrialised societies' and 'rich countries/regions'. I am aware that there are people living in so-called 'developed societies' in conditions of poverty and that in the poorest nations, some citizens live in luxury, but these general terms are necessary.

4. Other

Dummy	pacifier or soother
Teat	(artificial) nipple
Soya	Soy

appendix 1: the global strategy for infant and young child feeding: a summary (WHO and UNICEF 2003)

The Global Strategy for Infant and Young Child Feeding aims to revitalize efforts to promote, protect and support appropriate infant and young child feeding. It builds upon past initiatives, in particular the Innocenti Declaration and the Baby Friendly Hospital Initiative and addresses the needs of all children including those living in difficult circumstances, such as infants of mothers living with HIV, low-birth-weight infants and infants in emergency situations. The strategy calls for action in the following areas:

- All governments should develop and implement a comprehensive policy on infant and young child feeding, in the context of national policies for nutrition, child and reproductive health, and poverty reduction.
- All mothers should have access to skilled support to initiate and sustain exclusive breastfeeding for 6 months and ensure the timely introduction of adequate and safe complementary foods with continued breastfeeding up to two years or beyond.
- Health workers should be empowered to provide effective feeding counselling, and their services be extended in the community by trained lay or peer counsellors.
- Governments should review progress in national implementation of the International Code of Marketing of Breastmilk Substitutes, and consider new legislation or additional measures as needed to protect families from adverse commercial influences.
- Governments should enact imaginative legislation protecting the breastfeeding rights of working women and establishing means for its enforcement in accordance with international labour standards.

The strategy specifies not only responsibilities of governments, but also of international organisations, non-governmental organisations and other concerned parties. It engages all relevant stakeholders and provides a framework for accelerated action, linking relevant intervention areas and using resources available in a variety of sectors.

© World Health Organisation 2003. The full version is available from: www.who.int/entity/child_adolescent_health/documents/9241562218/en/ and was endorsed in the 2002 World Health Assembly Resolution WHA55.25

appendix 2: innocenti declaration 2005 on infant and young child feeding

*We who are assembled in Florence, Italy, on this Twenty-Second Day of November 2005 to celebrate the 15th Anniversary of the Innocenti Declaration on the Protection, Promotion and Support of Breastfeeding **declare that these actions are urgent and necessary to ensure the best start in life for our children, for the achievement of the Millennium Development Goals by 2015, and for the realisation of the human rights of present and future generations.***

In the 15 years since the adoption of the original Innocenti Declaration in 1990, remarkable progress has been made in improving infant and young child feeding practices worldwide. Nevertheless, inappropriate feeding practices – sub-optimal or no breastfeeding and inadequate complementary feeding – remain the greatest threat to child health and survival globally. Improved breastfeeding alone could save the lives of more than 3,500 children every day, more than any other preventive intervention.

Guided by accepted human rights principles, especially those embodied in the Convention on the Rights of the Child, our vision is of an environment that enables mothers, families and other caregivers to make informed decisions about optimal feeding, which is defined as exclusive breastfeeding* for six months followed by the introduction of appropriate complementary feeding and continuation of breastfeeding for up to two years of age or beyond. Achieving this vision requires skilled practical support to arrive at the highest attainable standard of health and development for infants and young children, which is the universally recognised right of every child.

Challenges remain: poverty, the HIV pandemic, natural and human-made emergencies, globalisation, environmental contamination, health systems investing primarily in curative rather than preventive services, gender inequities and women's increasing rates of employment outside the home, including in the non-formal sector. These challenges must be addressed to achieve the Millennium Development Goals and the aims of the Millennium Declaration and for the vision set out above to become reality for all children.

The targets of the 1990 Innocenti Declaration and the 2002 Global Strategy for Infant and Young Child Feeding remain the foundation for action. While remarkable progress has been made, much more needs to be done.

We therefore issue this Call for Action so that:

All parties
- Empower women in their own right, and as mothers and providers of breastfeeding support and information to other women.
- Support breastfeeding as the norm for feeding infants and young children.
- Highlight the risks of artificial feeding and the implications for health and

---

* Exclusive breastfeeding means that no other drink or food is given to the infant; the infant should feed frequently and for unrestricted periods.

development throughout the life course.
- Ensure the health and nutritional status of women throughout all stages of life.
- Protect breastfeeding in emergencies, including by supporting uninterrupted breastfeeding and appropriate complementary feeding, and avoiding general distribution of breastmilk substitutes.
- Implement the HIV and Infant Feeding – Framework for Priority Action, including protecting, promoting and supporting breastfeeding for the general population while providing counselling and support for HIV-positive women.

All governments
- Establish or strengthen national infant and young child feeding and breastfeeding authorities, coordinating committees and oversight groups that are free from commercial influence and other conflicts of interest.
- Revitalise the Baby-friendly Hospital Initiative (BFHI), maintaining the Global Criteria as the minimum requirement for all facilities, expanding the Initiative's application to include maternity, neonatal and child health services and community-based support for lactating women and caregivers of young children.
- Implement all provisions of the International Code of Marketing of Breastmilk Substitutes and subsequent relevant World Health Assembly resolutions in their entirety as a minimum requirement, and establish sustainable enforcement mechanisms to prevent and/or address non-compliance.
- Adopt maternity protection legislation and other measures that facilitate six months of exclusive breastfeeding for women employed in all sectors, with urgent attention to the non-formal sector.
- Ensure that appropriate guidelines and skill acquisition regarding infant and young child feeding are included in both pre-service and in-service training of all health care staff, to enable them to implement infant and young child feeding policies and to provide a high standard of breastfeeding management and counselling to support mothers to practise optimal breastfeeding and complementary feeding.
- Ensure that all mothers are aware of their rights and have access to support, information and counselling in breastfeeding and complementary feeding from health workers and peer groups.
- Establish sustainable systems for monitoring infant and young child feeding patterns and trends and use this information for advocacy and programming.
- Encourage the media to provide positive images of optimal infant and young child feeding, to support breastfeeding as the norm, and to participate in social mobilisation activities such as World Breastfeeding Week.
- Take measures to protect populations, especially pregnant and breast-feeding mothers, from environmental contaminants and chemical residues.
- Identify and allocate sufficient resources to fully implement actions called for in the Global Strategy for Infant and Young Child Feeding.
- Monitor progress in appropriate infant and young child feeding practices and report periodically, including as provided in the Convention on the Rights of the Child.

All manufacturers and distributors of products within the scope of the International Code
- Ensure full compliance with all provisions of the International Code and subsequent relevant World Health Assembly resolutions in all countries, independently of any other measures taken to implement the Code.

- Ensure that all processed foods for infants and young children meet applicable Codex Alimentarius standards.

Multilateral and bilateral organisations and international financial institutions
- Recognise that optimal breastfeeding and complementary feeding are essential to achieving the long-term physical, intellectual and emotional health of all populations and therefore the attainment of the Millennium Development Goals and other development initiatives and that inappropriate feeding practices and their consequences are major obstacles to poverty reduction and sustainable socio-economic development.
- Identify and budget for sufficient financial resources and expertise to support governments in formulating, implementing, monitoring and evaluating their policies and programmes on optimal infant and young child feeding, including revitalising the BFHI.
- Increase technical guidance and support for national capacity building in all the target areas set forth in the Global Strategy for Infant and Young Child Feeding.
- Support operational research to fill information gaps and improve programming.
- Encourage the inclusion of programmes to improve breastfeeding and complementary feeding in poverty-reduction strategies and health sector development plans.

Public interest non-governmental organisations
- Give greater priority to protecting, promoting and supporting optimal feeding practices, including relevant training of health and community workers, and increase effectiveness through cooperation and mutual support.
- Draw attention to activities which are incompatible with the Code's principles and aim so that violations can be effectively addressed in accordance with national legislation, regulations or other suitable measures.

The Global Strategy for Infant and Young Child Feeding
Operational Targets

Four operational targets from the 1990 Innocenti Declaration:
1. Appoint a national breastfeeding coordinator with appropriate authority, and establish a multisectoral national breastfeeding committee composed of representatives from relevant government departments, non-governmental organisations, and health worker associations.
2. Ensure that every facility providing maternity services fully practises all the "Ten steps to successful breastfeeding" set out in the WHO/ UNICEF statement on breastfeeding and maternity services [see Appendix 3].
3. Give effect to the principles and aim of the International Code of Marketing of Breastmilk Substitutes and subsequent relevant Health Assembly resolutions in their entirety.
4. Enact imaginative legislation protecting the breastfeeding rights of working women and establish means for its enforcement.

Five additional operational targets:
5. Develop, implement, monitor and evaluate a comprehensive policy on infant and young child feeding, in the context of national policies and programmes

for nutrition, child and reproductive health, and poverty reduction.

6. Ensure that the health and other relevant sectors protect, promote and support exclusive breastfeeding for six months and continued breastfeeding up to two years of age or beyond, while providing women access to the support they require – in the family, community and workplace – to achieve this goal.

7. Promote timely, adequate, safe and appropriate complementary feeding with continued breastfeeding.

8. Provide guidance on feeding infants and young children in exceptionally difficult circumstances, and on the related support required by mothers, families and other caregivers.

9. Consider what new legislation or other suitable measures may be required, as part of a comprehensive policy on infant and young child feeding, to give effect to the principles and aim of the International Code of Marketing of Breast-milk Substitutes and to subsequent relevant Health Assembly resolutions.

The Innocenti Declaration 2005 was adopted by participants at the event, "Celebrating Innocenti 1990-2005: Achievements, Challenges and Future Imperatives", held on 22 November 2005, in Italy, co-organised by the following organisations:

> The Academy of Breastfeeding Medicine
> International Baby Food Action Network
> International Lactation Consultants Association
> La Leche League International
> Regione Toscana, Italy
> UNICEF
> Wellstart International
> World Alliance for Breastfeeding Action
> World Health Organisation

Further information can be obtained from:
- Innocenti +15 www.innocenti15.net
- ABM www.bfmed.org
- ILCA www.ilca.org
- LLLI www.lalecheleague.org
- IBFAN www.ibfan.org/site2005/ (Code Watch Reports)
- UNICEF Adviser, Infant Feeding, smhossain@unicef.org, www.unicef.org/nutrition/index_breastfeeding.html
- Wellstart International www.wellstart.org
- WHO Department of Nutrition for Health and Development, nutrition@who.int, http://www.who.int/nutrition, Department of Child and Adolescent Health and Development, cah@who.int, www.who.int/child.adolescent.health
- WABA www.waba.org.my/innocenti15.htm

appendix 3: the ten steps to successful breastfeeding

Every facility providing maternity services and care for newborn infants should:

1. Have a written breastfeeding policy that is routinely communicated to all health care staff.
2. Train all health care staff in skills necessary to implement this policy.
3. Inform all pregnant women about the benefits and management of breastfeeding.
4. Help mothers initiate breastfeeding within half an hour of birth.
5. Show mothers how to breastfeed, and how to maintain lactation even if they should be separated from their infants.
6. Give newborn infants no food or drink other than breastmilk, unless medically indicated.
7. Practise rooming-in – that is, allow mothers and infants to remain together – 24 hours a day.
8. Encourage breastfeeding on demand.
9. Give no artificial teats or pacifiers (also called dummies or soothers) to breastfeeding infants.
10. Foster the establishment of breastfeeding support groups and refer mothers to them on discharge from the hospital or clinic.

Source: *Protecting, Promoting and Supporting Breastfeeding: The Special Role of Maternity Services*, a joint WHO/UNICEF statement published by the World Health Organization, 1989.

The Baby Friendly Hopsital Initiative was launched in 1991 as a strategy to implement the Ten Steps, the goal of the 2nd operational target of the 1990 Innocenti Declaration reiterated in 2005.

appendix 4: section from the convention on the rights of the child

The Convention on the Rights of the Child (CRC) was adopted by the annual Assembly of the United Nations on 20 November 1989. The following extract from the CRC (Article 24) is relevant to infant and young child feeding and the protection of parents and carers.

1. States Parties recognize the right of the child to the enjoyment of the highest attainable standard of health and to facilities for the treatment of illness and rehabilitation of health. States Parties shall strive to ensure that no child is deprived of his or her right of access to such health care services.

2. States Parties shall pursue full implementation of this right and, in particular, shall take appropriate measures:

(a) To diminish infant and child mortality;

(b) To ensure the provision of necessary medical assistance and health care to all children with emphasis on the development of primary health care;

(c) To combat disease and malnutrition, including within the framework of primary health care, through, inter alia, the application of readily available technology and through the provision of adequate nutritious foods and clean drinking-water, taking into consideration the dangers and risks of environmental pollution;

(d) To ensure appropriate pre-natal and post-natal health care for mothers;

(e) To ensure that all segments of society, in particular parents and children, are informed, have access to education and are supported in the use of basic knowledge of child health and nutrition, the advantages of breastfeeding, hygiene and environmental sanitation and the prevention of accidents;

(f) To develop preventive health care, guidance for parents and family planning education and services.

3. States Parties shall take all effective and appropriate measures with a view to abolishing traditional practices prejudicial to the health of children.

4. States Parties undertake to promote and encourage international co-operation with a view to achieving progressively the full realization of the right recognized in the present article. In this regard, particular account shall be taken of the needs of developing countries.

Author's note: The CRC is the most ratified convention in history. A Convention is stronger than any other international agreement because countries agree to be obligated to implement the provisions.

For further information on the CRC see: www.unicef.org/crc/

appendix 5: the united nations millennium development goals (MDGs) – target date 2015

GOAL 1   ERADICATE EXTREME POVERTY & HUNGER
Target 1   Reduce by half the proportion of people living on less than a dollar a day
Target 2   Achieve full and productive employment and decent work for all, including women and young people
Target 3   Reduce by half the proportion of people who suffer from hunger

GOAL 2   ACHIEVE UNIVERSAL PRIMARY EDUCATION
Target 1   Ensure that all boys and girls complete a full course of primary schooling

GOAL 3   PROMOTE GENDER EQUALITY AND EMPOWER WOMEN
Target 1   Eliminate gender disparity in primary and secondary education

GOAL 4   REDUCE CHILD MORTALITY
Target 1   Reduce by two thirds the under-five mortality rate

GOAL 5   IMPROVE MATERNAL HEALTH
Target 1   Reduce by three quarters the maternal mortality ratio
Target 2   Achieve universal access to reproductive health

GOAL 6   COMBAT HIV/AIDS, MALARIA AND OTHER DISEASES
Target 1   Halt and begin to reverse the spread of HIV/AIDS
Target 2   Achieve, by 2010, universal access to treatment for HIV/AIDS for all those who need it
Target 3   Have halted and begun to reverse the incidence of malaria and other major diseases

GOAL 7   ENSURE ENVIRONMENTAL SUSTAINABILITY
Target 1   Integrate the principles of sustainable development into country policies and programmes and reverse the loss of environmental resources
Target 2   Reduce biodiversity loss, achieving, by 2010, a significant reduction in the rate of loss
Target 3   Halve the proportion of the population without sustainable access to safe drinking water and basic sanitation
Target 4   Improve the lives of at least 100 million slum dwellers by 2020

GOAL 8   DEVELOP A GLOBAL PARTNERSHIP FOR DEVELOPMENT
Target 1   Address the special needs of least developed countries, landlocked countries and small island developing states
Target 2   Develop further an open, rule-based, predictable, non-discriminatory trading and financial system
Target 3   Deal comprehensively with developing countries' debt
Target 4   In cooperation with developing countries, develop and implement strategies for decent and productive work for youth
Target 5   In cooperation with pharmaceutical companies, provide access to affordable essential drugs in developing countries
Target 6   In cooperation with the private sector, make available benefits of new technologies, especially information and communications

See www.un.org/millenniumgoals

appendix 6: sources of information about mishaps, recalls and contaminants in infant feeding products

In previous editions of this book I included a list of adverse events. This is now too long to include. Below are some key sources of information on the internet and some documents that may be of particular interest:

The International Baby Food Action Network – www.ibfan.org
This site contains documents detailing violations of the code, studies and reports. When you visit the site please note:

- ICDC Product Recall List 2007–2008 as at September 30th/ICDC Product Recall List 2000–2006
  Both documents are detailed lists of incidents that have forced the companies to issue product recalls.
- INFOSAN – Food Safety and Nutrition During Pregnancy and Infant Feeding
- How Safe are Infant Formulas? (By JP Dadhich)
- 10 Reasons for informative labelling of powdered infant formulas
- 2005 Chronology of Withdrawal of Nestlé and other liquid milks due to ITX contamination
  A timeline of the discovery, withdrawal and fallout from an ITX contamination in Italy.
- Compilation of Official Action: Risk of Contamination of Powdered Infant Formula with Enterobacter sakazakii December 2004
- Update to compilation of official action on Enterobacter sakazakii January 2005

The World Health Organisation – www.who.int
- The latest research and policy announcements.
- WHO Guidelines for the safe preparation, storage and handling of powdered infant formula

Food and Agriculture Organization of the United Nations – www.fao.org
- FAO/WHO final report of expert meeting on 16–20 January 2006 to evaluate a quantitative risk assessment model for E. sakazakii in powdered infant formula.
  You can access web-based model to assess the risk associated with Enterobacter sakazakii in powdered infant formula. Use of this model does not require any specialist software other than an Internet platform.

National Alliance for Breastfeeding Advocacy – www.naba-breastfeeding.org
- List of recalls of infant feeding products
- A comprehensive rundown of recent infant formula recalls in the USA.

Baby Milk Action – www.babymilkaction.org
- Baby Milk Action's archive of articles on contaminants and infant feeding
  This archive falls into two main categories: 'Seeing behind the headlines about 'toxins in breastmilk' and 'Contaminants also impact on artificial feeding'.

for links see www.thepoliticsofbreastfeeding.com

appendix 7: infant feeding definitions

Exclusive breastfeeding: baby breastfed only (but may also receive expressed breastmilk). No other liquids or solids, except vitamins or medicines.

Predominant breastfeeding: breastmilk is baby's main source of nourishment, but also receives water, teas, or fruit juice, but not milk-based breastmilk substitutes.

Full breastfeeding: baby is fed mainly breastmilk, but occasionally receives a milk-based breastmilk substitute.

Partial breastfeeding: baby is fed breastmilk and regularly receives other milk-based breastmilk substitutes. Also called mixed feeding.

Artificial feeding: baby is fed milk or soy based breastmilk substitutes (infant formula). Can be exclusively artificially-fed, or partially breastfed and artificially-fed. Also called formula feeding.

Any breastfeeding: child receives breastmilk (combines exclusive and partially breastfed).

Breastmilk feeding: child receives expressed breastmilk.

Breastmilk substitute (BMS): in terms of marketing a BMS is any food being marketed or otherwise represented as a partial or total replacement for breastmilk, whether or not suitable for that purpose. In terms of nutrition, any food or drink given to a baby before six months of age, thereafter any food which replaces breastmilk in the diet to two years and beyond.

Complementary feeding: feeding of solid or semi solid foods in addition to breastmilk or infant formula. These foods may be manufactured by the food industry, big business or small local manufacture, or prepared at home. These foods are often called 'weaning foods'.

appendix 8: the convention on the elimination of all forms of discrimination against women

The Convention on the Elimination of All Forms of Discrimination against Women (CEDAW), adopted in 1979 by the UN General Assembly:

CEDAW has been called an international bill of rights for women. It defines what constitutes discrimination against women and sets up an agenda for national action to end such discrimination.

CEDAW defines discrimination against women as "...any distinction, exclusion or restriction made on the basis of sex which has the effect or purpose of impairing or nullifying the recognition, enjoyment or exercise by women, irrespective of their marital status, on a basis of equality of men and women, of human rights and fundamental freedoms in the political, economic, social, cultural, civil or any other field."

By accepting CEDAW, States commit themselves to undertake a series of measures to end discrimination against women in all forms,

CEDAW provides the basis for realizing equality between women and men through ensuring women's equal access to, and equal opportunities in, political and public life – including the right to vote and to stand for election – as well as education, health and employment. States parties agree to take all appropriate measures, including legislation and temporary special measures, so that women can enjoy all their human rights and fundamental freedoms.

CEDAW is the only human rights treaty which affirms the reproductive rights of women and targets culture and tradition as influential forces shaping gender roles and family relations. It affirms women's rights to acquire, change or retain their nationality and the nationality of their children. States parties also agree to take appropriate measures against all forms of traffic in women and exploitation of women.

CEDAW recognises the right to work as a human right, and one that women should enjoy on a basis of equality with men. To ensure this governments are called upon to, among other things:
- "prohibit ... dismissal on the grounds of pregnancy or maternity leave..."
- "introduce maternity leave with pay or with comparable social benefits without loss of former employment, seniority or social allowances"
- "encourage the provision of the necessary supporting social services to enable parents to combine family obligations with work responsibilities ... in particular through promoting the establishment and development of a network of child-care facilities."

For the full text of CEDAW see: www.un.org/womenwatch/daw/cedaw/

useful addresses

There are many more breastfeeding support organisations and campaigning groups than can be named here.

1. Breastfeeding support and information

Association of Breastfeeding Mothers (ABM)
PO Box 207, Bridgwater, Somerset, TA6 7YT, UK
t: +44 (0)444 122 949, e: counselling@abm.me.uk
web: www.abm.me.uk

Australian Breastfeeding Association (ABA)
1818-1822 Malvern Rd, East Malvern VIC 3145, Australia
ABN 64 005 081 523. t: +61 3 98850855, f: +61 3 98850866
e: info@breastfeeding.asn.au web: www.breastfeeding.asn.au

Australian Lactation Consultants Association
PO Box 4248, Manuka, ACT 2503, Australia
t: 02 6260 3099, f: 02 6282 7191 e: info@alca.asn.au web: www.alca.asn.au

The Breastfeeding Network (BfN)
PO Box 11126, Paisley, PA2 8YB, UK, t: +44 (0)844 412 4664
e: breastfeedingnetwork@googlemail.com
web: www.breastfeedingnetwork.org.uk

International Lactation Consultant Association (ILCA)
1500 Sunday Drive, Suite 102, Raleigh, North Carolina, 27607, USA
t: (919) 861 5577, f: (919) 787 4916
e: info@ilca.org, web: www.ilca.org

Lactation Consultants of Great Britain (LCGB)
PO Box 56, Virginia Water, Surrey, GU25 4WB, UK
e: info@lcgb.org web: www.lcgb.org

La Leche League Great Britain (LLLGB)
PO Box 29, West Bridgford, Nottingham, NG2 7NP, UK
t: +44 (0)845 456 1844
e: enquiries@laleche.org.uk, web: www.laleche.org.uk

La Leche League International (LLLI)
PO Box 4079, Schaumburg, IL 60168-4079, USA
t: 1 847 519 7730, f: 1 847 969 0460 web: www.llli.org

Little Angels
13-15 Railway Road, Darwen, Lancashire, BB3 2RJ, UK
t: 01254 772929, web: www.littleangels.org.uk

National Childbirth Trust (NCT)
Alexandra House, Oldham Terrace, London, W3 6NH, UK
Breastfeeding Helpline: +44 (0)300 330 0771
web: www.nctpregnancyandbabycare.org

Real Baby Milk CIC
t: 05601 536629, e: admin@realbabymilk.org, web: www.realbabymilk.org

UNICEF UK Baby Friendly Initiative
UNICEF House, 30a Great Sutton Street, London, EC1V 0DU, UK t:
020 7490 2388, web: www.babyfriendly.org.uk

Wellstart International
P.O. Box 602, Blue Jay, CA 92317, USA
e: info@wellstart.org, web: www.wellstart.org

World Alliance for Breastfeeding Action (WABA)
WABA Secretariat, PO Box 1200, 10850 Penang, Malaysia
t: 60 4 6584816, f: 60 4 6572655, e: waba@streamyx.com
web: www.waba.org.my

2. International Agencies

International Labour Organisation (ILO)
4 route des Morillons, CH-1211 Genève 22, Switzerland
t: +41 (0) 22 799 6111, f: +41 (0) 22 798 8685
e: ilo@ilo.org web: www.ilo.org

International Pediatric Association
1-3 rue de Chantepoulet, PO Box 1726, CH-1211 Genève 1, Switzerland
t: +41 (0) 22 906 9152, f: +41 (0) 22 732 2852
web:www.ipa-world.org

UNICEF
3 UN Plaza, 44th Street between 1st & 2nd Avenues, New York,
NY 10038, USA, t: (+1) 212 326 7000, f: (+1) 212 887 7465
web: www.unicef.org *or*
Palais des Nations, 1211 Genève 10, Switzerland
t: (+41) 22 909 5111, f: (+41) 22 909 5900, web: www.unicef.org

United Nations High Commission for Refugees (UNHCR)
Case Postale 2500, 1211 Genève 2 Dépot, Switzerland
t: (+41) 22 739 8111, web: www.unhcr.org

World Health Organisation (WHO)
Avenue Appia 20, 1211 Geneva 27, Switzerland
t: + 41 22 791 21 11 f: + 41 22 791 31 11, web: www.who.int
Relevant departments: WHO Department of Child and Adolescent
Health and Development (cah@who.int); WHO Department of
HIV/AIDS (hiv-aids@who.int); WHO Department of Nutrition for
Health and Development (nutrition@who.int)

3. International Baby Food Action Network – IBFAN.
Co-ordinating Offices:

IBFAN Africa
Centre Point, Cnr of Tin and Walker Streets, Mbabane, Swaziland
e: ibfanswd@realnet.co.sz

IBFAN Afrique Francophone
Co-ordination Régionale, 01 B.P 1776 Ouagadougou 01, Burkina Faso
e: ibfanfan@fasotnet.bf

IBFAN América Latina
Cefemina, Apartado Postal 5355, San Jose 1000, Costa Rica CA
e: cefemina@sol.racsa.co.cr

IBFAN Argentina
AV Corrientes 1922 V.P 12, Of 125 1045, Buenos Aires, Argentina
e: fvallone@intramed.net.ar

IBFAN Asia Pacific (Breastfeeding Promotion Network of India)
BP-33 Pitampura, Delhi 110088, India
e: agupta@bpni.org *and* ritarun@vsni.com

IBFAN Brasil
Caixa Postal 34, Paraguaçu-SP, Brazil
e: coordenacao@ibfan.org.br

IBFAN Caribbean
Co-ordinator Programa de Lactancia Materna, Secretaria del Estado
de Salud Publica, Av. Enriquillo No 58, Edif. Rhina, Apto 10,
Los Caciazagos, Santo Domingo, Dominican Republic
e: clavelsanchez@codetel.net.do

IBFAN Europe
IBFAN-GIFA, Avenue de la Paix 11, 1202 Geneva, Switzerland
T: (+41) 22 798 9164, F: (+41) 22 798 4443
e: info@gifa.org website: www.gifa.org

IBFAN North America
INFACT Canada,10 Trinity Square, Toronto M5G 1BI
Ontario PO Box 781, Canada
e: infact@ftn.net

Other relevant IBFAN groups:

Baby Milk Action
34 Trumpington Street, Cambridge, CB2 1QY, UK
t: (+44) 1223 464420, f: (+44) 1223 434471
e: info@babymilkaction.org, web: www.babymilkaction.org

IBFAN New Zealand
Infant Feeding Association of New Zealand, PO Box 35-252,
Christchurch 8640, New Zealand
t: 03 354 9249, f: 03 323 7179
e: info@ifanz-ibfan.org.nz

IBFAN Penang (International Code Documentation Centre – ICDC)
PO Box 19, 10700 Penang, Malaysia. e: ibfan@tn.net.my

National Alliance for Breastfeeding Advocacy (NABA)
254 Conant Road, Weston, MA 02493-1756, USA
f: 1 781-893-8608, web: www.naba-breastfeeding.org

4. Other Relevant Groups and Networks

Academy of Breastfeeding Medicine
140 Huguenot Street, 3rd floor, New Rochelle, New York 10801, USA
t: (800) 990 4ABM (USA toll free), (914) 740 2115
f: (914) 740 2101 Attn: ABM, e: abm@bfmed.org, web: www.bfmed.org

Baby Feeding Law Group (BFLG)
c/o Baby Milk Action, 34 Trumpington Street, Cambridge, CB2 1QY, UK
t: (+44) 1223 464420, f: (+44) 1223 434471
web: www.babyfeedinglawgroup.org.uk

Breastfeeding Manifesto Coalition
c/o Alexandra House, Oldham Terrace, London, W3 6NH, UK
t: (+44) 20 8752 2419
web: www.breastfeedingmanifesto.org.uk

Emergencies Nutrition Network (ENN)
32 Leopold Street, Oxford OX4 1TW, UK
t: (+44) 1865 324996, f: (+44) 1865 324997
e: office@ennonline.net, web: www.ennonline.net

Human Milk Banking Association of North America (HMBANA)
1500 Sunday Drive, Suite 102, Raleigh, North Carolina, 27607, USA
t: (919) 861-4530: info@hmbana.org, web: www.hmbana.org

UK Association for Milk Banking (UKAMB)
The Milk Bank, Queen Charlotte's and Chelsea Hospital,
Du Cane Road, Hammersmith, London W12 OHS, UK
t: +44 (0)20 8383 3559: info@ukamb.org, web: www.ukamb.org

Women's Environment Network (WEN)
PO Box 30626, London, E1 1TZ, UK
t: (+44) 207 481 9004, f: (+44) 207 481 9144
e: info@wen.org.uk, web: www.en.org.uk

5. Infant Feeding Industry Associations

The European Association of Dietetic Food Manufacturers (IDACE)
194, Rue de Rivoli, 75001 Paris, France
t: +33 1 53 45 87 87, f: +33 1 53 45 87 80
e: info@idace.org, web: www.idace.org

Infant and Dietetic Food Association (IDFA)
6 Catherine Street, London, WC2B 5JJ
t: 0207 836 2460, f: 0207 420 7119/ 7104
e: idfa@idfa.org.uk, web: www.idfa.org.uk

International Association of Infant Food Manufacturers (IFM/ ISDI)
no street address, contact form available on website
www.ifm.net

references and notes

Chapter 1: why breastfeeding is political

1 According to Professor Kim Michaelson, the International Society of Research in Human Milk and Lactation (ISRHML) classifies 50 to 60 relevant papers a month. Transcript of Witness Seminar on 'The Resurgence of Breastfeeding, 1975-2000' held by the Wellcome Trust Centre for the History of Medicine at UCL London, 24 April 2007.

2 Statement of baseball coach Tommy Lasorda, quoted by Peter Bowes, BBC Correspondent Los Angeles, 4 February 2004. US apoplexy over Jackson flash http://news.bbc.co.uk/1/hi/entertainment/music/3456497.stm

3 Global Industry Analysts, Inc. 'Worldwide Baby Foods and Infant Formula Sales to Reach US$20.2 Billion by 2010' 3 March 2008. www.strategyr.com/Baby_Foods_and_Infant_Formula_Market_Report.asp

4 BBC1 TV Look East Interview with CEO Avent 2003

5 WHO, Contemporary Patterns of Breastfeeding: a nine country study, 1991. Also: Attard Montalto S et al. Incorrect advice: the most significant negative determinant on breastfeeding in Malta. *Midwifery* 2008 doi:10.1016/j.midw.2008.06.002

6 Black RE, Morris SS & Bryce J. Where and why are 10 million children dying each year? *The Lancet* 2003;**361**:2226-34. The key to this statement is 'improving breastfeeding practices' which means supporting women to breastfeed exclusively for the first six months and to continue breastfeeding, together with nutrient-dense, complementary foods, for two years and beyond.

7 Confronting the US infant formula giants. *The Corporate Examiner*, July-August 1982; 2(7-8)

8 Costello A, Watson F, Woodward D. Human Face or Human Facade? Adjustment and the Health of Mothers and Children. Occasional paper London: Centre of International Child Health 1994.

9 I raised the issue in the first edition of *The Politics of Breastfeeding* (1988). Andrew Radford consolidated this theme in his paper, *The ecological impact of bottle feeding*. Cambridge: Baby Milk Action 1991.

Chapter 2: the right to call ourselves mammals: the importance of biology

1 Jelliffe DB & Patrice Jelliffe EF. *Human Milk in the Modern World: Psychological, Nutritional and Economic Significance*. Oxford: Oxford University Press 1978.

2 Prentice AM & Prentice A. Reproduction against the odds: Women in The Gambia Eat Too Little and Work too Hard But They Still Manage to Have Babies. *New Scientist* 1988;**118**:42-6

3 Anecdotal evidence from World War Two tells us that in prison camps and under forced labour, big men died more quickly than small ones, who could keep going on less food.

4 Elia I. *The Female Animal*. Oxford University Press 1985.

5 At least one in every three women has been beaten, coerced into sex or otherwise abused in her lifetime according to a study based on 50 surveys from around the world. In the USA women accounted for 85% of victims of domestic violence. WHO reports that 70% of female murder victims are killed by their male partners. www.amnesty.org.uk

6 Prentice AM & Whitehead RG. The energetics of human reproduction. In: Lowden ASI & Racey PA, eds. *Reproductive Energetics in Mammals* (Symposium of the Zoological Society of London). Oxford: Clarendon Press, 1987.

7 Vernelli T. *The Dark Side of Dairy*. Viva! 2005. Also: Lawrence F. *Eat your heart out*. Penguin 2008.

8 Atkins PJ & Brassley P. Mad Cows and Englishmen. *History Today* 1996;**46**(9):14-7. Atkins PJ. Mothers' milk and infant death in Britain, circa 1900-1940, *Anthropology of Food*. 2 September 2003.

9 Nestle M. Melamine taint – old problem has new urgency. *The San Francisco Chronicle*. 22 October 2008. See also Wilson B. *Swindled: from poison sweets to counterfeit coffee – The dark history of the food cheats*. John Murray 2008.

Chapter 3: how breastfeeding works – and how it was damaged

1 Widstrom A-M. Aren't Babies clever! Paper presented at Associates in Childbirth Education 'Breastfeeding–Baby Friendly!' Tour. September 1993.

2 There is evidence that men can and have lactated and suckled babies. See Marieskind H. Abnormal Lactation. *Journal of Tropical Pediatrics and Environmental Child Health* 1973;**19**:123-8. See also: Gould SJ. Male nipples and clitoral ripples. In: *Adam's navel*. London: Penguin 1995. Jones S. *Almost like a Whale: the origin of species updated*. Transworld Publishers 2000.

3 WHO. Evidence for the Ten Steps to Successful Breastfeeding. WHO Geneva 1998.

4 Anderson GC et al Early skin-to-skin contact for mothers and their healthy newborn infants (Review). The Cochrane Collaboration 2005 www.thecochranelibrary.com

5 Bystrova K et al. Skin-to-skin contact may reduce negative consequences of "the stress of being born": a study on temperature in newborn infants, subjected to different ward routines in St. Petersburg. *Acta Paediatrica* 2003;**92(3)**:320-6.

6 Dora Henschel CBE, Senior Midwife Tutor, Kings College London retired. Personal Communication 2001.

7 Ball HL et al. Randomised trial of mother-infant sleep proximity on the post-natal ward. *Archives of Disease in Childhood* 2006;**91**:1005-10. Published online 18 July 2006, doi: 10.1136/adc.2006.099416.

8 Cadogan W. *An essay upon nursing and the management of children, from birth to three years of age.* London: John Knapton 1748 (first ed).

9 Swaddling is an ancient custom still practised in much of the world, particularly Asia and Eastern Europe. It may have evolved as a means of carrying infants on horseback in cold climates. It keeps infants quiet or semi-comatose depending on your view and can cause death (Van Gestel 2002). It has been promoted by modern child care gurus who have little understanding of how breastfeeding works. Some small babies do 'settle' more with swaddling while others protest. A mother of breastfed twins told me how from early on one twin loved to be swaddled while the other hated it. Prolonged tight swaddling has negative consequences including increased rate of respiratory infection (Yurdakok K et al. Swaddling and ARI. *American Journal of Public Health* 1990;**80(7)**:873-5), cold feet (Bystrova K et al. Skin to skin contact may reduce negative consequences of the stress of being born: a study on temperature in newborn infants, subjected to different ward routines in St. Petersburg. *Acta Paediatrica* 2003; **92(3)**:272-3), Vitamin D deficiency (rickets), inhibitory effect on brain arousal (SIDS risk) (Gerard CM et al. Spontaneous arousals in supine infants while swaddled and unswaddled during rapid eye movement and quiet sleep. *Pediatrics* 2002 Dec;**110(6)**:e70) overheating (SIDS risk). Malocclusion (Personal communication Umit Kartoglu WHO).

10 Rendle-Short M. *Father of Childcare*. Bristol: Wright 1966.

11 The WHO Multicentre Growth Reference Study (MGRS) was undertaken between 1997 and 2003 in order to provide a single international reference that represents the best description of physiological growth for all children under five years of age and to establish the breastfed infant as the normative model for growth and development. The Who Multicentre Growth Reference Study. WHO standards based on length/height, weight and age. *Acta Pediatrica* 2006 **95**(Suppl. 450)76-85

12 Baird J, Fisher D, Lucas P, Kleijnen J, Roberts H, Law C. Being big or growing fast: systematic review of size and growth in infancy and later obesity. *British Medical Journal* 2005;**331(7522)**:929.

13 Ford G. *The New Contented Little Baby Book*. London: Vermilion 2002.

14 Griffiths DM. Do tongue ties affect breastfeeding? *Journal of Human Lactation* 2004;**20(4)**:409-14.

15 Prentice A et al. Evidence for local feedback control of human milk secretion. *Biochemical Society Transaction* 1989;**17**:122-3.

16 Edmond K et al. Delayed breastfeeding initiation increases the risk of neonatal mortality. *Pediatrics* 2006;**117**:380-6

17 WHO. Evidence for the Ten Steps to Successful Breastfeeding. WHO Geneva 1998. Also: Personal communication: nutritionist Rebecca Norton of GIFA Switzerland 2008. NS Working with the Baby Friendly Hospital Initiative and visiting maternity facilities in both rich and poor regions in the 21st century, I have found that the urge to give either artificial milk or glucose water to full term healthy babies persists despite evidence of negative effects.

18 Lunn PG. Maternal nutrition and lactational infertility: the baby in the driving seat. In: Dobbing J, ed. *Maternal Nutrition and Lactational Infertility*. Nestlé Nutrition, Raven Press, 1985. NB Lunn used the analogy for the contraceptive effect, but it is still an apt analogy for all aspects of breastfeeding. Apologies for using Nestlé reference.

19 Lang S. *Breastfeeding Special Care Babies*. 2nd ed. Elsevier 2005. Also: Jones E. *Feeding and Nutrition in the preterm infant*. Churchill Livingstone 2006.

20 Klaus MH & Kennell JH. *Maternal-infant bonding: the impact of early separation or loss on family development*. The CV Mosby Company, 1976.

21 Dr Albert Bandura (b 1925) of Stanford University, Cal. USA pioneered '*Social Learning Theory*' which shows that learning takes place through imitation and role models rather than reinforcement. The hiddenness of breastfeeding and the visibility of artificial feeding and the subsequent difficulties of re-establishing the normality of breastfeeding match these theories very well.

22 In 'Macbeth', Shakespeare alludes to Lady Macbeth having lost more than one child. This may explain her driven temperament.

23 Odent M. *The Nature of Birth and Breastfeeding*. Birgin and Garvey 1992. See also: www.birthworks.org/primalhealth ww.wombecology.com, www.michelodent.com

24 Uvnäs Moberg K. *The Oxytocin Factor*. Da Capo Press 2003.

25 Fisher C. Midwife and breastfeeding expert. Personal communication: 1996

Chapter 4: beauty, breasts and books

1 The American Society of Plastic Surgeons reports 564,635 procedures carried out by their members in 2006. One procedure (breast augmentation) increased by 55% since 2000.

2 Dyson L, McMillan B, Woolridge MW, Green JM Conner M, Clarke G, Bharj KK, & Renfrew MJ. Looking at infant feeding today: reducing inequalities in health among socio-economically disadvantaged and ethnic groups by increasing breastfeeding uptake: an examination of intentions and outcomes. *Final report to the UK Department of Health* 2003.

3 Renfrew M et al. The effectiveness of public health interventions to promote the duration of breastfeeding: systematic review. *National Insititute of Clinical Excellence (NICE)*, London 2005. www.publichealth.nice.org.uk. Also: Dyson L et al Promotion of breastfeeding initiation and duration: evidence into practice briefing. NICE London 2006. www.nice.org.uk.

4 The UK Infant Feeding Survey 2005 *The Statistics Office* 2007

5 Various sources cited in Walker M. *Still Selling out Mothers and Babies*. NABA 2007.

6 Rinker BD et al. The Effect of Breastfeeding upon Breast Aesthetics. *Aesthetic Surgery Journal* 2008;**28(5)**:534-37.

7 A hospital would not merit its baby friendly status if any member of staff asked this question.

8 Jelliffe DB and Jelliffe EFP, *Human Milk in the Modern World*, Oxford: Oxford University Press, 1978.

9 World Health Organisation (WHO), Child and Adolescent Health and Development (CAH), *Relactation: review of experience and recommendations for practice*. WHO Geneva. 1998.

10 Latham M. Statement made at workshop on 'Ethics and ideology in the battle against malnutrition'. *Fifth International Congress of Nutrition,* Brighton, 18-23 August 1985.

11 WHO. *Evidence for the Ten Steps to Successful Breastfeeding*. WHO Geneva 1998.

12 Koplick H. *The Diseases of Infancy and Childhood*. London: Henry Kimpton, 1903.

13 'Elastoplast' is a brand name commonly used in the UK for an adhesive surgical dressing or 'sticking plaster'. The brand name 'Band-Aid' is used in the USA.

14 Hogg T with Blau M. *Secrets of the baby whisperer. How to calm, connect and communicate with your baby.* London: Vermilion 2001.

15 *Mother & Baby* No1 pregnancy and baby mag. July 2008.

16 *Mother & Baby*, July 2008.

17 Cow & Gate website www.cowandgate.co.uk accessed 15th July 2008.

18 Nicoteri JAL & Farrell ML. *Quick Look Nursing: Nutrition*. Slack Inc, 2001.

19 Farrell ML & Nicoteri JAL. *Quick Look Nursing: Nutrition* (2nd edition) Jones and Bartlett 2007.

20 Conton L. Social, economic and ecological parameters of infant feeding in Usino, Papua New Guinea. *Ecology of Food and Nutrition* 1985;**16**(1):39-54.

Chapter 5: a taste of infant feeding

1 To explore the topic of attitudes to risk see: Bernstein PL. *Against the gods the remarkable story of risk*. John Wiley and Sons 1996. Also: Sutherland S. *Irrationality*. Pinter & Martin 2007.

2 Orent W. The White House vs mother's milk: the Bush administration squelched ads promoting the benefits of breastfeeding. *Los Angeles Times*, 30 September 2007.

3 This title was inspired by Berry NJ & Gribble KD. Breast is no longer best: promoting normal infant feeding. *Maternal and Child Nutrition* 2008;**4(1)**:74-79.

4 Waldmeir P. Third baby dies in China milk scandal. *Financial Times* 13 September 2008. See also http://www.who.int/csr/media/faq/QAmelamine/en/index.html.

5 American Academy of Pediatrics (AAP), Breastfeeding and the Use of Human Milk, *Pediatrics* 2005;**115**: 496-506.

6 Chen A and Rogan WJ, Breastfeeding and the risk of postneonatal death in the United States, *Pediatrics* 2004;**113**(5):e435-439.

7 American Academy of Pediatrics (AAP), Breastfeeding and the Use of Human Milk, *Pediatrics* 2005;**115**;496-506.

8 Hahn-Zoric et al. Antibody responses to parenteral and oral vaccines are impaired by conventional and low protein formulas as compared to breast-feeding. *Acta Paed Scandinavia* 1990;**79**:1137-1142.

9 Hanson LA. *Immunobiology of human milk: how breastfeeding protects babies*. Pharmasoft Publishing (now renamed Hale Publishing) 2004. Also: Kois WE. Influence of breastfeeding on subsequent reactivity to a related renal allograft. J of Surg Res 1989;**37**:89-93.

10 Kramer MS et al. Breastfeeding and child cognitive development: new evidence from a large randomised trial. *Arch Gen Psychiatry* 2008;**65**(5).

11 Codpietro L et al. Breastfeeding or oral sucrose solution in term neonates receiving heel lance: a randomized, controlled trial. *Pediatrics* 2008;**122**: e716-21.

12 Viggiano D et al. Breastfeeding, bottle feeding and non-nutritive sucking; effects on occlusion in deciduous dentition. *Arch Dis Child* 2004;**89**;1121-23.

13 Sobhy SM. The effect of early initiation of breastfeeding on the amount of vaginal blood loss during the fourth stage of labour. *Egypt Public Health Association* 2004;**79(1-2)**:1-12.

14 DeMaeyer E et al. Preventing and controlling iron deficiency anaemia through primary health care. A guide for health administrators and programme managers. WHO: Geneva 1989. Also: Dewey KG. Impact of breastfeeding on maternal nutritional status. *Adv Exp Med Biol* 2004;**554**:91-100.

15 Conde-Agudelo A. Effect of birth spacing on maternal and perinatal health: A systematic review and meta-analysis. *Report submitted to the CATALYST consortium*, October 2004. See also: Norton M. Birth spacing: 2004 evidence supports 3+ years. *Johns Hopkins Bloomberg School of Public Health*. Programs, information and knowledge for optimal health project (INFO), 16 May 2005.

16 Collaborative group on hormonal factors in breast cancer. Breast cancer and breastfeeding: collaborative reanalysis of individual data from 47 epidemiological studies in 30 countries, including 50,302 women with breast cancer and 96,973 women without the disease. *The Lancet* 2002;**360**:187-95.

17 Chiaffarino F et al. Breastfeeding and the risk of epithelial ovarian cancer in an Italian population. *Gyynecol Oncol* 2005;**98**;304-8.

18 Karlsson MK et al. Maternity and mineral density. *Acta Orthopaedica 2005*;**76**:2-13. See also: Paton LM et al. Pregnancy and lactation have no long-term deleterious effect on measures of bone mineral in healthy women: a twin study. *Am J Clin Nut* 2003;**77**:707-14.

19 Stuebe AM et al. Duration of lactation and incidence of type 2 diabetes. *JAMA* 2005;**294**:2601-2610

20 Karlson EW et al. Do breastfeeding and other reproductive factors influence future risk of rheumatoid arthritis? Results from the Nurses' Health Study. *Arthritis & Rheumatism* 2004;**50**:3458-3467.

21 Liu B, Beral V, Balkwill A on behalf of the Million Women Study Collaborators. Childbearing, breastfeeding, other reproductive factors and the subsequent risk of hospitalization for gall bladder disease. *Int J Epi* 2008;Doi:10.1093/ije/dyn174.

22 Zaidi AK et al, Hospital–acquired neonatal infections in developing countries,

Lancet 2005;**365**:1175-88 cited in Otto Cars and colleagues, Meeting the challenge of antibiotic resistance, Analysis *BMJ* 2008;(337) 726-728.

23 Edmond KM et al. Delayed breastfeeding initiation increases risk of mortality. *Pediatrics* 2006;**117**:380-86.

24 A calorie is the common term for a unit of energy. It comes from kilocalorie (kcal) which though now officially replaced by kilojoule (kJ) is still in common use. Labels use both units. 1kcl=4.184 kJ; 1kJ = 0.239 kcal.

25 Horta BL et al. Evidence of the long-term effects of breastfeeding: systematic reviews and meta-analyses. WHO (CAH), 2007.

26 Bryson B. *A Short History of Nearly Everything*: Black Swan 2004. BB provides an entertaining discussion of when humans 'began' and the dates of when they moved north.

27 Bender DA. Fat-soluble vitamins. In: Geissler C and Powers H, eds. *Human Nutrition.* Elsevier Churchill Livingstone 2005; 217-222. See also: Scientific Advisory Committee on Nutrition. Paper for discussion: Vitamin D deficiency in Children. *Subgroup on maternal and child nutrition.* Agenda Item 2. SMCN/03/02. http://www.sacn.gov.uk/. See also: HM Rhein, Vitamin D deficiency is widespread in Scotland. *BMJ* 2008;**336**:1451 (28 June), doi:10.1136/bmj.39619.479155.3A.

28 Williams C. The composition of breastmilk and how it compares with formula and cows' milk. *WHO Consultancy Review Paper*. Breastfeeding: Practice and Policy Course, UCL Centre for International Health and Development, Institute of Child Health, London. June 2005.

29 Lozoff et al. Neurodevelopmental Delays Associated With Iron-Fortified Formula for Healthy Infants, Presented at *Pediatric Academic Societies (PAS) and Asian Society for Pediatric Research Joint Meeting* 2008. Also: Hallberg L et al. Iron, zinc and other trace elements. In Garrow JS et al, eds. *Human Nutrition and Dietetics*. Churchill Livingstone 2001.

30 Lawrence RA & Lawrence RM. *Breastfeeding a guide for the medical profession.* Mosby 1999. See also: Kiles RV et al. Vitamin K content of maternal milk: influence of the stage of lactation, lipid composition and vitamin K supplements given to the mother. *Pediatric Research* 1987; 22:513-17. Also: Discussion with Professor Michael Crawford. Director of the Institute of Brain Chemistry and Human Nutrition, London, UK.

31 Duce M et al. Suspected Thiamine Deficiency in Angola. *Field Exchange* 2003;**20**:26-28. Also: Allen LH. Maternal micronutrient malnutrition: effects on breastmilk and infant nutrition, and priorities for intervention. *SCN News* 1994;**11**:21-24

32 International Vitamin A Consultative Group (IVACG) Secretariat. Report of XIX IVACG Consultative Group Meeting. *Vitamin A and other micronutrients: biologic interactions and integrated interventions.* Durban South Africa. 8-11 March 1999.

33 Butte N, Lopez-Alarcon MG & Garza C. Nutrient adequacy of exclusive breastfeeding for the term infant during the first six months of life. WHO, Geneva 2002. See also: Prentice AM et al. Body Mass index and lactation performance. *European Journal of Clinical Nutrition*. 1994;**48** (Suppl.3: S78-S89). Also: Prentice AM and Prentice A. Reproduction against the odds. *New Scientist* 18 April 1988;**1608**:42-46

34 Prentice AM & Prentice A. Can maternal dietary supplements help in preventing infant malnutrition. *Acta Paediatr Scand* (Suppl) 1991;**374**:67-77.

35 Picciano MF, Pregnancy and lactation: Physiological adjustments, nutrition requirements and the role of dietary supplements. *Journal of Nutrition* 2003;**133**:1997S-2002S. NB: an example of the energy values of a typical helping of a south Asian diet might be: 60g rice = 240kcal (1005.6kJ); 30g lentils = 120kcal (502.8kJ); half a banana = 90kcal (377.1kJ); teaspoon (5ml) of oil= 50 kcal (209.5kJ).

36 Baumslag N. *J Hum Lact* 2005;**21**:6-7 Also: Hilpern Kate. A lifetime of Denial *The Guardian* 29.4.2008 [Dr Diana Brighouse, who suffered from anorexia nervosa and worked with other sufferers, breastfed each of her four children for a year.]

37 Barker DJP. *Mothers, babies and disease in later life*. BMJ Publishing House, London 1994.

38 Hanson, LA, Non-breastfeeding: the most common Immunodeficiency. *ALCA*

Galaxy December 1998;**9(3)**:15-17.

39 Ngom PT et al. Improved thymic function in exclusively breastfed babies is associated with IL-7. *Am J Clin Nutr* 2004.

40 Hanson LA. *Immunobiology of human milk: how breastfeeding protects babies.* Pharmasoft Publishing 2004.

41 Hahn-Zoric et al. Antibody responses to parenteral and oral vaccines are impaired by conventional and low protein formulas as compared to breast-feeding. *Acat Paed Scandinavia* 1990;**79**:1137-42.

42 Van de Perre P et al. Infective and anti-infective properties of breastmilk from HIV 1-infected women. *The Lancet* 1993;**341**:914-918.

43 www.who.int/child-adolescent-health 25 June 2008.

44 Weyerman M et al. Duration of breastfeeding and risk of overweight in childhood: a prospective birth cohort study from Germany. *Int J Obesity.* 28 February 2006.

45 Sachs MA. *'Following the Line': An ethnographic study of the influence of routine baby weighing on breastfeeding women in a town in the Northwest of England.* PhD thesis submitted to the University of Central Lancs. 2005.

46 WHO. The optimal duration of exclusive breastfeeding: a systematic review. *WHO/FCH/CAH/01.23* and *WHO/NHD/01.08.* WHO Geneva 2002

47 Defined as less than 2500g irrespective of gestational age. The great majority (96%) of the 25 million LBW babies are born (annually) in developing countries.

48 Klaus MH & Kennell JH. *Maternal-infant bonding: the impact of early separation or loss on family development.* CV Mosby Company 1976.

49 Williams AF. Human Milk and the Preterm Infant. Chapter 3 in *'Current Topics in Neonatology' Volume 3.* Edited by: Hanson TN and McIntosh N. WB Saunders & Co. London 1999.

50 Martinez GH, Rey SE, Marquette CM. The mother kangaroo programme. *Int Child Health* 1992;**3**:55–67.

51 Bergman N. Restoring the original paradigm and Rediscover the natural way. www.kangaroomothercare.com 2005. See also: WHO Department of Reproductive Health and Research. *Kangaroo mother care: a practical guide.* WHO Geneva 2003.

52 Conde-Aguledo et al, Kangaroo mother care to reduce morbidity and mortality in low birth weight infants. *Cochrane Database of Systematic Reviews* 2003, Issue 2. Art No: CD002771. DOI: 10.1002/14651858. CD002771.

53 Michel Odent, lecture at La Leche League UK Annual General Meeting and Conference. April 2004.

54 Pattinson RC et al. Does kangaroo mother care save lives? *J Trop Peds* 5 July 2006. Also: Van Rooyen E (Department of Paediatrics, University of Pretoria, MRC Unit for Maternal and Infant Health Care Strategies, Kalafong Hospital, Pretoria, South Africa.) Presentation at Breastfeeding: advocacy and practice course, Nutrition Directorate of South Africa Infant Feeding Consortium, Pretoria 2004. Also: Van Rooyen E. An Ongoing Audit of the Kangaroo Mother Care Unit at Kalafong Hospital. *Proceedings: 25th Conference on Priorities in Perinatal care in Southern Africa*, March 2006, Champagne Castle, South Africa.

55 Moster D, Lie RT, Markestad T. Long-term medical and social consequences of preterm birth. *N Engl J Med.* 2008;**359(3)**:262-73.

56 Quotation by Malan cited in Van Rooyen E et al. The Value of the KMC Unit at Kalafong Hospital, Geneeskunde *The Medical Journal*, April 2002.

57 WHO. The optimal duration of exclusive breastfeeding. Geneva 2001. Also: Kramer MS and Kakuma R. The optimal duration of exclusive breastfeeding: A systematic review. *Cochrane Library* 2002.

58 Rattigan S, Ghisalberti AV & Hartmann PE. Breastmilk production in Australian women. *British Journal of Nutrition 1981*; **45**:243-9. Also: Personal communication: Professor Peter Hartmann of the University of Western Australia.

59 Rapley G, Baby-led weaning. In: Hall Moran V and Dykes F, eds. *Maternal and Infant Nutrition Controversies and Challenges.* Quay Books 2006.

60 Goodall J. Hans Gadow Lecture, 26 November 1987, University of Cambridge. Also:Goodall J. *In the Shadow of Man* London: Collins 1971.

61 Dettwyler KA. A Time to Wean: The Hominid Blueprint for the Natural Age of Weaning in Human Populations. In Stuart-Macadam P & Dettwyler KA, eds. *Breastfeeding Biocultural Perspectives.* Aldine de Griyter 1995.

62 Most iron-rich foods, or foods which facilitate iron-absorption, are also rich in zinc.

63 Jones M. Feast: why humans share food OUP 2007 [NB Boxgrove man was not homo sapiens but homo heidelbergensis.]

64 Hallberg L et al. Iron, zinc and other trace elements. In Garrow JS, James WPT & Ralph A, eds. *Human Nutrition and Dietetics*. Churchill Livingstone, 2001: p177-210.

65 The small amount of iron in breastmilk is much more bioavailable than larger amounts in infant formulas and other foods. Giving other milks with meals too early may inhibit the absorption of iron in solid foods. Excess iron is dangerous so any pharmaceutical supplementation must be done with caution. See: Lozoff et al. Neurodevelopmental Delays Associated With Iron-Fortified Formula for Healthy Infants, Presented at *Pediatric Academic Societies (PAS) and Asian Society for Pediatric Research Joint Meeting* 2008.

66 Chaparro CM et al, Effect of timing of umbilical cord clamping on iron status in Mexican infants: a randomised control trial. *www.thelancet.com* 17 June 2006.

67 Dunn Peter, Clamping the umbilical cord, *AIMS Journal* 2004/5;**16(4)**:8-10

68 48 http://www.gainhealth.org/improving-nutrition accessed November 2008.

69 Williams C et al. CODEX needs to tread with caution on fortified foods. Letter to *The Lancet*. To be published 2008.

70 Wilson AC et al. Relation of infant diet to childhood health: seven-year follow-up of cohort of children in Dundee infant feeding study. *BMJ* 1998, **316**(7124), 21-5.

71 Drummond, Jack Cecil, *The Englishman's Food*. London: Jonathan Cape 1958 p.375.

72 UBIC Consulting. Ingredients for the world formula market: update 2008. ubi@ubicc-consulting.com 2008.

73 Vallaeys C. DHA/ARA Replacing Mother- Imitating Human Breastmilk in the Laboratory. Novel Oils in Infant Formula and Organic Foods: Safe and Valuable Functional Food or Risky Marketing Gimmick? *The Cornucopia Institute* January 2008. www.cornucopia.org

74 EFSA Statement August 2008. See also: Baby Milk Action. EFSA: tough on claims? *Baby Milk Action Update*. 2008 Issue 41.

75 Sartori C, Arnoldi A & Johnson SK. Phytoestogens: End of a Tale? *Annals of Medicine*. 2005;**37**:423-428. Also: Nestlé www.verybestbaby.com 05/10/2005 Also: Daniel KT. The Whole Soy Story: The Dark Side of America's Favorite Health Food. 505-984-2093 Issue 124: May/June 2004 www.wholesoystory.com Also: www.soyonlineservice.co.nz

76 Weir E. Powdered infant formula and fatal infection with Enterobacter sakazakii. *CMAJ* 2002;166.

77 USFDA. Health professionals' letter on Enterobacter sakazakii infections associated with use of powdered (dry) infant formula in neonatal intensive care units. 10 October 2002.

78 Van Acker et al. Outbreak of NEC associated with Enterobacter sakazakii in powdered infant formulas. *J Clin Microbiol* 2001;**39**:293-97.

79 FAO/WHO. *Enterobacter sakazakii* and other microorganisms in powdered infant formula. Meeting Report, Geneva Switzerland, 2-5 February 2004.[FAO/WHO] *Microbiological Risk Assessment Series No.6*

80 Muytjens HL et al. Quality of powdered substitutes for breastmilk with regard to members of the family *Enterobacteriacae*. *JClin Microbiol* 1988;**26**:743-746.

81 WHO/FAO. Safe preparation, storage and handling of powdered infant formula Guidelines. 2006. Also: Baby Milk Action. You can't trust company carelines. *Baby Milk Action Update* Issue 40; November 2007. See also Forsythe S. *Enterobacter sakazakii* and other bacteria in powdered infant formula. *Mother and Child Nutrition* 2005;**1**(1):44-50.

82 Koletzko B & Shamir R. Standards of infant formula milk. Commercial interest may be the strongest driver of what goes into infant formula. *Br Med J* 2006;**332**:621-622.

83 Codex Alimentarius Commission. Joint FAO/WHO Food Standards Programme. Codex Committee on Nutrition and Foods for Special Dietary Uses. 28th Session. Proposals of Working Group for Sectors on Food Additives. CX/NFSDU 06/28/4-Add 2. September 2006. www.codexalimentarius.net

84 Nottingham S. *Eat your genes: how genetically modified food is entering our diet.* Zed Bools 2003.

85 Whelan J. "Making formula milk more like mum's" *New Scientist* 14 July 2008; 2664. Also: Transgenic goats' milk offers hope for tackling children's intestinal

disease. *Science Daily* 4 August 2006.

86 BBC TV World Service. Hard Talk: Interview with Dr Ferid Murad by Tim Sebastian. 1998.

87 Baby Milk Action. Melamine contamination deaths in China show need for regulations. *Baby Milk Action Update* November 2008; 41: 16-17. See also: Nestle M. Melamine taint – old problem has new urgency. *San Francisco Chronicle* 22 October 2008;F1

88 Baby Milk Action. Bisphenol A: new danger. *Baby Milk Action Update* November 2008;41:7.

89 Black RE et al. Where and why are 10 million children dying every year? *The Lancet* 2003; 361: 2226-2234. Jones G et al and the Bellagio Child Survival Study Group. How many deaths can we prevent this year? *The Lancet* 2003;**362**:65-71. WHO Collaborative Study Team on the Role of Breastfeeding on the Prevention of Infant Mortality. Effect of breastfeeding on infant and child mortality due to infectious diseases in less developed countries: a pooled analysis. Cesar JA et al. Impact of breastfeeding on admission for pneumonia during the postneonatal period in Brazil: nested case-control study. *BMJ* 1999;**318**:1316-1320. Arifeen S et al. Exclusive breastfeeding reduces acute respiratory infection and diarrhoea deaths among infants in Dhaka slums. *Pediatrics* 2001;108:E67.

90 Aldrin, DDT, chlordane, dieldrin, endrin, heptachlor, hexachlorobenzine, mirex, toxaphene, polychlorinated (pc) biphenyls, pc dibenzodioxins, pc dibenzofurans.

91 Zetterström R. Child health and exposure to persistent organic chlorines. *Annals Nestlé* 2004; 62:74. Apologies to readers for citing a Nestlé publication, but it was a good article that taught me a lot. Please will Dr Zetterström (of the renowned Karolinska University, Sweden) use his relationship to remind N to reform its marketing practices.

92 Vreugedenhill HJI et al. Prenatal exposure to polychlorinated biphenols and breastfeeding: opposing effects on auditory P300 latencies in 9-year old Dutch children. *Develop Med & Child Neurol* 2004; 46: 398-405. Also: Lakind JS, Berline CM & Mattison DR. *Breastfeeding Medicine* 2008;3(4):251-259.

93 Van Tram D et al. Survey on immunisation, diarrhoeal disease and mortality in Quang Ninh Province, Vietnam. *Journal of Tropical Paediatrics* 1991;**37**:280-5.

94 Arendt M. Review: Communicating human biomonitoring results to ensure policy coherence with public health recommendations: analyzing breastmilk whilst protecting, promoting and supporting breastfeeding. *Environmental Health* 2008 & (Suppl 1):56.

95 WHO. Fourth WHO-Coordinated Survey of Human Milk for Persistent Organic Pollutants in Cooperation with UNEP, Guidelines for Developing a National Protocol. WHO Geneva 2007.

96 Lakind JS, Berlin CM & Mattison DR. The heart of the matter on breastmilk and environmental chemicals: essential points for healthcare providers and new parents. *Breastfeeding Medicine* 2008;**3(4)**:DOI:10.1089/bfm.2008.0121.

97 A diet with high consumption of meats, dairy products, sugar and saturated fats.

98 Koppe JG. Nutrition and breastfeeding. *European Journal of Obstetrics & Gynecology and Reproductive Biology* 1995:**61**:73-78.

99 Greer FR & Shannon M. Infant methemoglobinemia: the role of dietary nitrate in food and water. *Pediatr* 2005;**116**:784-786.

100 Personal Communication: Palmer J MCI WEM, Water Engineer. The pollution incidents occurred in Cambridgeshire UK, a well-monitored region. Such pollution is often not discovered because there is insufficient monitoring, or the incident is never publicly documented.

101 www.infactcanada.org Canada moves to ban bisphenol A in baby bottles. 18.10.2008.

102 Salvucci F. Sustainable Urban Mobility-Transport solutions for the 21st century. 2nd Annual Lecture Series in Sustainable development. *Cambridge University Department of Engineering,* 28 April 2004. Fred Salvucci alerted me to the heroic work of Clair Patterson who devoted his life trying to get lead out of petrol (gas). See Bryson B. Chapter 10 in *A short history of nearly everything.* Black Swan 2004.

103 Dorea, José G. Mercury and lead during breastfeeding. *Br J Nutr* 2004;92,21-40.

104 Fernandez-Lorenzo JR et al. Aluminium contents of human milk, cows' milk and infant formulas. *J Paediatr Gastroenterol Nutr* 1999;**28**:270-275.

105 Except for one woman who had eaten an unusually large amount of local fish and

reindeer meat. *Swedish National Institute of Radiation Protection*, Box 60204, S-10401 Sweden, May 1987.

106 Di Lallo D et al. Radioactivity in breastmilk in Central Italy in the aftermath of Chernobyl. *Acta Paediatrica Scandanavica* 1987; **76**:530-1. Also: Haschke E et al. Radioactivity in Austrian Milk after the Chernobyl accident (letter). *New Eng. J Med.* 1987;7:409-10.

107 Baby Milk Action Newsletters 1987/1988.

Chapter 6: it's not just the milk that counts

1 Gerhardt S. *Why Love Matters: how affection shapes a baby's brain*. Routledge 2004.

2 Film footage of a father suckling his child is shown in the Margaret Mead and Gregory Bateson 1951 film 'A Balinese Family'.

3 Lvoff NM, Lvoff V & Klaus MH. Effect of the baby-friendly initiative on infant abandonment in a Russian Hospital. *Archives of Pediatrics & Adolescent Medicine* 2000;**154(5)**:474-477 (**ISSN** 1072-4710). Also: Kennell JH & Klaus MH. Bonding: recent observations that alter perinatal care. *Pediatrics in Review* 1998;**19(1)**:4-12. Also: Dr Keiko Teruya reports that in the 1970s after the establishment of breastfeeding supportive practices in Hospital Guilherme Alvaro in Santos, Sao Paulo, Brazil, abandonment fell from 47 cases to nine in one year. Personal communication and thanks to Dr Vilneide Serva of IMIP, Recife Brazil 2008

4 Cusk R. *A life's work: on becoming a mother.* Fourth Estate 2001

5 Klaus MH and Kennel JH. *Maternal-infant bonding: The impact of Early Separation or Loss on Family Development*. The CV Mosby Company, 1976

6 Karolinska Institute. *Breastfeeding: the Baby's Choice*. Sweden: Karolinska Institute 1991.

7 Stratheam L et al. Does breastfeeding protect against substantiated child abuse and neglect? A 15-year cohort study. *Pediatrics* 2009;**123(2)**:483-493

8 Goodall J et al. *The Chimpanzees of Gombe*. Cambridge: Harvard University Press 1986.

9 UK Department of Health Policy is based on Fleming P et al. Sudden Unexpected Deaths in Infancy CESDI/SUDI-Stationery Office. London 2000.

10 Shaikh T. Inquiry into Bringing up Baby nanny. *The Guardian* 27 October 2008.

11 Gould SJ. Males nipples and clitoral ripples. In: *Adam's navel.* Penguin 1995. Also: Marieskind H. Abnormal lactation. *J Trop Peds and Environ Child Health* 1973;19:123-8

12 Turner-Maffei C. Lactation Consultant (IBCLC) and Coordinator of BFHI US. Personal Communication 2007.

13 Myr R. Midwife and Lactation Consultant (IBCLC). Personal communication 2007.

14 Lori Brown S et al. Breast Pump Adverse Events: Reports to the FDA. *J Hum Lact* **21**(2) 2005.

15 Consultant's Corner. Manual Expression of Breastmilk. *J Hum Lact* 21(2), 2005.

16 Becker GE, McCormick FM, Renfrew MJ. Methods of milk expression for lactating women. *Cochrane Database of Systematic Reviews* 2008, Issue 4. Art. No.: CD006170. DOI: 10.1002/14651858.CD006170.pub2

17 Lang S. Midwife and researcher. Personal Communication. 2008

18 I am indebted to Dr Helen Ball for explaining this concept to me. Also to Dr Tomoko Seo and many Japanese midwives and mothers who shared their knowledge and experience.

Chapter 7: your generous donations could do more harm than good

1 Different agencies use different definitions. The Centre for Research on the Epidemiology of Disasters (CRED) only enter a disaster on their database if at least one of the following has happened: 10 or more people reported killed; 100 people reported affected; declaration of state of emergency; call for international assistance. The term 'complex emergency' has been used in recent years for major humanitarian crises of a multicausal, essentially political nature that requires a system-wide response. Thanks to Marie McGrath for these explanations.

2 Figures from International Federation of the Red Cross and the Red Crescent Societies (1994-98 =428 per year; 1999-2003=707 per year) cited in http://www.goinginternational.org/pdf/Brennan-Gutschow_e.pdf. Also: International Displacement Monitoring Centre (IDMC) figures for end of 2007.

Also: United Nations High Commission for Refugees (UNHCR) Press release 17 June 2008. 31.7 million people entitled to UNHCR support (excluding 4.6 million Palestinian Refugees helped by UN Relief and Works Agency for Palestinian Refugees in the Near East); 647,200 asylum or refugee status requests submitted to governments and UNHCR offices in 154 countries during 2007.There are an estimated 12 million stateless people worldwide.

3   Jakobsen M et al. Breastfeeding status as a predictor of mortality among refugee children in an emergency situation in Guinea-Bissau. *Tropical Medicine & International Health* 2003;8(11):992-996

4   De Waal A. *Famine that kills*. Oxford Clarendon Press 1989 and (updated) Oxford University Press 2004

5   Kelly M. Infant feeding in emergencies. *Disasters* 1993;**17(2)**

6   Personal communication from field staff of Save the Children UK. 1996.

7   Maclaine A. Infant Feeding in Emergencies – Lebanon September 2006. *Final Report to Save the Children UK* April 2007.

8   CNN July 2006

9   Van Rooyen M. Twelve Myths and Misconceptions in Disaster Response. *Harvard Public Health on line*. 1 February 2008. Also: Jaspars S. From food crisis to fair trade: livelihoods analysis, protection and support in emergencies. *ENN Special Supplement Series No 3* March 2006.

10   Cow & Gate (sponsor). Advertisement appeal for Feed the Children. *GMTV* 28 June 1994.

11   McGrath M et al. Meeting the nutritional needs of infants during emergencies: recent experiences and dilemmas. *Report of an international workshop*. November 1999 Save the Children UK. Institute of Child Health, London.

12   Borrel A et al. From Policy to Practice: challenges in infant feeding in emergencies during the Balkan crisis. *Disasters*, 2001;**25(2)**:149-163

13   Fisher C. Midwife and breastfeeding expert. Unpublished report and personal communication. 1996.

14   The agency was IsraAid. I received the Press Photo electronically in January 2005.

Chapter 8: HIV and breastfeeding

1   BBC1 The Dying Game. *Panorama* 17 April 2000.

2   Coovadia HM, Rollins CR, Bland RM, Little KE, Coutsoudis A, Bennish ML, Newell ML, Mother- to- child transmission of HIV-1 infection during exclusive breastfeeding in the first 6 months of life: an intervention cohort study. *www.thelancet.com* 31 March 2007;**369**. Also Bland RM, Little K, Coovadia HM, Coutsoudis A, Rollins CR, Newell ML. Intervention to promote exclusive breastfeeding in the first 6 months of life in a high HIV prevalence area. *AIDS* 2008;**22**:883-891

3   This statement was made in an email discussion group I took part in when working at UNICEF Headquarters in November 2000. I have withheld the identity of the participant who said this.

4   WHO Collaborative Study Team on the Role of Breastfeeding on the Prevention of Infant Mortality. Effect of breastfeeding on infant and childhood mortality due to infectious deseases in less developed countries: a pooled analysis. *The Lancet* 2000;**355**:451-455

5   Nigel Rollins. Infant feeding practices to prevent HIV transmission. Presentation at Meeting on Management of Severe Malnutrition, Institute of Child Health (ICH), London 20 March 2007.

6   The ARV drug story shames the powerful. Big Pharma exploited international trade rules (GATT, TRIPS) to block the donations or sales of cheap generic ARVs to poor countries. It is beyond the scope of this book. See Lawson L. *Side Effects*. Double Storey Books, Capetown, 2008.

7   One third of Nigerian state medical graduates migrated to USA, UK or Canada within ten years. Fact from Review by *International Department BMA* London cited in: Roberts O. Tackling global shortages in health workers. *BMJ* 2008;**337**:a1971. Also: McColl K. International action on migration of health workers. *BMJ* 2008;**337**:a2065. Also: Zarocostas J. Globalisation spurs migration of healthcare workers from poor nations. *BMJ* 2008;**337**:a2841. Also: *"There are more Ethiopian doctors on the east coast of America than there are in Ethiopia."* says

leading Kenyan scientist, Professor Miriam Ware in 'Africa: Health Worker Migrations 'Crimes Against Humanity' 12 May 2008 *African Path* website.

8   UNICEF/WHO/UNAIDS Guidelines on HIV and Infant Feeding WHO 1992.

9   UNICEF/WHO/UNAIDS Guidelines on HIV and Infant Feeding WHO 1998.

10 Doherty T et al. Effect of the HIV epidemic on infant feeding in South Africa: "When they see me coming with the tins they laugh at me". *Bulletin of WHO* February 2006;**84(2)**. NB The mix of sugar, salt and water is home-made oral-rehydration fluid. Promoted by UNICEF and other child health agencies during the 1970s and 80s, it enabled mothers to save babies from the dehydration of diarrhoea. Its use, together with water, juices and teas became routine for all babies, whether ill or not, and undermined exclusive breastfeeding.

11 Sachs M. Reflections on HIV and feeding babies in the UK. On: Hall Moran V & Dykes F, eds. *Maternal and Infant Nutrition controversies and challenges*. Quay Books 206:p165-203.

12 White E. *Breastfeeding and HIV/AIDS: the Research, the Politics and the Women's Responses*. McFarland & Co. Jefferson. 1999.

13 The Royal College of Midwives/Department of Health Seminar Recommendations of which Point 6 states: *"HIV infected women who feel strongly committed to breastfeeding should be assisted to explore ways to reduce the risks of doing so."* Page 13 of Department of Health. *HIV and Infant Feeding, Guidance from the UK Chief Medical Officer's Expert Advisory Group on AIDS*, updated 2004.

14 The UN Guidelines on HIV and Infant Feeding 2004 state: *"When replacement feeding is acceptable, feasible, affordable, sustainable and safe, avoidance of all breastfeeding by HIV-infected mothers is recommended. Otherwise exclusive breastfeeding is recommended during the first months of life."* For Sara (not her real name) replacement feeding was not acceptable or feasible for the early period after birth.

15 UNICEF undertook the commissioning and production process in 1998/1999.

16 Walker M. *Still selling out mothers and babies*, National Association for Breastfeeding Advocacy 2007; p12.

17 Doherty T et al. Effect of the HIV epidemic on infant feeding in South Africa: "When they see me coming with the tins they laugh at me". *Bulletin of WHO* February 2006;84(2).

18 De Wagt, A & Clark D. A Review of UNICEF Experience with the Distribution of Free Infant Formula for Infants of HIV-Infected Mothers in Africa. *Presentation at the LINKAGES Art and Science of Breastfeeding Series*. 14 April 2004 Academy for Educational Development, Washington DC, USA.

19 WHO/FAO Safe preparation, storage and handling of powdered infant formula (PIF) 2007.

20 PMTCT Advisory Group. Evaluation of infant feeding practices by mothers at PMCT and non PMTCT sites in Botswana. Report, Botswana Food and Nutrition Unit. Family health Division. MOH Bostswana 2001.

21 Articles and summaries of published research. *Field Exchange*. December 2006**(29)**;22-25. Also: IBFAN Monitoring 2003

22 Noel F et al. Contribution of bacterial sepsis to morbidity in infants born to HIV-infected Haitian mothers. *J Acquir Immune Defic Syndr* 2006;**43(3)**:313-9

23 Nduati R et al. Effect of breastfeeding and formula feeding on transmission of HIV-1: a randomised clinical trial. *JAMA* 2000;**283**:1167-74

24 Nduati R. Presentation at UNICEF Meeting on HIV and Infant Feeding, Nairobi, Kenya, October 2000.

25 WHO. New data on PMTCT of HIV and their policy Implications: Technical Consultation, UNFPA/UNICEF/WHO/UNAIDS Inter-agency team on MTCT of HIV, Geneva, 11-13 October 2000. Conclusions and recommendations. 2001. WHO Geneva. WHO/RH/)1.28

26 Illiff P, Piwoz E, Tavengwa NV et al. Early exclusive breastfeeding reduces the risk of HIV transmission and increases HIV-free survival. 2005. Also: Coovadia HM, Rollins NC, Bland RM, Little K, Coutsoudis A, Bennish ML, Newell, M-L. Mother-to-child transmission of HIV-infection during exclusive breastfeeding in the first 6 months of life: an intervention cohort study. *The Lancet* 2007;**369**:1107-116

27 Bhandari et al. Effect of community-based promotion of exclusive breastfeeding on diarrhoeal illness and growth: a cluster randomised controlled trial. *The Lancet*

2003;**361**:1418-23 cited in Holmes W and Savage F. Exclusive breastfeeding and HIV (Letter) *www.the lancet.com* 369 pp1065-1066.31.3.2007. Also: Bland RM, Little K, Coovadia HM, Coutsoudis A, Rollins CR, Newell ML. Intervention to promote exclusive breastfeeding in the first 6 months of life in a high HIV prevalence area. *AIDS* 2008;**22**:883-891

28 WHO HIV and Infant Feeding Technical Consultation held on behalf of the Inter-agency task team (IATT) on prevention of HIV infections in pregnant women, mothers and their infants. WHO Geneva. 25-27 October 2006.

29 Hohnson W et al. The challenge of providing adequate infant nutrition following early breastfeeding cessation by HIV-positive mothers, food insecure Mozambican mothers. *16th International AIDS Conference*. Toronto, Canada 13-18 August 2006.

30 Professor and paediatrician, Anna Coutsoudis who was an initiator of the exclusive breastfeeding research set up the first human milk bank in Africa to help orphaned and abandoned HIV+ babies in the iThemba Lethu orphanage.in Durban, South Africa 2006.

Chapter 9: life, death and birth

1 Barker DJP. Mothers, Babies and Disease in Later Life. London: *BMJ* 1994. Also: Dykes F & Hall Moran V. Transmitted nutritional deprivation from mother to child. In: Hall Moran V & Dykes F, eds. *Maternal and Infant Nutrition and Nurture Controversies and Challenges*. Quay Books 2006: p6-39.

2 Kaati G, Bygren LO, Pembrey M & Sjöström M. Transgenerational response to nutrition, early life circumstances and longevity. *Eur J of Hum Gen*. 2007;1-7. www.nature.com/ejhg

3 Still GF. The History of Paediatrics. London: Oxford University Press 1931: p135.

4 Babies die from lack of breastfeeding in industrialised countries. See: Chen A and Rogan WJ, Breastfeeding and the Risk of Postneonatal Death in the United States. *Pediatrics* 2004;**113(5)**:e435-439

5 This is because the majority of humans live in poverty. Three billion live on less than \$2 per day and millions more live in conditions where artificial feeding is high risk. See Glenn JC, Gordon TJ and Florescu E. 2008 State of the Future. World Federation of UN Associations Millennium Project 2008.

6 Cars O and colleagues. Meeting the challenge of antibiotic resistance. *BMJ* 2008;**337**:726-728

7 Malaria kills 8% of children under 5 years (cf 19% pneumonia, 3% AIDS, 4% measles). Breastfeeding does not prevent malaria. Prevention includes sleeping under a mosquito net, especially one treated with insecticide, and regular use of anti-malarial drugs (AMDs). In Africa about 16% of children under five use nets, half of which are treated ones. About 43% receive anti-malarial drugs. Source: UNICEF: The State of the World's Children, 2008.

8 Information comes from OXFAM, UNDP, UNFPA, UNICEF, UNIFEM, WHO, WaterAid, Women Aid International. See their websites and publications. View http://www.un.org/millenniumgoals Also: Glenn JC, Gordon TJ and Florescu E. 2008 State of the Future. World Federation of UN Associations Millennium Project 2008. Thanks to water and sanitation engineers Professor Sandy Cairncross of LSHTM and John Palmer MCIWEM for guidance.

9 WHO/FAO. Safe preparation, storage and handling of powdered infant formula Guidelines. 2006. See also Forsyth S. Enterobacter sakazakii and other bacteria in powdered infant formula. *Mother and Child Nutrition* 2005; **1(1)**:44-50. NB Bottled water must be boiled in exactly the same way. Bottled 'mineral' waters must not be used for babies because the minerals (particularly sodium) are dangerous for babies. Bottled waters are no safer than well-regulated tap water. They contain micro-organisms which may increase during storage. Also: De Wagst A & Clark, D. A Review of UNICEF Experience with the Distribution of Free Infant Formula for Infants of HIV-Infected Mothers in Africa. *Presentation at the LINKAGES Art and Science of Breastfeeding Series*. 14 April 2004 Academy for Educational Development, Washington DC.

10 Information comes from Oxfam, Save The Children UK, UNDP, UNFPA, UNICEF, UNIFEM, WHO, WaterAid, Women Aid International. See their websites and publications. View http://www.un.org/millenniumgoals Also: Glenn JC, Gordon TJ and Florescu E. 2008 State of the Future. World Federation of UN Associations

Millennium Project 2008. Also: Von Hove T. More than one billion people call urban slums their home. City Mayors' Website 2003. Also: UN-HABITAT, The challenge of the slums: Global Report on Human Settlements 2003. Also: George R. The Big Necessity: Adventures in the World of Human Waste. Portobello Books 2008.

11 Agencies cited in references 8 and 10. Also: Report (2005) from Integrated Research for Action and Development (IRADe) New Delhi, India www.irade.org Also: The World Bank. World Development Report 2004: Making services work for poor people. Also: Parikh J. Home and Hearth. *Business Standard* 13 October 2005 (which cites IRADe study). Also: Gilman RH and Skillicorn P. Boiling of drinking water: can a fuel-scarce community afford it? *Trop Dis Bull* 1986;**83(3)**

12 Information from Save The Children UK, UNICEF and IBFAN. Gupta K and Khanna K. Economic value of breastfeeding in India. *Nat Med J of India* 1999;**12(3)**:123-127. FAO/WHO. How to prepare formula for cup-feeding at home. WHO 2007. Booklet to accompany FAO/WHO .Safe preparation, storage and handling of powdered infant formula Guidelines. 2007. Available at: http://www.who.int/foodsafety/ publications/micro/pif2007/en. Also IBFAN monitoring reports: Breaking the Rules and The State of the Code by Country. www.ibfan.org

13 UNICEF State of the World's Children 2008. Also: The Millennium Development Project Goals Report 2008. Education for All Global Monitoring Report 2009. See UNESCO Press Release 2008-115.

14 Countdown 2008 Equality Analysis Group. Mind the gap: equity and trends in coverage of maternal, newborn, and child health services in 54 Countdown countries. www.thelancet.com; 371: 12 April 2008. Bagchi S. Telemedicine in Rural India. *Public Library of Science Medicine* 2006;3(3);e82. Also: Costello A, Watson F & Woodward D. Human Face or Human Façade? Adjustment and the Health of Mothers and Children. London:Centre for International Child Health, Institute of Child Health 1994.[This documents the ill-effects of structural adjustment on healthcare.] Ouendo EM et al. Healthcare Access in Benin; poverty and community aid networks. *Santé* 2004;*14(4)*:217-21. UNICEF State of the World's Children 2008. http://www.un.org/millenniumgoals

15 Countdown 2008 Equality Analysis Group. Mind the gap: equity and trends in coverage of maternal, newborn, and child health services in 54 Countdown countries. *www.thelancet.com*; 371: Also: 12 April 2008. World Development Movement. http://www.wdm.org.uk/about/ accessed 23 July 2008. World's richest men in July 2008 were Warren Buffet ($62 billion); Carlos Slim Helu ($60 billion); Bill Gates ($58 billion). Source: Elizabeth Nelson http://business-success-stories.suite101.com/article.cfm/worlds_richest_men. Also: Save the Children UK, Running on Empty: Poverty and Child Malnutrition, 2007.

16 Ronsmans C & Graham W, Lancet Maternal Survival Campaign. Maternal Mortality: who, when, where and why. *The Lancet* 2006;**368**:1189-1200. NB The comparison with jumbo jet crashes was suggested by Dr Malcolm Potts, CEO of Familiy Health International.

17 Türmen T. Foreword in Murray SF, ed. *Midwives and Safer Motherhood.* Mosby 1996.

18 Save the Children, State of the World's Mothers 2006: Saving the lives of Mothers and Newborns. *Save the Children* 2006;p14-18 Also: Black RE et al. The Maternal and Child Undernutrition Study Group. Maternal and Child Undernutrition 1, Maternal and child undernutrition: global and regional exposures and health consequences. *www.thelancet.com* 17 January 2008. Also: WHO Making Pregnancy Safer Initiative http://www.who.int/making_pregnancy_safer/publications/standards/en/index.html.

19 Boseley S. Special Report Saving Grace 'From despair to fragile hope'. *The Guardian*, 7 June 2008.

20 Lucas S. Maternal death, autopsy studies and lessons from pathology. *Public Library of Science.* 2008.

21 UK Department of International Development (DFID). Maternal Health November 2007 www.dfid.gov.uk/mdg/health.asp. Also: Countdown Writing Group on behalf of the Countdown to 2015 Core Group. Countdown to 2015 for maternal, newborn and child survival: the 2008 report on tracking coverage of interventions. www.thelancet.com Vol 371 12 April 2008. Also: Factsheets at

http://www.un.org/millenniumgoals
22 Davidson JRT & Foa EB. *Posttraumatic Stress Disorder*: DSM-IV and Beyond. Washington, DC: American Psychiatric Press 1993. Also: Gerhardt S. *Why love matters: how affection shapes a baby's brain*. Routledge 2004. Also: Creamer M, O'Donnell ML & Pattison P. Amnesia, traumatic brain injury and posttraumatic stress disorder: a methodological inquiry. *Behaviour Research and Therapy*; 143 (10) October 2005.
23 Cassidy T. *Birth A History*. Chatto and Windus 2007. Also: Wagner M. *Pursuing the Birth Machine*. Ace Graphics 1994. Also: Oakley A. *The Captured Womb: a history of medical care of pregnant women*. Oxford: Basil Blackwell 1984.
24 Röckner G. *Reconsideration of the use of episiotomy in primiparas: A study in obstetric care*. Department of Obstetrics and Gynecology, Karolinska Institute, Huddinge University Hospital, Huddinge, Sweden 1991. Also: Williams A. Third-degree perineal tears; risk factors and outcome after primary repair. *Journal of Obstetrics and Gynaecology* 2003;**23**(6):611-614
25 Kroeger M with Smith LJ, *Impact of Birthing Practices on Breastfeeding*, Jones and Bartlett, 2004.
26 Walker M. Do Labor medications affect breastfeeding? *J Hum Lact* 1997;**13**(2). Also: Hale T. The effects on breastfeeding of anaesthetic medications used during labour. *Paper presented at Passage to Motherhood Conference* Brisbane Australia 1998. Also: Hale T. Medications and mothers' milk. Hale Publishing 2007.
27 Scott K, Laus PH & Klaus M. The obstetrical and post-partum benefits of continuous support during childbirth. *J Women's Health and Gender-based Medicine* 1999;**8(10)**:1257-1264
28 Odent M. *The farmer and the obstetrician*. Free Association Books 2002.
29 Klaus MH, Kennell JH & Klaus PH. *The Doula Book: How a trained labour companion can help you have a shorter, easier and healthier birth*. A Merloyd Lawrence Book 2002 (2nd ed).
30 WHO/UNICEF *Promoting, protecting and supporting breastfeeding: the special role of the maternity services*. Geneva WHO 1989.
31 Edmond KM et al. Delayed Breastfeeding Initiation Increases Risk of Neonatal Mortality. *Pediatrics* 2006;**117**;380-386. Also: Perez-Escamilla R et al. Infant feeding policies in maternity wards and their effect on breastfeeding success: an analytical overview. *American Journal of Public Health* 1994;**84(1)**:89-97
32 The following are publications which provide broad information about birth, particularly in relation to breastfeeding: Buckley SJ. Labour and birth: undisturbed birth – nature's hormonal blueprint for safety, ease and ecstasy. *MIDIRS Midwifery Digest* 2004;**14(2)**:203-209. Also: Buckley SJ. Labour and birth; What disturbs birth. *MIDIRS Midwifery Digest* 2004;**14(3)**:353 -359. Also: Walsh D. *Evidence-based care for normal labour and birth*. London: Routledge 2007. Odent M. *The nature of birth and breastfeeding*, Bergin & Garvey 1992. Also: Kroeger M with Smith LJ, *Impact of Birthing Practices on Breastfeeding*. Jones and Bartlett, 2004. Also: Klaus MH, Kennell JH & Klaus PH. *The Doula Book: How a trained labour companion can help you have a shorter, easier and healthier birth*. A Merloyd Lawrence Book 2002 (2nd ed).

Chapter 10: population, fertility and sex

1 Figures from The Office of the Deputy Prime Minister (UK), cited in Shelter website 2006. *Against the Odds* Shelter Report 2006.
2 Mirkin B. Statement of the 38th Session of the Commission on Population and Development World Demographic Trends: Report of the Secretary General Agenda Item 7. Programme Implementation and Future Programme of Work of the Secretariat in the Field of Population. 6 April 2005. Also: Hart SL. Beyond agreeing: strategies for a sustainable world. *Harvard Business Review* Jan/Feb 1997. Also: 'Human Footprint'. National Geographic Channel TV. Broadcast 13 April 2008.
3 Most taxes are not paid by the rich who hire clever lawyers and accountants to help them avoid taxation. Wealthy corporations are also adept tax avoiders, especially through the persuasion of governments to provide 'tax breaks'. For an example of ordinary tax payers funding schemes which benefit the elite in both donor and recipient countries see coverage of the UK Department for International Development's CDC (formerly the Commonwealth Development

Corporation). *Private Eye* 2008; Issues:1199 to 1125.

4 Monbiot G. Population growth is a threat. But it pales against the greed of the rich. *The Guardian* 29 January 2008.

5 Man-made famine. Channel 4. May 1985.

6 Raman Kutty V. Historical analysis of the development of health care facilities in Kerala State, India. *Health policy and planning* 2000;**15.1**:103-109

7 Levine R. Reducing Fertility in Bangladesh. In: Peterson PG *Millions Saved: Proven Successes in Global Health.* Institute for International Economics 2004.

8 Tanner JM. *Foetus into Man: physical growth from conception to maturity* (2nd ed). Castlemead Publications 1989 (update 1999); p161. Also: Leung AW et al. Evidence for a programming effect of early menarche on the rise of breast cancer incidence in Hong Kong. *Cancer Detect Prev* 2008;**32(2)**:156-61. Epub 2008 Jul 16. Also: Kvåle G, Heuch I & Ursin G. Reproductive Factors and Risk of cancer of the uterine corpus: a prospective study *Cancer Research* 1988;**48**:6217-6221

9 Singhal A & Lucas A. Early origins of cardiovascular disease. Is there a unifying hypothesis? *The Lancet* 2004;**363**:1642-45 Also: Singhal A et al. Is slower early growth beneficial for long-term cardiovascular disease? *Circulation* 2004;**109**:1108-1113. Also Singhal A et al. Promotion of faster weight gain in infants born small for gestational age: is there an adverse effect on later blood pressure? Also: Ziegler A-G et al. Early Infant Feeding and Risk of Developing Type 1 Diabetes-Associated Autoantibodies. *JAMA* 2003;**290**:1721-1728

10 Sandra Steingraber. *The Falling Age of Puberty*. 2007. www.breastcancerfund.org.

11 Tan, Karen A L et al, Infant feeding with soy formula milk: effects on puberty progression, reproductive function and testicular cell numbers in marmoset monkeys in adulthood. *Hum Reprod* (Advance Access originally published online on 13 February 2006). *Hum Reprod* 2006;**21(4)**:896-904; doi:10.1093/humrep/dei421

12 Kois WE. Influence of breastfeeding on subsequent reactivity to a related renal allograft. *J of Surg Res* 1984;37;89-93

13 Hanson LA. *Immunobiology of Human Milk*. Pharmasoft 2004.

14 Bongaarts J & Greenhalgh S. An alternative to the one child policy in China. *Population and Development Review* 1985;**11(4)**

15 Potts M & Short R. *Ever since Adam and Eve: the evolution of human sexuality.* Cambridge University Press 1999. See also: Becker S, Rutstein S & Labbock M. Estimation of births averted due to breastfeeding and increases in levels of contraception needed to substitute for breastfeeding. *J Biosc Sci* 2003;**35**:559-74. Also: Personal Communication: Professor Roger Short, University of Melbourne, Victoria, Australia. 2007.

16 Conde-Agudelo A. Effect of birth spacing on maternal and perinatal health: A systematic review and meta analysis. *Report submitted to the CATALYST consortium*, October 2004. See also: Norton M. Birth spacing: 2004 evidence supports 3+ years. Johns Hopkins Bloomberg School of Public Health. Programs, information and knowledge for optimal health project (INFO), 16 May 2005. Also: Catalyst Consortium September 2005.

17 USAID Maternal and Child Health, Birth Spacing: 2004 Evidence Supports 3+ Years 4 August 2004.

18 www.un.org/millenniumgoals/

19 Agency for Healthcare Research and Quality (AHRQ), Breastfeeding and maternal and infant health outcomes in developed countries. Evidence Reports and Summaries No 153, April 2007. www.ahrq.gov/clinic/tp/brf/outtp/ Also: Becker S, Rutstein S & Labbok M. Estimation of births averted due to breastfeeding and increases in levels of contraception needed to substitute for breastfeeding. *J Biosoc Sci* 2003;**35**:559-574

20 Cadogan W. *An essay upon nursing and the management of children, from birth to three years of age.* London: John Knapton 1748 (first ed).

21 Blair PS et al and the CESDI SUDI research group. Babies sleeping with parents: case-control study of factors influencing the risk of the sudden infant death syndrome. *British Medical Journal* 1999;**319**(7223):1457-1462

22 Ball H. Breastfeeding, dummies and bed sharing. Presentation at All-Ireland Conference '*Breastfeeding: making a difference*'. Northern Ireland Health Promotion Agency and Health Service Executive in Ireland, King's Hall, Belfast October 2008.

23 McKenna JJ, Ball HL & Gettler LT. Mother-infant cosleeping, breastfeeding and sudden infant death syndrome: what biological anthropology has discovered about normal infant sleep and pediatric sleep medicine. *Am J Phys Anthropol* 2007;Suppl45:133-61 Also:McKenna JJ. *Sleeping with your baby: a parents' guide to cosleeping.* Platypus Media 2007.
24 McNeilly AS. Professor at MRC human reproductive science unit, Edinburgh. Personal communication 1987. Also: McNeilly AS, Tay CC & Glasier A. Physiological mechanisms underlying lactational amenorrhoea. *Annals of the NY Academy of Sciences* 1994;709:145-155. Also: Diggory P, Teper S & Potts M. *Natural human fertility: Social and biological mechanisms.* London: Macmillan 1988.
25 Labbok M. Breastfeeding, fertility and family planning. *Global library of women's medicine.* 2008 (ISSN: 1756-2228) 2008; DOI 10.3843/GLOWM.10397. Also: Linkages: LAM FAQ. September 2001.
26 Konner M & Worthman C. Nursing frequency, gonadal function and birth spacing among !Kung hunter-gatherers. *Science* 1980;**207**:788-791. Also: Shostak M. *Nisa the life and words of a !Kung woman.* Vintage Books 1983. Also: Ellison PT. Breastfeeding, fertility and maternal condition. In: Stuart-Macadam P & Dettwyler K, eds. *Breastfeeding: biocultural perspectives.* Aldine de Gruyter 1995:p.305-345
27 *The Guinness Book of Records* 1984:p.17.
28 Lunn PG. Maternal nutrition and lactational infertility: the baby in the driving seat. In: Dobbing J, ed. *Maternal nutrition and lactational infertility.* Nestlé Nutrition, Raven Press 1985. Also: McNeilly AS, Tay CC & Glasier A. Physiological mechanisms underlying lactational amenorrhoea. *Annals of the NY Academy of Sciences* 1994;**709**:145-155. Also: Howie PW & McNeilly AS. Effect of breastfeeding patterns on human birth intervals. *Journal of Reproduction and Fertility* 1982;**65**:545-557. Also: Perez A, Labbok MH & Queenan JT. Clinical study of the lactational amenorrhoea method for family planning. *The Lancet* 1992;**339**:18
29 Gerhardt S. *Why love matters: how affection shapes a baby's brain.* Routledge 2004.
30 I thank Marjorie Jack and Malcolm Jack for this and other observations of parent child behaviour. Both worked and travelled in Nepal and Bhutan during the 1980s and 90s..
31 McKenna JJ. *Sleeping with your baby: a parents' guide to cosleeping.* Platypus Media 2007 Also: Barbieri A. The sleep of Reason. *The Guardian* 24 November 2004.
32 King FT. *The feeding and care of baby. New Zealand 1913* (further editions up to 1945. Also: King FT. *The expectant mother and baby's first month.* London: Macmillan 1924.
33 Taylor SE, *The Tending Instinct*, Henry Holt 2002. Also: Hrdy SB. *Mother nature: a history of mothers, infants and natural selection.* Pantheon 1999. Also: Odent M. *The farmer and the obstetrician.* Free Association Books 2001.
34 Shaikh T. Inquiry into Bringing up Baby nanny. *The Guardian* 27 October 2008.
35 Van Esterick P. Infant feeding options for Bangkok professional women. *Cornell International Nutritional Monograph, Series No.10.* Cornell University Press 1982.
36 Morley D. *Paediatric Priorities in the Developing World.* London: Butterworths 1978.
37 Thompson F. *Lark Rise to Candleford.* Oxford University Press 1968 (first published 1939): p139
38 Masters WH & Johnson VE. *Human Sexual Response.* Boston: Little Brown 1966. Comment: the evidence for this statement is very weak because breastfeeding rates were so low in the 1960s in the USA that it would have been impossible to compare two groups of women who were similar in other respects.
39 Alder EM et al. Hormones, mood and sexuality in lactating women. *British Journal of Psychiatry* 1986;**148**:74-9
40 Dyson L, McMillan B, Woolridge MW, Green JM Conner M, Clarke G, Bharj KK, & Renfrew MJ Looking at infant feeding today: reducing inequalities in health among socio-economically disadvantaged and ethnic groups by increasing breastfeeding uptake: an examination of intentions and outcomes. *Final Report to the UK Department of Health* 2003.
41 *Living Magazine.* February 1986.
42 Based on the 1972 novel by Ira Levin: two film versions one directed by Brian Forbes 1974, the second by Frank Oz 2004.

43 Edwina Currie, UK Junior Health Minister in PM Margaret Thatcher's government 1987.
44 Trish S. Marriage and social change in the liberated zones of Eritrea controlled by the Eritrean People's Front. *Paper presented at conference of the Review of Political Economy.* University of Liverpool, 26-27 September 1986.

Chapter 11: from the stone age to steam engines: a gallop through history

1   Many of the facts in this chapter are drawn from Lee RB and Daly R, eds. *The Cambridge Encyclopaedia of Hunters and Gatherers.* Cambridge University Press 2002.
2   *'Of the 80 billion humans who have walked this earth, 90% have been hunter-gatherers'.* Richard B Lee in ref1.
3   A UK politician, Jenny Tonge, has been caught up in a debate about land use in Botswana. She offended the First People of the Kalahari (FPK) by calling them primitive and suggesting that the women wanted to leave their gatherer/hunter lives and live in government resettlement camps. *The Guardian* 23 March 2006. Representatives of FPK have stated that *'women in our communities are some of the strongest speakers about wanting to go home and have gone to court to get our land back.'* (letter to The Guardian 23 March 2006) The land where FPK have lived for generations has the potential for mineral mining.
4   I am referring here to 'homo sapiens' but other types of 'humans' such as Neanderthal and those who used Acheulan tools existed long before then and would have hunted and gathered food.
5   http://www.survival-international.org/about
6   Mead M. *Male and Female.* Penguin Books 1950.
7   Endicott K in Lee RB and Daly R, eds. *The Cambridge Encyclopaedia of Hunters and Gatherers.* Cambridge University Press 2002.
8   The 2006 Plan of Action from the United Nations Standing Committee on Nutrition (SCN) cites the modern problem of excess consumption of energy-dense and micronutrient-poor food as the major nutrition problem in the world. People everywhere are getting fatter and more malnourished. SCN 33rd Session. *Tackling the double burden of malnutrition: a global agenda.* 13-17 March 2006: Geneva Switzerland. http://www.unsystem.org/scn/ My comment: When habitats are not sabotaged (eg by land control or recreational hunting by tourists)the gatherer-hunter diet contains excellent nutrition quality.
9   Truswell AS. Diet and nutrition of hunter-gatherers. In: *Health and disease in tribal societies.* Ciba Foundation Symposium No.49. Elsevier-Excerpta Medica, North Holland 1977.
10 Sahlins MD: *Stone-age economics.* London: Tavistock 1974.
11 Woodburn JC. Sex roles and the division of labour in hunter-gatherer societies. *Paper presented at First International Conference on hunter-gatherer societies.* Paris June 1978. Also: many discussions with James and Lisa Woodburn who have contributed much to my education.
12 Jelliffe DB et al. The children of the Hadza hunters. *Journal of Pediatrics* 1962;60(6)
13 *'Of the 80 billion humans who have walked this earth, 90% have been hunter-gatherers'.* Richard B Lee. See references 1 and 2 above.
14 Farb P & Armelagos G. The food connection: new crops and increased production allow populations to soar. *Natural History* September 1980:p26-30.
15 Keegan J. *The History of Warfare.* First Vintage Books 1994.
16 More energy does not necessarily mean better nutrition. Though staple grain and root crops have their value, their dominance in the diet would have led to a decrease in important micronutrients found in the more diverse gatherer-hunter diet.
17 Conton L. Social, economic and ecological parameters of infant feeding in Usino, Papua New Guinea. *Ecology of Food and Nutrition* 1985;16:39-54
18 Norway has the highest rate of breastfeeding of industrialised countries. In 2003 99% of women were breastfeeding at one week and 80% at six months. Frigitt 28. March 2003 Statistics Norway.
    http://www.ssb.no/vis/emner/03/01/kostspe/main.html
19 Lampman J. New fight, old foe: slavery. Some 27 million men, women, and children are in unpaid servitude, the UN says-200,000 of them in the US. *Christian Science Monitor* 21 February 2007. Also: Cox C and Marks J. *This Immoral Trade*

slavery in the 21st century. Monarch Books 2006. Also: Bales K. *Disposable People: new slavery in the global economy.* Berkeley: University of California Press 2004. Also: Snyder L. Contemporary child slavery in Mauritania. *The American Anti-Slavery Group* http://www.iabolish.org/

20 In 2005, just 47% of women in the developed world were in 'non-agricultural wage employment'. In Southern Asia this figure is 18%. The 'non-agricultural' definition means these statistics exclude the many women engaged in family and subsistence agriculture. Source: *The Millennium Development Goals* Report 2007.

21 This lack of rights for women regarding property and/or child custody exists in several countries in Sub-Saharan Africa.

22 Holland J. *Misogyny: the world's oldest prejudice.* London: Robinson 2006.

23 King J and Ashworth A. Changes in infant feeding practice in the Caribbean: an historical review. *Occasional Paper No.8. Department of Human Nutrition 1987.* The London School of Hygiene and Tropical Medicine.

24 In 1976 in the UK expectation of life was 69.7 years for males and 75.8 years for females. In 2003 the UK figure was 76.3 for males and 80.7 for females.

25 For a depiction of Romanian life in these conditions see Cristian Mungiu's 2007 film, '*4 Months, 3 Weeks, 2 days*'.

26 Jacobson P. Lee's tight little island. *The Sunday Times* 1984.

27 Brin H. President of The National Union of Family Associations (France).

28 Ballantyne J. Europe: France pays mothers to have more children. *News Weekly (Australia)* 8 October 2005.

29 ILO Maternity Protection Convention C183 2000. ILO Maternity Protection Recommendation R191 2000.

30 Bryan B, Dadzie S & Scafe S. *The heart of the race: black women's lives in Britain.* Virago 1985.

31 In 2003 the infant mortality rate for non-Hispanic black mothers was significantly higher than for all other groups. Source: Mathews TJ & Mac Dorman MF. Infant mortality statistics from the 2003 period linked brith/infant death data set. *Natl Vital Stat Rep* 2006;54(15) cited in *CDC MMWR Weekly* 23 June 2006/55(24);683

32 US Department of Health and Human Services. HRSA *Maternal and Child Health Bureau.* Rockville, Maryland 2006. Also: Chen A & Rogan WJ. Breastfeeding and the risk of postneonatal death in the United States. *Pediatr* 2004;113:e435-e439

33 Jane Austen's novel *Pride and Prejudice* (pub.1813) gives readers the impression that most women of that era did not work. Her characters represent a certain sector of society but not the great majority.

34 Laslett P. *The world we have lost – further explored.* London: Methuen 1983.

35 See Save the Children UK website and UNICEF website for links on this subject.

36 Pollock LA. *Forgotten children: parent-child relationships from 1500 to 1900.* Cambridge University Press 1983.35

37 Fildes V. *Breasts, bottles and babies: a history of infant feeding.* Edinburgh University Press 1986.

38 Walker M, CEO NABS: Personal Communication 2007.

39 Cock J. *Maids and madams: domestic workers under apartheid.* Women's Press Ltd 1990. Also: Fildes V. *Wet nursing: a history from antiquity to the present.* Basil Blackwell 1988.

40 Fildes V. *Breasts, bottles and babies: a history of infant feeding.* Edinburgh University Press 1986. Also: Smith FB. *The People's Health* 1930 to 1916. London: Croom Helm 1979.

41 McLaren D. Nature's contraceptive: wet nursing and prolonged lactation: the case of Chesham, Bucks. 1578-1601. *Medical History* 1979;**23**:426-41

42 Pollock LA. *Forgotten children: parent-child relationships from 1500 to 1900.* Cambridge University Press 1983. p35.

43 Fildes V. *Breasts, bottles and babies: a history of infant feeding.* Edinburgh University Press 1986.

44 Infant mummy and feeding bottle (exhibit photos 28 and 29). Ca 800 BCE (Zhou Dynasty). In collection of Xinjiang Uygar Autonomous Regional Museum.In: *Archeological Treasures of the Silk Road in Xinjiang Uygar Autonomous Region.* Shanghai Translation Publishing House. Illustration reproduced with permission of exhibition directors. Shanghai Museum 1998.

45 No evidence indicates transmission of syphilis via breastmilk in the absence of a breast or nipple lesion'. Statement in Lawrence, Ruth, A. and Lawrence, Robert, M. *Breastfeeding: A Guide for the Medical Profession*, Mosby, 5th ed 1999. p606. Also: Fildes V. Syphilis as an occupational disease of wet nurses: an international review 1490s to 1980s. Paper presented to *The Society for the Social History of Medicine*. London 5 February 1988.

46 Fildes V. *Breasts, bottles and babies: a history of infant feeding*. Edinburgh University Press 1986.

47 Khodel J & Van de Walle E. Breastfeeding, fertility and infant mortality: an analysis of some early German data. *Population Studies* 1967;**21**:109-31

48 Infantile mortality. *British Medical Journal*. 23 November 1889 p1198.

49 Scrimshaw NS et al. Interaction of nutrition and infection. *WHO Monograph* No.29 1968

50 Broström G et al. The impact of breastfeeding patterns on infant mortality in a 19th century Swedish parish. *Newsletter No.1, Demographic Data Base*. Umeå University, Sweden.

51 Fildes V. *Breasts, bottles and babies: a history of infant feeding*. Edinburgh University Press 1986:p330

52 Broström G et al. The impact of breastfeeding patterns on infant mortality in a 19th century Swedish parish. *Newsletter No.1, Demographic Data Base*. Umeå University, Sweden.

53 Spencer M. Is breast really best? *The Observer* 8 June 2008.

Chapter 12: other women's babies: wet nursing

Many of the facts in this chapter are drawn from: Fildes V. *Wet nursing: a history from antiquity to the present*. Basil Blackwell 1988; Maher V (ed). *The Anthropology of Breastfeeding*. Berg 1992; Apple R. *Mothers and Medicine.* The University of Wisconsin Press 1987. All points that are not referenced can be found within these books.

1 Still GF. *The history of paediatrics*. Oxford University Press 1931 p.141.

2 Hanson LA. *Immunobiology of human milk: how breastfeeding protects babies.* Pharmasoft Publishing 2004.

3 Fildes V. p51.

4 Shakespeare W. *Romeo and Juliet.* Probably first written 1595.

5 In 2006 Italy reintroduced a modern version of these 'tours' to cope with an increasing problem of abandoned babies. Owen R. Hospital to bring back abandoned baby wheel. *The Times* 7 September 2005.

6 Laslett P. *The world we have lost – further explored*. Methuen 1983.

7 The poet Alexander Pope (1688-1744) built an elaborate memorial to his wet nurse, Mary Beach. This can be seen at the Church of St Mary, Twickenham, Middlesex, UK.

8 Jenkins L. Mix-up babies back with the right parents. *The Daily Telegraph*. September 1986.

9 Fred Attewill and agencies. Czech mate - DNA tests show hospital mixed up babies. *www.guardian.co.uk* 10 October 2007.

10 This was due to many reasons, including the infuence of William Cadogan through his writings and the theories of French thinker Jean-Jacques Rousseau (1712-1778) who changed ideas about child-rearing.

11 Fildes, V. *Breasts, Bottles and Babies*. Edinburgh University Press 1986. p86.

12 Apple R. *Mothers and Medicine*. The University of Wisconsin Press 1987 p56.

13 Laverty M. *No more than human*. Longmans, Green & Co 1944.

14 Chung AW. Breastfeeding in a developing country. The People's Republic of China. In: Raphael D, ed. *Breastfeeding and Food Policy in a Hungry World*. Academic Press 1979.

15 Feng Deming and his wife Sun Feng Dan became my friends when I lived in Shanghai from 1997-1999. Feng Deming is now in his 80s.

16 UN Guidelines on HIV and Infant Feeding 2004.

17 Bear L. The Hollywood wet nurses. *Eve* June 2007

Chapter13: the industrial revolution in britain: the era of progress?

1 I do not provide detailed references for this opening overview of history. It is

based on decades of reading. However the authors I cite when referring to specific points have influenced my ideas.

2   The risk in a developed country now is less than one in 10,000. See Chapter 9 for more on risks.

3   Puerperal or childbed fever was caused by blood poisoning (septicaemia) occurring shortly after childbirth, due to infection often introduced by medical staff and general bad hygiene practices. Improved hygiene and antibiotics have reduced the incidence dramatically in the rich world, but this still occurs in poor countries where women give birth in bad conditions. See Chapter 9.

4   Porter R. *The greatest benefit to mankind. A medical history of humanity from antiquity to the present*. Harper Collins 1997 p711-12. Also: Woods R & Woodward J. *Urban disease and mortality in 19th century England*. London: Batsford 1984. Also: Cassidy T. *Birth: a history*. Chatto and Windus 2007. Also: Oakley A. The Captured Womb: a history of medical care of pregnant women. Oxford: Basil Blackwell 1984.

5   Laslett P. *The World we have lost-further explored*. London: Methuen 1983.

6   Thompson B. Infant mortality in 19th century Bradford. In: Woods R& Woodward J. *Urban disease and mortality in 19th century England*. London: Batsford 1984. NB Diarrhoeal deaths are the ones most easily prevented by exclusive breastfeeding and are, in the absence of modern hygiene and health services, indicate inadequate infant feeding practices.

7   Edwin Chadwick, (1800-1890), the innovator of piped water and the removal of sewage through pipes, had a major influence on public health. Ferriman A. BMJ readers choose the "sanitary revolution" as greatest medical advance since 1840. *BMJ* 2007;**334**(7585):111 (20 January), doi:10.1136/bmj.39097.611806.DB

8   Lewis J. *Women in England* 1870-1950. Wheatsheaf Books 1984.

9   Reid G. Infant mortality and the employment of married women in factories. *BMJ* 1901:410-12

10 Lewis J. *Women in England* 1870-1950. Wheatsheaf Books 1984.

11 Infantile mortality and the occupation of married women. *BMJ* 1901;**2(2123)**:634

12 Reid G. Infant mortality and the employment of married women in factories. *BMJ* 1901:410-12

13 Asby HT. *Infant mortality*. Cambridge University Press 1915: p45

14 Thompson F. *Lark Rise to Candleford*. Oxford University Press 1968 (first published 1939).

15 Dunicliff J and the Tean and Checkley Historical Society. *Making History*. BBC Radio 4, 17 June 2008.

16 Reid G. Infant mortality and the employment of married women in factories. *BMJ* 1901:410-12

17 Rivers J. *The health of nations*. Open University Press 1985: p127.

18 The Barker hypothesis vindicates the authorities' conclusions. Barker DJP. *Mothers, babies and disease in later life*. London: BMJ Publishing House 1994.

19 Bunting M. Baby, this just isn't working for me. *The Guardian*. 1 March 2007.

20 The ILO was formed in 1919, in the wake of the First World War, to pursue a vision based on the premise that universal, lasting peace can be established only if based on the decent treatment of working people. The ILO became the first specialized agency of the UN in 1946. www.ilo.org/global

21 Western feminists have sometimes written as though they had discovered women's physical strength. Though cultural norms vary, even where men do arduous tasks, women still perform hard physical work everyday in Africa, Asia and Latin America. Women may carry as much as 30kg weight (66lbs [30 litres of water weighs 30kg]) on their heads, sometimes over long distances (several kilometres). They win no prizes nor gain any glory for these daily feats of strength. When machines are introduced men usually are the first to use them. This sometimes applies in Europe too. In 2006 I witnessed older women in Northern Portugal carrying 25kg to 30kg sacks of newly-harvested maize to silos while younger men sat on tractors.

22 Morgan CE. *Women Workers and Gender Identities, 1835-1913: The Cotton and Metal Industries in England*. Routledge 2001. Also: John AV. *By the Sweat of Their Brow: Women Workers at Victorian Coal Mines*. McGraw Hill Professional 2006.

23 In the UK rape in marriage was made a crime in 1991. See www.rapecrisis.org..

24 Llewellyn Davies M, ed. *Maternity: letters from working women. Collected by the*

Women's Cooperative Guild. London: Virago 1978 (first pub. By G. Bell & Sons 1915).

25 Buffle JC. *Dossier N comme Nestlé*. Alain Moreau 1986.

26 Coutts FJM. *Inquiry into condensed milks with special reference to their use as infants' foods*. Local Government Board Reports: Food Report No.15. London: HMSO 1911. Also Coutts FJM. On the use of proprietary foods for infant feeding and analysis and composition of some proprietary foods for infant feeding. Food Report No.20 London: HMSO 1914.

27 Atkins PJ. Mother's milk and infant death in Britain, circa 1900-1940. *Anthropology of Food*. 2 September 2003. Milk was the medium of transmission from diseased cattle to unwitting consumers that led to approximately 500,000 deaths amongst infants in the period 1850-1950, and up to 30 per cent of all deaths from tuberculosis before 1930 (Atkins 2000a). The hazard was only brought under control gradually as milk was increasingly pasteurized in the 1930s and 1940s.

28 Oakley A. *The Captured Womb: a history of medical care of pregnant women*. Oxford: Basil Blackwell 1984: p60.

29 Enock AG. *This milk business: a study from 1895-1943*. London: H K Lewis & Co.Ltd 1943. Also Lewis J. *The politics of motherhood*. London: Croom Helm 1980: p65. Also:Atkins P & Brassley P. Mad Cows and Englishmen. *History Today*. September 1996;46. Bovine tuberculosis caused over 800,000 deaths in Britain 1850-1950. Children who drank milk were particularly vulnerable. Post-mortems on children in late 19th C London showed 30-40% had TB - most would have been of bovine origin.

30 Chamberlain M. *Fenwomen: a portrait of women in an English village*. London: Ruutledge & Kegan Paul 1983: p74-5. [First pub. Virago 1975]. The woman who spoke these words had brought her children up just after the First World War.

31 Frame Food advertisement in *Nursing Times* 16 June 1906;12(59).

32 Lee L. *Cider with Rosie*. Harmondsworth: Penguin Books 1986: p123 (First published 1959).

33 *The Infant's Magazine*. Annual for 1913. London: SW Partridge & Co. Ltd. Also: James Joyce (1882-1941), in his novel *Ulysses* (first published 1922) described the hero Leopold Bloom as carrying a tin of Neave's Food. The death of his baby is a central theme but there is no awareness that the artificial food might be implicated in the death.

34 The Russian Imperial Family (the Romanovs) led by Czar Nicholas II were shot by the Bolshevik authorities in July 1918.

35 *Maternity and Child Welfare*. No1 January 1917.

Chapter 14: markets are not created by god

1 With family unit labour, individual members can replace each other for whatever reason; the employer is indifferent as long as the works gets done. This still occurs in parts of the world for example, in tea estates.

2 Conyington M. Report on condition of women and child wage-earners in the US, vol18. *Employment of women and children in selected industries*. Washington: Government Printing Office 1913. Also: Vol 13 *Infant mortality and its relation to the employment of mothers*. The Fall River Study 1912.

3 Winikof B & Laukaren VH. Breastfeeding and Bottle Feeding Controversies in the Developing World: Evidence from a Study in Four Countries. *Social Science and Medicine* 1989;29:859-868. This research found that most artificial feeding was done by women who stayed at home and women who worked outside the home were more likely to be breastfeeding.

4 Cassidy T. *Birth: a history*. London: Chatto & Windus 2007. Also Carter J & Duriez T. *With child: birth through the ages*. Edinburgh: Mainstream Publishing 1986. Also: Porter R. *The greatest benefit to mankind. A medical history of humanity from antiquity to the present*. Harper Collins 1997.

5 Ehrenreich B & English D. *Complaints and disorders: the sexual politics of sickness*. The Feminist Press 1973. See also: Gilman CP. *The yellow wallpaper*. Small, Maynard & Company 1901; for an account of male attitudes to women's 'nervous conditions'.

6 Apple R. *Mothers and medicine: a history of infant feeding from 1850-1950*. Madison: University of Wisconsin Press 1887: p21. Also: Rotch TM. A discussion on the modification of milk in the feeding of infants. *BMJ* 6 September 1902:653

7 Hardyment C. *Dream babies: childcare from Locke to Spock*. Oxford University Press 1984: p127. Also: Apple R. *Mothers and medicine: a history of infant feeding from 1850-1950*. Madison: University of Wisconsin Press 1887.

8 Apple RD. "To be used only under the direction of a physician" – commercial infant feeding and medical practice – 1870-1940. *Bull Hist Med* 1980;**54(3)**:402-417. Also: Apple RD. "Advertised by our loving friends": the infant formula industry and the creation of new pharmaceutical markets 1870-1910. *Journal of the History of Medicine and Allied Sciences* January 1986;**41(1)**

9 All quotations in this section are drawn from the two citations above (ref 8), Rima Apple's book and Dr.Rotch's *BMJ* article (ref 6). I am indebted to Rima Apple for her groundbreaking research and have drawn substantially on her work.

10 Davis WH. Statistical comparison of the mortality of breastfed and bottle-fed infants. *American Journal of Diseases in Childhood* 1913;**5**:234-47. Also: Woodbury RM. The relation between breast and artificial feeding and infant mortality. *American Journal of Hygiene* 1922;**2**:668-87

11 WHO Collaborative Study Team on the role of breastfeeding in the prevention of infant mortality. Effect of breastfeeding on infant and child mortality due to infectious diseases in less developed countries: a pooled analysis. *The Lancet* 2000;**355**:451-455

12 Grulee CG et al. Breast and artificial feeding, JAMA 8 September 1934; 16(80):735-9. Also: *JAMA* 1 June 1935;**104(22)**:1988-90

13 Relucio-Clavano N. The results of a change in hospital practices – a paediatrician's campaign for breastfeeding in the Philippines. In: *Assignment Children: Breastfeeding and Health.* Geneva: UNICEF 1981: p139-65

14 De Carvalho M etal. Effect of frequent breastfeeding on early milk production and infant weight gain. *Pediatrics* 1983;72(3):307-311

15 For three months in the early summer of 2008, the AAP journal, the web issue of *Pediatrics*, published e-advertising by Nestlé which violated the Code and also AAP policy. Dr Marco Kerac of the Institute of Child Health, London and other concerned health professionals wrote to the AAP expressing their concern. See also: Walker M. *Selling out mothers and Babies*. NABA 2007.

16 Baby Milk Action. Melamine contamination deaths in China show need for regulations. *Baby Milk Action Update* 41 November 2008: p16.

17 Cunningham AS. Letter to Jane McNeil, Acting Director of Supplemental Foods Division, Food and Nutrition Services, USDA, Washington DC 1979. Also: Palmer G. Who helps health professionals with breastfeeding? *Midwives Chronicle*. May 2003.

18 Horta B, Bahl R, Martines JC & Victora CG. Evidence on the long-term effects of breastfeeding: systematic reviews and meta-analyses. WHO 2007.

19 Deeny J. Epidemiology of infantile enteritis. *The Lancet* 1942;**253**(23):284-5. Also: *Journal of the Medical Association of Eire* 1946;**19**:146

20 Meredith D. The Empire Marketing Board 1926-32. *History Today*. January 1987:30-36. Also: Source of money equivalents: The House of Commons Library. *Inflation: the value of the pound 1750-2005*. Research Paper 06/09. 13 February 2006.

21 Rubber teats were first patented in the USA in 1845 but leather and animal teats were in use long after this date. Hardyment C. *Dream Babies: Childcare Advice from John Locke to Gina Ford*. France: Lincoln Ltd 2008.

22 Malaysia: women plantation workers' conditions in oil palm plantations. *World Rainforest Bulletin* Issue No.105 April 2006 [Rubber trees were replaced with oil palms. Women forced to become herbicide sprayers or lose employment.] Sangaralingam M. Plantation workers face poverty and poison. *Consumers' Association of Penang*.http://www.socialwatch.org/en/informesNacionales/437.html

23 Consumers' Association of Penang (CAP) Malaysia. *The other baby killer*. CAP 1981.

24 King J and Ashworth A. Changes in infant feeding practice in Malaysia: an historical review. *Occasional Paper No.7. Department of Human Nutrition*. The London School of Hygiene and Tropical Medicine 1987.

25 Manderson L. Bottle-feeding and ideology in colonial Malaya: the production of change. *International Journal of Health Services* 1982; **12**(4):597-616

26 Consumers' Association of Penang (CAP) Malaysia. *The other baby killer*. CAP 1981.

27 Williams C. *Milk and Murder*. Address to the Singapore Rotary Club 1939. Allain A

(ed) Penang: IOCU, PO Box 1045, 10830 Penang, Malaysia.

28 Letter from GA Raffé, General Manager of Nestlé UK to Miss June Thompson, Public Relations Manager of the UK Health Visitors' Association, 9 February 1983.

29 King J and Ashworth A. Changes in infant feeding practice in Malaysia: an historical review. *Occasional Paper No.7. Department of Human Nutrition 1987*. The London School of Hygiene and Tropical Medicine.

30 Jelliffe DB & Jelliffe EFP. *Human milk in the modern world*. Oxford University Press 1978: p189. Jeanine Klaus of ILCA suggested to me in the 1990s that the lactation suppressant drug bromocriptine might trigger infant abuse because it inhibited prolactin production. Prolactin is associated with mothering behaviour. Mothers who do not breastfeed still have circulating prolactin for some time after birth.

31 Nestlé Thailand '71. *Bulletin Nestlé* No.3 1971. Cited in Van Esterick P. Infant feeding options for Bangkok women. *Cornell International Nutrition Monograph Series* No.10. Cornell University Press 1982.

32 For an overview of the causes and treatment of severe malnutrition see: Golden MHN and Golden BE. Severe Malnutrition. In Garrow JS, James WPT and Ralph A, eds. *Human Nutrition and Dietetics* (10th edition) Edinburgh: Churchill Livingstone 2001.

33 McLaren DS. The great protein fiasco. *The Lancet* 1974;2:93-6

34 Rush D et al. A randomized controlled trial of prenatal nutritional supplementation in New York City. *Pediatrics* 1980;65:683

35 Singhal A et al. Promotion of faster weight gain in infants born small for gestational age: is there an adverse effect on later blood pressure? *Circulation* 16 January 2007:**115**(2):213-20. Epub December 18 2006.

36 Davidson S et al. *Human Nutrition and Dietetics*. Edinburgh: Churchill Livingstone 1979: p683.

37 Trinidad Nutrition Commission 1938. Cited in King J and Ashworth A. Changes in infant feeding practice in the Caribbean: an historical review. *Occasional Paper No.8. Department of Human Nutrition 1987*. The London School of Hygiene and Tropical Medicine.

38 King J and Ashworth A. Changes in infant feeding practice in Nigeria: an historical review. *Occasional Paper No.9. Department of Human Nutrition 1987*. The London School of Hygiene and Tropical Medicine.

39 King J and Ashworth A. Changes in infant feeding practice in the Caribbean: an historical review. *Occasional Paper No.8. Department of Human Nutrition 1987*. The London School of Hygiene and Tropical Medicine.

40 King J and Ashworth A. Changes in infant feeding practice in Malaysia: an historical review. *Occasional Paper No.7. Department of Human Nutrition 1987*. The London School of Hygiene and Tropical Medicine.

41 EC Dairy Facts and Figures 1992.

42 UNICEF. The State of the World's Children 2008.

43 Clark C. *UNICEF for beginners*. New York: Writers and Readers Publishing Inc 1996. This delightful book gives a cartoon history of UNICEF, delicately describing its travails, successes and errors. The author Christian Clark is a cartoonist and writer who used to work on the TV show Sesame Street.

44 Punjab Lok Sujag. *The political economy of milk in the Punjab: a people's perspective*. Lahore, Punjab Lok Sujag 2003. www.loksujag.org

Chapter 15: the lure of the global market

1 Apple RD. "To be used only under the direction of a physician" – commercial infant feeding and medical practice – 1870-1940. *Bull Hist Med* 1980;**54(3)**:402

2 Williams C. Interview in the *Lansing Star*, 18 October 1978.

3 Orwell S & Murray J. Infant feeding and health in Ibadan. *Journal of Tropical Paediatrics and Environment and Child Health* 1974;**20**:205-19

4 Chetley A. *The Baby Killer Scandal: a War on Want investigation into the promotion and sale of powdered baby milks in the Third World*. London: War on Want 1979.

5 Willat N. How Nestlé adapts products to its markets. *Business Abroad* June 1970: p31-3.

6 George S. *How the other half dies: the real reasons for world hunger*. Harmondsworth: Penguin 1979: p180.

7 Jelliffe DB. Commerciogenic malnutrition? *Food Technology* 1971;25(55) Also: Wennen van der May CAM. The decline of breastfeeding in Nigeria. *Tropical and Geographical Medicine* 1960;21:93

8 Ashworth Hill A. Emeritus Professor of Community Nutrition LSHTM: Personal communication 1985.

9 Chetley A. *The politics of baby foods: successful challenges to an international marketing strategy*. London: Frances Pinter 1986. Also: *WHO Collaborative Study on Breastfeeding*. Geneva: WHO 1979.

10 Action now on baby foods. *New Internationalist* 10 August 1973. Also: Muller M. *The Baby Killer*. London: War on Want 1973.

11 Jelliffe DB & Jelliffe EFP. *Human milk in the modern world*. Oxford University Press 1978.

12 Post JE & Baer E. Demarketing infant formula: consumer products in the developing world. *Journal of Contemporary Business* 1979;7(4)

13 Arbeitsgruppe Dritte Welt (AgDW) or Third World Working Group.

14 INFACT. *Nestlé in the USA: Giant in Disguise*. INFACT 1978.

15 Furer A. Chief Executive Officer of Nestlé quoted in Chetley A. *The politics of baby foods: successful challenges to an international marketing strategy*. London: Frances Pinter 1986: p45.

16 Reverend W Beaver of Interfaith Centre for Corporate Accounts: Personal communication 1984.

17 Bader M. Breastfeeding: the role of multinational corporations in Latin America. *International Journal of the Health Service* 1976;6(4):609-26. Also: Greiner T. The promotion of bottle-feeding by multinational corporations: how advertising and the health professionals have contributed. *Cornell Internal Nutritional Monograph Series No. 2*. Cornell University Press 1975.

18 Chetley A. *The Baby Killer Scandal: a War on Want investigation into the promotion and sale of powdered baby milks in the Third World*. London: War on Want 1979: p50-2.

19 Kreig P. *Bottle Babies*. Workers' Film Association 1975.

20 Buffle JC. *Dossier N comme Nestlé*. Alain Moreau 1986.

21 Laskin CR & Pilot LJ. Defective infant formula: the Neo-Mul-Soy/Cho-Free incident. In: Moss HA, Hess R & Swift C, eds. *Early interventions for infants, vol.1(4), Prevention in Human Services*. New York: Harworth Press 1982: p97-106. Also: Minchin M. *Breastfeeding matters*. Alma Publications 1985 (updated edition 1998).

22 Laskin CR & Pilot LJ. Defective infant formula: the Neo-Mul-Soy/Cho-Free incident. In: Moss HA, Hess R & Swift C, eds. *Early interventions for infants, vol.1(4), Prevention in Human Services*. New York: Harworth Press 1982: p97-106.

23 IBFAN Asia. *Babies, breastfeeding and the Code*. Report of the IBFAN Asia Conference. Sam Phran, Thailand 5-12 October 1986: p22. Also: Walker M. *Selling Out Mothers and Babies*. National Alliance for Breastfeeding Advocacy, Research, education and legal branch (NABA REAL), 2001.

24 Willoughby A et al. Developmental outcome in children exposed to chloride deficient formula. *Pediatrics* 1987;79(6): p851-7. Also: Malloy MH et al. Hypochloremic metabolic alkalosis from ingestion of chloride deficient formula: outcome 9 and 10 years later. *Pediatrics* 1991;87(6):811-22. Also: Federal Administration Washington HQ/Division of Regulatory Guidance: telex refusing permission for Syntax request to donate for export recalled formula, 29 September 1979.

25 Debbie's symptoms were similar to those related to infection with enterobacter Sakazakii, a pathogen which has been found in infant formula and is difficult to eliminate in the manufacturing process. This and some other pathogens come into the category of 'intrinsic contamination'.

26 Makil LP & Simpson M. *Seven infant deaths*. IPC Working Paper. Institute of Philippine Culture, Ateneo de Manila University, Quezon City, 28 Septmber 1984. Also: National Coalition for the Promotion of Breastfeeding and Childcare(BUNZO) Information Pack, Quezon City. 1985.

27 Vaughn VC et al, eds. *Nelson Textbook of Pediatrics*. Philadelphia: WB Saunders 1979: p203.

28 Baby Milk Action. Melamine contamination deaths in China show need for regulations. *Baby Milk Action Update 41*, November 2008. Also: China's baby-milk scandal. *The Economist* 18 September 2008. Also: Food regulations in China. *The*

Economist 25 September 2008. Also: Land of Milk and Money. *The Economist* 3 October 2008.

29 Cohen R et al. Comparison of maternal absenteeism and infant illness rates among breastfeeding and formula-feeding women in two corporations *American Journal of Health Promotion* 1995;**10**:148-153. Also: Rental Roundup. The State of Breastfeeding Legislation in the United States – November 1999. *Medela Inc.* Also Ehrenreich B. *Nickel and dimed: undercover in low-wage USA.* Granta Books 2002.

30 UNICEF The State of the World's Children 1992. Also Fides L. The silent slaughter. In: Aldaba-Benitez CH, ed. *Unmasking a giant.* IBON Philippines Databank and Research Centre 1992.

31 *Fortune* 13 February 1978: p.81. Also: Buffle JC. *Dossier N comme Nestlé.* Alain Moreau 1986. Also: Monbiot G. *"Hill and Knowlton, the public relations company famous for the unsavoury nature of its clients."* Quotation from: A bully in ermine. In: Monbiot G. *Bring on the Apocalypse.* Atlantic Books 2008. George Monbiot cites http://www.hillandknowlton.com/index/case_studies/our results/10

32 Chetley A. *The politics of baby foods: successful challenges to an international marketing strategy.* London: Frances Pinter 1986: p52-4.

33 McComas M et al. *The dilemma of Third World nutrition, Nestlé and the role of infant formula.* Nestlé USA 1985: p12.

34 Angst CL. The social responsibility of the food industry. *Consumer Affairs.* September/October 1985: p51.

35 Korten DC *When corporations rule the world.* West Hartford CT; Kumarian Press 1995, cited in Richter, Judith. *Holding Corporations Accountable.* Zed Books 2001.

36 Hunt EK. *Property and prophets: the evolution of economic institutions and ideologies.* New York: Harper &Row (5th ed) 1986.

37 Galbraith, JK. *The Economics of Innocent Fraud Truth for our Time.* Allen Lane Penguin Books 2004.

38 Richter J. Engineering of Consent: uncovering corporate PR. *Corner House Briefing Paper No.6* March 1998. Also: Richter J. *Holding Corporations Accountable.* Zed Books 2001.

39 Individuals in the artificial milk companies may grumble about the Code and its restrictions but the International Council of Infant Food Industries (ICIFI) proposed the idea. According to the Nestlé account, the ICIFI director (Ian Butler of Cow & Gate) suggested to Senator Edward Kennedy that WHO should be the forum for creating an international Code. The companies were involved in the entire drafting process.

40 The annual World Health Assembly (WHA) is the meeting of UN Member State representatives for debate and decision (votes) on health issues. The World Health Organisation (WHO) is the secretariat whose role is to support the implementation of the decisions of the member states.

41 Argentina, Japan and South Korea abstained. In 2008, Argentina has the Code as law; Japan a mix of law and voluntary measures, South Korea few voluntary measures. All three nations have agreed to WHA Resolutions which include the Code.

42 Hertz, Noreena. *The Silent Takeover. Global Capitalism and the Death of Democracy,* William Heinemann London 2001: p4. NB: This brand of capitalism has been based on neo-liberal economics, an ideology based on the thinking of Professor Milton Friedman (1912-2006) of the Chicago School of Economics based at the University of Chicago, USA.

43 Chetley A. *The politics of baby foods: successful challenges to an international marketing strategy.* London: Frances Pinter 1986.

Chapter 16: what is the code?

1 WHO/UNICEF. The International Code of Marketing of Breastmilk Substitutes. Geneva: WHO 1981. NB A breastmilk substitute is any fluid or food, whether suitable or not, that is given to a baby before six months of age. After six months, anything which replaces the breastmilk component of child's diet, for two years or beyond, is a breastmilk substitute. [Source: UNICEF]

2 Codex Alimentarius Commission. Joint FAO/WHO Food Standards Programme. Codex Committee on Nutrition and Foods for Special Dietray Uses. 28th Session. Proposals of Working Group for Sectors on Food Additives. CX/NFSDU 06/28/4-Add 2. September 2006. www.codexalimentarius.net

3   All infant formulas will have to be redesigned because WHO research (WHO 2005) has shown that the growth charts WHO endorsed for the past 40 years were based on artificially fed US babies. Infants on high energy-high protein artificial milks grow too fast and too much with possible detrimental consequences to long-term health. See: Singhal A et al. Is slower early growth beneficial for long-term cardiovascular disease? *Circulation* 2004;**109**:1108-1113

4   Dana J and Loewenstein G. A social science perspective on gifts to physicians from industry. *JAMA* 2003;**290**:252-255

5   WHO/FAO. Safe preparation, storage and handling of powdered infant formula Guidelines. 2006.

6   A friend from Pakistan who was quite unaware of the risks of artificial feeding. I do not want to give his name.

7   Thomas Baumgartner et al. Oxytocin Shapes the Neural Circuitry of Trust and Trust Adaptation in Humans. *Neuron* 2008;**58(4)**:470

8   Sterken E. Personal communication. Also: Walker M. Selling out mothers and Babies. NABA 2007.

9   The original article (6.6), permitting free supplies for institutions, was intended for orphanages. The companies rarely provided continuous supplies for orphanages but flooded maternity units with enough milk to artificially feed all babies and provide take-home samples.

10 WHA39.28 1986.

11 WHA47.5 1984.

12 IBFAN monitoring and reports: www.ibfan.org

13 Clavano NR. The results of a change in hospital practices - a paeditrican's campaign for breastfeeding in the Philippines. A Case Study. *Assignment Children* 55/56, UNICEF, 1981. NB Dr Clavano was a witness at the 1978 US Senate Hearing.

14 *China Daily* 17 October 2005. Interview with Peter Brabeck Letmanthe (Nestlé CEO) who was reported to say: "Nestlé is giving out samples and stationing doctors in Beijing supermarket chains to answer customer concerns." This occurred after recalls of Nestlé Gold 3 and Chenchang infant formulas with higher than permitted iodine levels. Cited in *Campaign for Ethical Marketing*, Baby Milk Action Update 2005.

15 Baby Milk Action Update 40, November 2007.

16 Dana J and Loewenstein G. A social science perspective on gifts to physicians from industry. *JAMA* 2003;290:252-255

17 Walker M. *Selling Out Mothers and Babies*. National Alliance for Breastfeeding Advocacy, Research, Education and Legal branch (NABA REAL) 2001.

18 Dr Thomas Hale, Associate Professor of Pharmacology Texas Tech University School of Medicine: personal communication 2001.

19 WHA49.15 1996; WHA58.32 2005. WHA Resolutions can be obtained from WHO Geneva www.who.int or IBFAN Code Documentation Centre (ICDC), IBFAN Penang, Malaysia www.ibfan.org

20 INFACT Canada. Scientific fraud and child health. How Nestlé-funded research supported deceptive "hypoallergenic" claims. *INFACT Canada Newsletter*. Winter 2006.

21 WHO/FAO. Safe preparation, storage and handling of powdered infant formula Guidelines. 2006.

22 The Mark Thomas Product. *Channel 4 TV 5 October 1999*. Also Channel 4 TV 13 January 2000.

23 Cow & Gate. What every midwife should know. *Midwives: The Official journal of The Royal College of Midwives* December 2007;20(11):502-3. The citation in this advertisement is: Arsanoglu S & Moro G et al. Early dietary intervention with a mixture of prebiotic oligo saccharides reduces the incidence of allergy associated symptoms and infections during the first two years of life. Oral presentation OP3-06. Presented at ESPGHAN 2007, Barcelona, Spain, 9 -12 May 2007. See also: Fugh-Berman A, Alladin A & Chow J. Advertising in medical journals: should current practices change? *PLoS Medicine* June 2006;**3(6)**:e130

24 Rea, Marina Ferreira. A review of breastfeeding in Brazil and how the country has reached ten months' breastfeeding duration. *Cad Saúde Pública* 2003, vol.19 suppl.1, p.S37-S45. ISSN 0102-311X.

25 Monitoring by Baby Milk Action 2008.

26 In Haiti infant formula costs US$56 a month. A factory wage is less than US$2 a day. *Newsletter of the Hôpital Albert Schweitzer Alumni Association*. Summer 2005.

27 In the 1980s and 1990s in Germany there were about lawsuits brought against Milupa concerning the damage to children's teeth from the use of sweetened 'teas' For more information contact Aktionsgruppe Babynahrung (AGB) www.babynahrung.org

28 WHA39.28 1986

29 National Opinion Poll (NOP). Research on behalf of the UK Department of Health 2005. MORI Poll on behalf of UNICEF UK and the National Childbirth Trust 2005.

30 IBFAN-ICDC Press Statement. The Sanlu Fiasco: risks of formula feeding. 20 September 2008.

31 IBFAN State of the Code by Country 2006. www.ibfan.org

32 Biddulph J Impact of legislation restricting the availability of feeding bottles in PNG. *Nutrition and Development* 1980;3:2

33 Gerber was bought by Sandoz for US$3.7 billion in 1994. Sandoz merged with CIBA and became Novartis (Swiss pharmaceutical company). In 2007 Nestlé bought Novartis for US$5.5 billion. Owning Gerber makes Nestlé the leader in the US complementary food market. See also: Minei A. Evaluation of implementation of the International Code in PNG. Presentation at Code Training Course. ICDC, Penang April 1992.

34 Sokol EJ. Guatemala: a case study for full Code implementation by legislation. In: *The Code Handbook*. Penang: ICDC 1997.

Chapter 17: power struggles

1 Milton Friedman (1912-2006). The 'no free lunch' has been attributed to other writers and speakers before Milton Friedman but he still gained fame for the use of the phrase.

2 The Global Compact: www.unglobalcompact.org

3 Personal Communication, Dr Elisabet Helsing, The First European Conference on Nutrition, Budapest, Hungary, November 1989.

4 WHO Constitution (established 1948) in basic documents 46th edition. WHO 2007. These quotations were originally taken from: WHO. *Introducing WHO*. Geneva WHO 1976.

5 Childers E. *In a time beyond warnings: strengthening the UN system*. CIIR 1993.

6 Women's Health in a Free Market Economy. The Corner House Briefing 31, June 1994. www.thecornerhouse.org.uk Also: Costello A, Watson F and Woodward,D, *Human Face or Human Façade? Adjustment and the Health of Mothers and Children,* Centre for International Child Health 1994.

7 World Bank World Development Report 2000.

8 UNICEF *Adjustment with a Human Face*. Cornia GA, Jolly R, and Stewart F (eds), UNICEF/Clarendon Press Oxford 1988. Also: Ed: Emmerij E et al. Ahead of the Curve? Overview of the Intellectual History Project. 2001.

9 Richter J. *Public-private partnerships and international health policy-making. How can public interests be safeguarded?* Helsinki: Ministry for Foreign Affairs of Finland (Development Policy Information Unit) 2004.

10 Canadian Health Coalition. *Public Private Partnerships or Private Exploitation of the Public?* Talking notes for Kathleen Connots RN, *Global Health is a Human Right* 2003: Ottawa 21-22 May 2003.

11 Dr Roger Shrimpton was at that time director of Nutrition Section, UNICEF New York.

12 Letter from Nestle Vice President Carl Angst to Lisa Woodburn, European Coordinator of the International Nestlé Infant Boycott Committee (INBC) cited in Andrew Chetley, *The Politics of Baby Foods* Frances Pinter 1986.

13 The European Economic Community was founded in 1957, at some time it dropped the middle 'E' and became the European Community. In 1993 it became the European Union.

14 Taylor A and Costello A, Violations of the International Code of Marketing of BMS: Prevalence in Four Countries. *BMJ* 11 April 1998;**316**:1117-1122

15 Dr Mary Manandhar, Nutritionist with MSF: Personal Communication 1991.

16 Baby Milk Action Update No.18 March 1996.

17 Civil Society Meeting with EU Commissioner for Trade Pascal Lamy. Written

answers to Baby Milk Action:

Baby Milk Action Question 1: Do Member States have the sovereign right to bring in and retain legislation which they believe is necessary for human rights and health protection?

Commission Answer 1: "Yes, if non-discriminatory, and ultimately, science-based."

Q2: Does the Commission agree that trade agreements should not be allowed to undermine implementation of the International Code and subsequent relevant WHA Resolutions?

A2:"In principle yes: the Commission subscribes to the view that international agreements, particularly, but not exclusively those related to protection of the environment or human health, and international trade rules should be mutually supportive."

Q3: In matters of health will WTO defer to the decisions of the World Health Assembly?

A3:"International agreements/ organisations should be mutually supportive, and their relationship clarified where necessary and useful."

Q6: For the optimum health in infants everywhere, EU legislation should be brought into line with the International Code and WHA Resolutions.

A6:"To the extent that the EU and its Member States subscribe to them - to a large extent, these are issues of Member State competence."

http://www.babymilkaction.org/update/update30.html

18 David Clark, Legal Officer Nutrition Section UNICEF New York. Personal communication 2002.

19 *Protection, promotion and support of breastfeeding in Europe: a Blueprint for Action. Developed and written by Participants in the Project. Promotion of Breastfeeding in Europe* (N.SPC 2002359). European Commission, Directorate of Public Health and Risk Assessment, IRCCS Burlo Garofolo, Trieste, Italy, Unit for Health Services and International Health, WHO Collaborating Centre for Maternal and Child Health. Presented at EU Conference on Promotion of Breastfeeding in Europe, Dublin Castle, Ireland 2004.

Chapter 18: dying for the Code

1 Liv Ullmann Address to UK Committee for UNICEF Press lunch. 16 June 1983.

2 Correspondence between Dr Marilen Danguilan of the Philippines' Ministry of Health and Professor David Morley of The Institute of Child Health London. Professor Morley consulted Gabrielle Palmer of Baby Milk Action. All three actors communicated with each other. 1992

3 *Formula for Disaster* (film) UNICEF 2007. May be viewed online at www.babymilkaction.org.

4 *Philippine Daily Inquirer*. Armand N Nocum, 'P1M* for info on OSG man's slay'. *1 million Philippine dollars reward. 14 December 2006.

5 AC Nielsen, cited by Marical E Estevillo, 14th July 2006. Business World, Philippines cited in 'George Monbiot, *Breast Beating*. http://www.monbiot.com/archives/2007/06/05/breast-beating/ Also: Connie Levett, 3 February 2007. Formula for profit seen as recipe for disaster. *Sydney Morning Herald*. http://www.smh.com.au/news/world/formula-for-profit-seen-as-recipe-for-disaster/2007/02/02/1169919531018.html as cited in Monbiot G.

6 UNHCR, 26 February 2007. UN Special Rapporteur Appalled with the Deceptive Tactics of Milk Companies in the Philippines. www.unhcr.ch/huricane/huricane.nsf/ view01/3035D668F9E92329C125728F00294A69 NB This section on the Philippines is also based on information from Baby Milk Action (IBFAN UK), IBFAN Philippines, Alessandro Iellamo and articles by George Monbiot in *The Guardian* 5 June 2006 and on http://www.monbiot.com/archives/2007/06/05/breast-beating/

7 *Yorkshire Television*, First Tuesday Series, "Vicious Circles" 5 June 1990. Also: IBFAN, Breaking the Rules 1991. UNICEF State of the World's Children 1992. Also: Conde-Agudelo A. Effect of Birth Spacing on Maternal and Perinatal Health: A Systematic Review and Meta-Analysis. Report submitted to the *CATALYST Consortium*, October 2004.

8 Baby Milk Action Update. Milking Profits. How Nestle puts sales ahead of infant health. February 2000. Also Baby Milk Action Press Releases throughout 2000

www.babymilkaction.org Also: Personal communication with Baby Milk Action staff. Also: The Network, Feeding Fiasco 1998, available from IBFAN

9   *New York Times*, Infant Diarrhea Kills Hundreds Yearly in US: a report of JAMA study by Dr Mei-Shang Ho 9 December 1988. Also Ryan AS et al, Recent declines in breastfeeding in the US, 1984 through 1989. *Pediatrics* 1990;**88(4)**;719-27 Also: Chen A and Rogan WJ, Breastfeeding and the Risk of Postneonatal Death in the US, *Pediatrics* 2004:**113(5)**:e435-439

10 Lawrence F. *Eat your heart out, why the food business is bad for the planet and for your health*. Penguin Books 2008

11 Margen S et al. *Infant Feeding in Mexico*. NIFAC Washington.

12 Baby Milk Action Update November 1991.

13 Nestlé UK. Nestlé and Baby Milk. Nestlé UK 1992.

14 The Interagency Group on Breastfeeding Monitoring (IGBM), *Cracking the Code*, 1997. Also: Taylor A. *Violations of the international code of marketing of breast milk substitutes: prevalence in four countries*, BMJ 1998;**316**;1117-1122

15 Allain A. *Fighting an old battle in a new world: how IBFAN monitors the baby food market*. Offprint from Development Dialogue: The Dag Hammarskjöld Foundation 2005.

16 Nestlé's Little Problem. *Marketing Week* 11 January 1999.

17 Report to the Director General World Health Organisation. Nestlé implementation of the WHO Code (International Code of Marketing of Breastmilk Substitutes), Official Response of Governments. July 1999.

18 *Business World* 30 September 1999. Also: Baby Milk Action Campaign for Ethical Marketing. October 1999.

19 Letter to Peter Brabeck-Letmathe Nestlé CEO from Carol Bellamy UNICEF Executive Director. 31 December 1999.

20 François Perroud, Nestlé public relations director. *You and Yours*, BBC Radio 4, 1988.

21 Baby Milk Action, Boycott News, July 2002.

22 IBFAN. Breaking the Rules Stretching the Rules, 2007.

23 *INFACT CANADA Newsletter*. Nestlé Scientist's False Claims Exposed, 12/02/06 www.infactcanada.com

24 *Food Industry News*. Nestlé: Nutrition Division to be Significant Growth Driver; Infant Nutrition Segment to Play Major Role. FLEXNEWS 20 June 2008. http://www.flex-news-food.com. Also: IBFAN. Breaking the Rules Stretching the Rules, 2007.

25 Christiansen N, Creating Shared Value through Basic Business Strategy. *Development Outreach*. June 2008.

26 Global Industry Analysts Inc. www.strategyr.com Accessed 7 August 2008.

27 UNICEF. The State of the World's Children 2008.

28 IBFAN-ICDC Press Statement. The Sanlu fiasco: risks of formula feeding. 20 September 2008.

29 *Associated Press* (AP). China dairy boss appeals sentence in milk scandal. 2 February 2009.

30 Wilson B. *Swindled: from poison sweets to counterfeit coffee – the dark history if the food cheats.* John Murray 2008.

31 Yardley J. Infants in Chinese city starve on protein short formula. *New York Times* 5 May 2004.

32 Agostini C et al. How much protein is safe? International Journal of Obesity 2005;**29**:s8-s13. Also: Singhal A et al. Is slower early growth beneficial for long-term cardiovascular health? *Circulation* 2004;**109**:1108-1113

33 Israeli milk facts from: IBFAN/ICDC. Regulations in a fix over sub-standard formula and non-compliant labeling. *ICDC Legal Update*; Issue 8: December 2006. Chinese milk story and Mr Chai Shauqiu's statement from: Wilson B. *Swindled: From Poison Sweets to Counterfeit Coffee – The Dark History of the Food Cheats* John Murray 2008.

34 Global Industry Analysts Inc. www.strategyr.com Accessed 7 August 2008. The USA has approximately 20 million under five year olds, Canada has around one million. Source: UNICEF State of the World's Children 2008.

35 The Personal Responsibility and Work Opportunity Reconciliation Act (PRWORA) 1996.

36 Haider S, Jacknowitz A & Schoeni RF, Welfare Work Requirements and Child Well-

Being: Evidence from the Effects on Breastfeeding. *Demography* August 2003;**40(3)**;479-497

37 Kent G, WIC's promotion of infant formula in the United States. *International Breastfeeding Journal* 2006; 1:8 http://www.internationalbreastfeedingjournal.com/content/1/1/8. Also: Walker M. Still selling out mothers and babies: marketing of breast milk substitutes in the USA. NABA REAL, 2007

38 Dietz WH. Breastfeeding may help prevent childhood overweight. *JAMA* 2001;**285**:2506-7

39 Caldwell, Karen and Turner-Maffei, Cindy. Promoting breastfeeding in the USA: what can we learn? Presentation at UNICEF UK BFI Annual Conference Cardiff, UK, 28-29 November 2006.

Chapter 19: documents and declarations

1 Comment by Dr Alan Court of UNICEF at Innocenti Declaration Meeting, Florence, Italy, November 2005.

2 Protecting, Promoting and Supporting Breastfeeding, The Special Role of the Maternity Services. A Joint WHO/UNICEF Statement WHO Geneva 1989.

3 www.un.org/news2005

4 There are three Maternity Protection Conventions (No 3 1919; No 103, 195; No 183, 2000) and two Maternity Protection Recommendations (No 95, 1952, No 191 2000).

5 Labbock, MH et al , Trends in Exclusive Breastfeeding: Findings from the 1990s. *J Hum Lact* 2006;**22(3)**

6 http://www.childinfo.org/breastfeeding_overview.html

7 WHO Collaborating Centre for MCH, Unit for Health Services Research and International Health, Protection, promotion and support of breastfeeding in Europe: current situation, December 2003.

8 Michaelsen KF et al. Feeding of Infants and Young Children. WHO Europe 2003.

9 Walker M. Still selling out mothers and babies: marketing of breast milk substitutes in the USA. NABA REAL, 2007.

10 Jones, G et al and the Bellagio Child Survival Study Group. How many child deaths can we prevent this year? *The Lancet* 2003;**362**:65-71

11 Goldenberg P. *Repensando a desnutrição como questão social*. Cortez Editora Unicamp 1988.

12 Dr Mirian Silveira: personal communication. I thank Dr Vilneide Serva of IMIP who facilitated for Dr Silveira to tell me her story. With thanks to Dr Silveira.

13 Rea, MF. A review of breastfeeding in Brazil and how the country has reached ten months' duration. (in Portuguese). *Cadernos de Saúde Pública* v.19 supl.1Rio de Janeiro 2003. Also: IBFAN Case studies: Using international tools to stop corporate malpractice - does it work? IBFAN 2004. Also: Personal Communication: Tereza Toma, Vilneide Serva, Mike Brady.

14 *Breaking the Rules*. p71, IBFAN International Code Documentation Centre (ICDC) 2007.

15 Nestlé Infant Nutrition Centre Product Information: "GOOD START®" infant formula milk (cited 7 June 2008).

16 AAP, Breastfeeding and the Use of Human Milk. Pediatrics 2005;**115**;496-506

17 Dana J and Loewenstein G. A social science perspective on gifts to physicians from industry. *JAMA* 2003;**290**:252-255

Chapter 20: work, economics and the value of mothering

1 Berg A. *The Nutrition Factor*. Washington DC: Brooking Institute 1973.

2 Smith, Julie P. Human milk supply in Australia. *Food Policy 24* 1999;71-91

3 Jelliffe DB & Jelliffe EFP. *Human milk in the modern world*. Oxford University Press 1978.

4 Rohde JE. Mother milk and the Indonesian economy: a major national resource. *Journal of Tropical Paediatrics* 1982;**28(4)**:166-74

5 Hosken F P. Review of Raphael D and Davis F, *Only Mothers Know*. In: *Women's International Network News: Women and Health*. 1985.

6 Canton Appenzell Innerrhoden. The majority of men were still against women's right to vote and held out until a ruling from the Swiss Supreme Court forced them to change in 1990. Two other cantons had suffered the same overturning of male authority in 1989.

7   Rich A. *Of women born*. Bantam Books 1977.
8   Oakley A. *Essays on women, medicine and health*. Edinburgh University Press 1993.
9   Shulamith Firestone. *The dialectic of sex: the case for feminine revolution*. New York: William Morrow 1970.
10 Haider R. Discussion Paper prepared for and presented at *WHO/UNICEF Meeting on Infant and Young Child Feeding*. Geneva WHO 2000. Unpublished.
11 More so in North America. In Scandinavia women seemed at ease with the coexistence of their reproductive and mothering roles and their ability to compete in the so-called male world.
12 Koonz, C, *Mothers in the Fatherland: Women, the Family and Nazi Politics*. Methuen 1988.
13 Menon L. & Patel V. Grinding Realities: Women and breastfeeding in the informal sector. WABA 2005 and PG Dept. of Economics, SNDT Women's University of India, 2005.
14 Coronel FK & Unterreiner F. Increasing the impact of remittance on children's rights. *Philippines working paper* UNICEF 2007.
15 Ehrenreich, B, *Nickel and Dimed, Undercover in Low-wage USA*. Granta Books 2002. Toynbee P, *Hard Work: Life in low-pay Britain*. Bloomsbury 2003.
16 You cannot be both an illegal immigrant and an asylum seeker. The latter means your status has not been defined.
17 This account is based on correspondence with those involved and Melissa Benn's report: First Person. *The Guardian* 24 November 2007.
18 Greenwald R. *Walmart. The High Cost of Low Price* (film) 2005.
19 The UN research Institute for Social Development (UNRISD). *States of disarray: the social effects of globalisation*. UNRISD 1995 [p70 350,000 illegal nannies in the USA.] Also: Parreñas R. *The Global Servants: (Im)Migrant Filipina Domnestic Workers in Rome and Los Angeles* PhD dissertation, Dpt. Of Ethnic Studies, UCal, Berkeley, 1999, in Hochschild AR, *Love and Gold* in Ehrenreich B and Hochschild AR, *Global Women, Nannies, Maids and Sex workers in the New Economy*. Granta Books 2003.
20 Campbell CE. Nestlé and breast vs bottle-feeding: mainstream and Marxist perspectives. *International Journal of Health Services* 1984;**14**(**4**):547-66
21 Correspondence between UNICEF employees based in Former Yugoslavia and Nutrition Section UNICEF New York. 1997.
22 Smith JP and Ingham LH. Mothers' milk and Measures of Economic Output, *Feminist Economics* March 2005;**11**(**1**):41-62
23 Weimer J. *The Economic Benefits of Breastfeeding: A Review and Analysis*. Food and Rural Economics Division, Economic Research Service, US Department of Agriculture. Food Assistance and Nutrition Research Report No13, March 2001. The three illnesses are otitis media (ear infections), gastroenteritis (diarrhoea) and the often fatal bowel disease of low birth weight babies, necrotizing enterocolitis (NEC).
24 Bisqeura JA et al. Impact of NEC on length of stay and hospital discharge in VLBW infants. *Pediatrics* 2002;**109**: 423-8. In: Williams AF, Kingdon CC and Weaver G. *Banking for the future: investing in human milk* www.archdischild.com 7 July 2008.
25 UNICEF UK/National Childbirth Trust/Save the Children UK. A weak formula for legislation: how loopholes in the law are putting babies at risk. 2006
26 The UK National Breastfeeding Working Group 1995.
27 Walker, Marsha. *Still Selling Out Mothers and Babies*. p41, NABA Real 2007.
28 Cigna Press Release. http://www.csrwire.com/PressRelease.php?id=241 *Corporate Social Responsibility News*, 15 June.2000. Cigna is one of the health insurance companies cited for unethical practices in Michael Moore's 2007 film Sicko.
29 Titmuss, Richard. *The Gift Relationship*. LSE Books, 1997.
30 Personal communication: Gillian Weaver, Director of the UK Human Milk Banking Association (UKAMB) 2008.
31 Personal communication by email from Gretchen Flatau, Director of the Human Milk Bank, Austen, Texas, USA. 2008.
32 Arnold LD. The Cost-effectiveness of using banked donor milk in the neonatal intensive care unit: prevention of necrotizing enterocolitis. *J Hum Lact* 2002;18(**2**):172-177
33 Number of human milk banks (HMBs) worldwide: Europe 135 plus; Brazil 190; rest of Latin America 12 plus more planned; USA 10 (larger quantities of milk collected than is usual in other countries); Canada 1 plus 1 planned; Australia 3; Africa:

Cameroon 5; South Africa 5; India 25 (according to WHO); China: many BFHI (55% of all) hospitals have in-house HMBs. These data do not reflect quality of regulation and management procedures nor quantities of human milk used. Personal Communication: Gillian Weaver, Director UKAMB Summer 2008.

34 Aguayo VM & Ross J. The monetary value of human milk in Francophone West Africa: a profile for nutrition policy communication. *Food and Nutrition Bulletin* 2002;**23**(2):153-161

35 Save the children UK. *Running on empty*. 2007.

36 Todd H., *Women at the Center, Grameem Bank Borrowers after one decade*. Mohiuddin Ahmed, The University Press Ltd, Red Crescent Building, 114 Motijheel C/A, GPO Box 2611, Dhaka 1000, Bangladesh, 1996.

37 Waring, Marilyn. *If women counted, a new feminist economics*. Macmillan 1988. Also an expanded and updated version of this book. *Counting for nothing: What men value and what women are worth*. University of Toronto Press 1999.

38 Smith JP and Ingham LH. Mothers' milk and Measures of Economic Output, *Feminist Economics* March 2005;11(1):41-62

39 Galbraith, JK, *The Economics of Innocent Fraud Truth for our Time*. Allen Lane 2004.

40 BBC News website August 2005 'Move to commercialise breast milk'.

41 Weaver G & Williams SA. A mother's gift: the milk of human kindness. In: Titmuss RM. *The Gift Relationship*. LSE Books 1997. NB Both the chapter and the entire book are relevant. Originally published in 1970, Ann Oakley (daughter of Richard Titmuss and John Ashton) edited this new version which includes the chapter on breastmilk.

42 Clyde H Farnsworth, Quebec Bets on Subsidised Milk, Mother's Kind. *Montreal Journal* 5 April 1994.

43 Galtry, Judith. The Impact on Breastfeeding of Labour Market Policy and Practice in Ireland, Sweden and the USA. *Social Science and Medicine*, 2003;**57**(1);167-177

44 Birth intervals of less than 15 months are associated with a 150% increase in maternal death. Conde-Aguledo A and Belizan JM. Maternal morbidity and mortality associated with interpregancy interval: cross-sectional study. *BMJ* 18 November 2000;**321(7271)**:1255

45 Department of International Development (DFID) Press Release. UK Government aid contributes to dramatic decline in women dying in childbirth in Bangladesh and Nepal. 1 July 2008. http://www.dfid

46 Dummy Mummy. *Private Eye*. Issue 1205, 7 April 2008.

47 Talking points: New salvos over maternity leave. *The Sunday Times*. 20 July 2008.

48 Landes D. *The Wealth and poverty of nations*. Little, Brown and Company, 1998.

49 Layard R. *Happiness Lessons From a New Science*. Allen Lane 2005.

50 Sen A. *Poverty and Famines: An essay on entitlement and deprivation*. Oxford University Press 1981.

51 Chossudovsky, M. Sowing the Seeds of famine in Ethiopia. *Global Research 10* September 2001.

52 Talking points: New salvos over maternity leave. *The Sunday Times*. 20 July 2008.

53 Schwartz Cowan R. More work for mother. Basic Books 1983. Also: Ehrenreich B & Engish D. *For her own good: 150 years of experts' advice to women*. Anchor Books 1989.

54 Leach P. *Children First: What society must do – and is not doing – for children today*. Penguin Books 1994.

55 Gerhardt S. *Why Love Matters: how affection shapes a baby's brain*. Routledge 2004.

56 Gerhardt S. Cradle of civilisation. *The Guardian*, 24 July 2004.

57 Hospital Paediatrician in the Sultanate of Oman, Personal Communication 1994.

58 Anubhuti M. AIDWA Organises convention on home-based workers. *People's Democracy* 2008;**32(16)** Also:Shah M & Trivedi S. Don't forget the home-based workers. *Labour File* 2004;**2(5)**:58-60

59 Huws A. *Action Programme for the Protection of Home-based workers: ten case studies from around the world*. Geneva:ILO 1995 This trend was first noted in Mitter S. *Common Fate, Common Bond: Women in the Global Economy*. London, Pluto Press 1986.

60 Agland P. *Baka: People of the Rainforest*. DJA River Films for *Channel 4*, January 1988.

61 *Baka women claim their rights*. http://www.plan-uk.org/wherewework/westafrica/cameroon/bakarights

Chapter 21: ecology, waste and greed

1   States which have ratified international conventions are legally bound to fulfil them: 191 states have ratified CRC and 161 CEDAW. The CRC Committee is not a policing body but exists to assist governments to fulfil their obligations.

2   Martin A. How green is my orange? *New York Times* 21 January 2009. Calculations were made by PepsiCo in conjunction with Columbia Earth Institute. See also: http://actonco2.direct.gov.uk Also: Uvnäs Moberg K. *The oxytocin factor*. Da Capo Press 2003

3   Department of Nutrition. MOH, Maputo, Mozambique 1982. One litre is needed for mixing feeds plus two litres for boiling bottles, teats or cups and preparation equipment.

4   Radford A. The ecological impact of bottle feeding. *Baby Milk Action* 1991.

5   Elston S. Banning the bottle. www.infactcanada.com 25 April 2008.

6   AVENT spokesperson on *BBC1 TV news 'Look East'* 2003. Cited in Palmer G. Feminism and breastfeeding in: Stewart M, ed. *Pregnancy, birth and maternity care: feminist perspectives*. Books for Midwives: Elsevier Science 2004: p.85-105.

7   Stanway P. *Green Babies*. London: Random Century 1990. Also: San Antonio Breast Cancer Symposium, Dec. 14-17, 2006. Michael Gnant, MD, Medical University of Vienna, Austria. Kathy Albain, MD, professor of medicine, Loyola University of Chicago Medical Center.

8   Booth R. Come on in but watch out for the sewage, tampons and cotton buds. The Guardian 23 August 2008.

9   Tim Lang Professor of Food Policy, City University, London.

10 Yaqoob T. British seafood shipped to Thailand – and back – just to have the shells removed. *Daily Mail website* 16 November 2006.

11 Food Safety Authority of Ireland (FSAI). Ireland: a natural source of infant nutrition. *FSAI News* May/June 2007; Issue 3

12 Trivedi B. Dinner's dirty secret. *New Scientist* 13 September 2008.

13 USDA. Economic effects of US dairy policy and alternative approaches to milk pricing. *Report to Congress* 2004.

14 Lawrence F. *Not on the label*. Penguin Books. 2004. Also: Lawrence F. *Eat your heart out*. Penguin Books 2008. Sallie J. Milking the customers: the high cost of US dairy policies. *The Cato Institute* 9 November 2006.

15 Sallie J. Milking the customers: the high cost of US dairy policies. *The Cato Institute* 9 November 2006.

16 Woods TE. *The politically incorrect guide to American history*. Regnery Publishing 2004.

17 USDA. Economic effects of US dairy policy and alternative approaches to milk pricing. *Report to Congress* 2004.

18 Lawrence F. *Eat your heart out: why the food business is bad for the planet and your health*. Penguin Books 2008.

19 Mathiason N. Who's milking it? *The Observer* 26 June 2005.

20 Richter J. *Holding corporations accountable*. Zed Books 2001. Also: Richter J. *Public-private partnerships and international health policy-making*. Ministry of Foreign Affairs of Finland 2004.

21 Hertz N. *The silent takeover: global capitalism and the death of democracy*. William Heinemann 2001.

22 Hyde M. It's Davos, but where is the Bono of financial crisis? *The Guardian* 31 January 2009. See also: http://www.taxjustice.net

23 Toynbee P. It's time to rattle and bang in protest at this outrage. *The Guardian* 31 January 2009.

24 I am keeping this informant anonymous because this information was given in private correspondence.

25 Punjab Lok Sujag. *The political economy of milk in the Punjab: a people's perspective*. Punjab Lok Sujag August 2003.

26 Trivedi B. Dinner's dirty secret. New Scientist 13 September 2008.

27 Nestle M. *Food politics: how the food industry influences nutrition and health*. University of California Press 2003.

28 Waring M. The Value of Death, Chapter 7. In *Counting for nothing: what men value and what women are worth*. University of Toronto Press 1999. MW writes: "Since the possibility of our dying more than once is slightly ridiculous this means that for

every living person on this planet (in 1999), there has been an expenditure of $700 million to kill us once. The real expenditure on killing us has been $700 m x 12."

29 Personal Communication: Lord Tim Garden (1944-2007), defence expert and author of *Can Deterrence Last?* Buchan & Enright 1984 and *The Technology Trap: science and the military.* Brasseys 1989.

30 Thomas M. *As used on the famous Nelson Mandela.* Ebury Press 2006.

31 Galbraith JK. *The economics of innocent fraud.* Allen Lane 2004.

32 Hertz N. *The silent takeover: global capitalism and the death of democracy.* William Heinemann 2001.

33 Save the Children UK. *Running on empty: poverty and child malnutrition.* Save the Children UK 2007.

34 Chant S. Children in female-headed households: interrogating the concept of an intergeneratiomnal transmission of disadvantage with particular reference to the Gambia, the Philippines and Costa Rica. London School of Economics, *Gender Institute New Working paper Series* Issue 19; February 2007

35 Longmate N. *How we lived then: a history of everyday life during the Second World War.* Arrow Books 1971.

36 Korten DC. *The post-corporate world: life after capitalism.* Kumarian Press and Berrett-Koehler Publishers 1999.

37 Dawkins R. *The Selfish Gene.* Oxford University Press 1976.

38 Firestone S. *The dialectic of sex: the case for feminine revolution.* William Morrow 1970.

39 http://www.prolacta.com/ accessed 7 February 2009.

40 Williams AF. Human Milk and the Preterm Infant. In: Hanson TN & McIntosh N eds. *Current Topics in Neonatology: Volume 3.* London WB Saunders & Co 1999.

41 WHO Department of Reproductive health and Research. *Kangaroo mother care: a practical guide.* WHO Geneva 2003.

42 Weaver G & Williams SA. A mother's gift: the milk of human kindness. In: Titmuss RM. *The Gift Relationship.* LSE Books 1997. NB Both the chapter and the entire book are relevant. Originally published in 1970, Ann Oakley (daughter of Richard Titmuss) and John Ashton edited this new version which includes the chapter on breastmilk. Also: Huxley A. Brave New World. Doubledau, Doran & Co 1932.

43 Hochschild AR. *The commercialisation of intimate life.* University of California Press 2003.

44 Chant S. Children in female-headed households: interrogating the concept of an intergenerational transmission of disadvantage with particular reference to the Gambia, the Philippines and Costa Rica. London School of Economics, *Gender Institute New Working paper Series* Issue 19; February 2007.

45 Professor Sylvia Rumball (Massey University), leading New Zealand bio-ethicist: personal communication 1988.

46 Hansen M. The mealy bug gets stung. In: Institute for Consumer Policy Research Consumers' Union (ICPRCU). *Escape from the pesticide treadmill: alternatives to pesticides in developing countries.* ICPRCU 1987.

47 Baby Milk Action. Nestlé's claims on water bottling operation in Brazil demonstrably untrue, says Baby Milk Action. Press release, 2 March 2006.

Epilogue

1 William Least Heatmoon in www.pbs.org/lewisandclark/inside/saca.html

2 Michaelsen K. Comment in: Christie DA & Tansey EM, eds. **The Resurgence of Breastfeeding 1975-2000.** Draft transcript of a witness seminar held at the Wellcome Trust centre for the History of Medicine at UCL, London, 24 April 2007. Vol 34 Breast[1].DOC02/08/2007: p.75

3 If compared with average wages of the time, US$500.00 was roughly equivalent to US$239,000.00 in today's money. If compared with what goods could be purchased at the time, it was worth US$8,756.00. This was because manufactured goods were relatively more expensive in those days. However we compare the sums, this was a high fee and a decent spread of land for her husband.

index

Page numbers followed by *i* mean that there is an illustration on the subject.

also by **Gabrielle Palmer** *from* **Pinter & Martin**

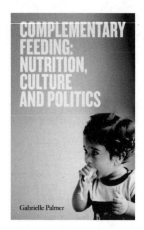

Complementary Feeding:
Nutrition, Culture and Politics

Gabrielle Palmer's groundbreaking book *The Politics of Breastfeeding* highlighted the controversies surrounding the aggressive promotion of breastmilk substitutes. She now turns her attention to complementary feeding – the first foods that a child eats besides milk.

For most of human existence, children went without industrially processed foods and branded food products. Can we applaud the progress of the way children are fed today? In our unequal world one billion people risk their health through overconsumption while two billion people are hungry. The health problems of both groups start in early childhood.

The power and influence of the food industry has increased dramatically in recent decades. Seductive and often unethical modern marketing methods have led to the promotion of unsuitable, unnecessary and sometimes harmful baby foods. Yet not all industrially processed foods are bad and not all 'natural' foods are good. Both poor and rich children may be inappropriately fed.

What lessons can we learn from history? How do cultural and religious beliefs influence the choice of food? Can government initiatives have any effect? How can we provide good nutrition for all infants? This brief, compassionate and thought-provoking new book will be of interest to anyone who is curious about the world, its children and their nutrition, and will stimulate discussion and debate as part of the campaign to create a world where health for all is a true goal.

pinter
&
martin

visit **www.pinterandmartin.com**
for further information, extracts and special offers